About the Author

Tony Robertson is a retired gynaecologist. He was born in England but has lived in Africa from the age of six. He obtained his medical degree from the University of Cape Town and is a Fellow of the Royal College of Obstetricians and Gynaecologists in England. Married to Fiona they live in Zimbabwe. Tony has taught and lectured publicly for many years. He was a lecturer at the University of Zimbabwe before spending the last 40 years in private medical practice.

Dedication

To those who appreciate the truth fairy rather than the toothed one.

Tony Robertson

QUACKERY, THE 20 MILLION DOLLAR DUCK

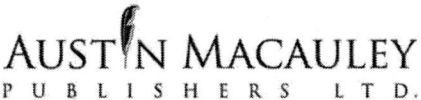

Copyright © Tony Robertson (2015)

The right of Tony Robertson to be identified as author of this work has been asserted by him in accordance with section 77 and 78 of the Copyright, Designs and Patents Act 1988.

All rights reserved. No part of this publication may be reproduced, stored in a retrieval system, or transmitted in any form or by any means, electronic, mechanical, photocopying, recording, or otherwise, without the prior permission of the publishers.

Any person who commits any unauthorized act in relation to this publication may be liable to criminal prosecution and civil claims for damages.

A CIP catalogue record for this title is available from the British Library.

ISBN 978 1 78455 454 5 (Paperback)
ISBN 978 1 78455 456 9 (Hardback)

www.austinmacauley.com

First Published (2015)
Austin Macauley Publishers Ltd.
25 Canada Square
Canary Wharf
London
E14 5LB

Printed and bound in Great Britain

Acknowledgments

To my teachers and mentors who encouraged me to think, always to question and only to accept where there is good evidence.

Contents

Chapter one - Quackery - General 11

Chapter two - Quackery - Hormones 17

Chapter three - Quackery - Complementary and Alternative medicine (CAM) 30

Chapter four - Quackery - Homeopathy 87

Chapter five - Quackery - Traditional Chinese medicine 123

Chapter six - Quackery - Miracle cures 165

Chapter seven - Quackery - Medical quackery 173

Chapter eight - Quackery - Research misconduct 195

Chapter nine - Quackery - Food Supplements and vitamins 228

Chapter ten - Quackery - Pharmaceutical companies 257

Chapter eleven - Quackery - Top Health Frauds 275

Chapter twelve - Evidence-based Medicine 289

Chapter thirteen - Change 315

Chapter fourteen – Management 326

CHAPTER ONE - QUACKERY - GENERAL

On the walls of Les Trois Frères cave in the Pyrénées, there is a rock painting of a man, wrapped in the skin of an animal, with his legs and arms painted in stripes and with the antlers of a stag fixed on his head. The artist, who lived in the Aurignacian age, between 40,000 and 28,000 years ago, has provided an authentic portrait of a contemporary witchdoctor in his professional dress, and it is from the witchdoctor that the medical man of today is descended.[1] Quackery is not new.

The word "quack" is derived from the archaic "quacksalver", an early-modern Dutch word. It referred to someone who sold home and other remedies to gullible purchasers by fast talking patter or "quacking". By the time the customers found that the medicines they had purchased were worthless; the "quack" had disappeared. These days, gullible people still buy worthless medicines, but the vendors do not disappear, they merely become richer. "For every quack who later proves to be a genius, there are 10,000 quacks that prove later only to be quacks"[2]. By no means are all of them shysters; many are very intelligent and write or speak persuasively and with great authority.

Conversely many of the discoverers of very important advances in medicine were originally thought to be quacks before their discoveries or treatments were proven to work. Gynaecologists of today use a colposcope to look at the cervix of the uterus and a hysteroscope to look through the cervix into the cavity of the uterus. A laparoscope is used to investigate the abdominal cavity. The Italian-German Philip Bozzini[3] was the physician credited with the first significant attempt to visualize the interior body, earning him the title of *the* father of endoscopy. He first started to do this using candles and mirrors with an apparatus called a "lichtleiter" at the beginning of the 19th century.

Bozzini was frustrated by the then-standard technique of "blind palpation" or fingertip exploration. This was the only means of examination in gynaecology. A common saying at that time was that "the eye of the obstetrician should be located in his fingertips." Bozzini, was heavily censured by almost all his eminent contemporaries for "undue curiosity." His most vigorous critic; Dr. Andreas Josef von Stifft, head of the opposing Viennese medical centre, dismissed the new apparatus, with its candlelight and mirrors, claiming that even if Bozzini improved the optics "the judgment of a reasonable doctor and the finger of an experienced examiner will still remain, as in the past, the sole means from which the patient … can expect … fitting treatment." Within a few short decades of course, Bozzini was vindicated.[4]

The resistance to change and personal rivalries of colleagues has been a persistent problem affecting pioneers throughout the history of medicine. An official *Imperial Resolution* signed by the Kaiser banned the use of Bozzini's "lichtleiter." This was probably at the instigation of a Dr. Stifft, Bozzini's most powerful critic and rival, who just happened to be the personal physician to the Kaiser. Influence rather than any shortcomings of the actual device may have had more to do with this decree. In what was an unfortunate and untimely demise Bozzini succumbed to typhoid fever on April 4th, 1809, a month before his 36th birthday and just three years after his first test with the apparatus. He did not live to see the ban revoked.[5]

Within only three short years from its first testing in 1806 until his passing in 1809 Bozzini's "lichleiter", attracted the attention of some of the most important medical centers of the world. In comparison even in the 20th century the value of the discovery of penicillin by Alexander Fleming in 1928 took over ten years to be recognised by the scientific community.

Kenneth Walker, the author of *The Story of Medicine,* distinguishes the quack from the physician by considering their predominant motive rather than the nature of their treatment. The most common motive of the quack by far, is his or her personal gain whilst that of the physician by contrast, is the welfare of his or her patient. This does not imply that the physician is completely indifferent to his own profit. It means only that his personal gain is not the sole key to his actions.[6]

The relationship between doctor and patient is a very special one. Unlike the quack, the doctor's own profit and convenience must often be sacrificed to those of the patient. He must put the interests of his patient first but there are defaulters in the medical profession as there are defaulters in every other walk of life, men who put their own interests first and who are ready to make profit out of their patients' gullibility.

Why do people listen to quacks? Francis Bacon wrote: "We see the weakness and credulity of men is such as they will often prefer a mountebank or witch to a learned physician."[7] This is as true today as it was true of Bacon's time, because the quack has the great attraction that he promises his patient what the "learned physician" is quite unable to offer him; a quick cure without any complications. The "learned physician" may only be able to recommend an operation for the removal of his cancer, the quack knows how to remove it with tablets, an infinitely preferable proceeding. The honest physician may require all sorts of inconveniences from the patient. He may request that the patient stops smoking or abandons other bad habits. He may require a hospital stay in an expensive nursing home. The quack, on the other hand, can promise the earth. It is no wonder that they never lack patients.

The intellectual is particularly partial to quackery. He or she is very often convinced that it is professional jealousy alone which prevents the medical profession from recognising quacks. Bernard Shaw had a very strong bias in the direction of the unorthodox practitioner. He accused the medical profession, in the preface to *The Doctor's Dilemma*, of being "the strongest and the most reactionary of all the trade unions."[8] According to Shaw it was jealousy alone which prevented the Royal Colleges of Physicians and Surgeons from recognising quacks.

The first Act in Britain to suppress unlicensed practice was passed in the year 1511.[8] The College of Physicians was founded seven years after the passing of this licensing Act, and this College was given powers for the suppression of quacks and impostors. These powers were not sufficient however, to stop quackery. Thomas Gale,[9] an army surgeon, complained in 1544 that while visiting St.Thomas's and St. Bartholomew's hospitals in London, he saw three hundred people so severely damaged by "mischief" brought about "by witches, by women, and by counterfeit javels (worthless fellows) that take upon themselves the use of art, not only robbing them of their money, but of their limbs and perpetual health."

Life was not always plain sailing for the quack. Even before the passing of the Act of 1511 in the U.K. some foreign rulers had adopted their own private measures to curtail quackery. In 1140, Roger II of Sicily issued an edict forbidding anyone from practising medicine without producing satisfactory credentials and punishing infringement of this law by imprisonment. Mathias, King of Hungary went further. In 1464, he proclaimed that any person who could "cure him of his arrow wound" would be richly rewarded but that if this proved unsuccessful, then the practitioner himself would be put to death. This was an arrangement discouraging even to a *bona fide* surgeon and still less attractive to the quack.[10]

Foreign practitioners have often had a reputation far beyond that deserved.[11] Dr. Abraham of Groningen was an example of the special popularity enjoyed by the foreign quack in the seventeenth and eighteenth centuries. He claimed that he could perform many fine and curious manual operations "not before heard of" and that he had many excellent remedies for curing disease "which others have not yet found out." These two examples were typical of the quack; that he knew what other doctors did not know, and he could do what other doctors could not do. He possessed special knowledge and skill beyond the reach of ordinary men. Another example of the selling techniques used by the typical quack is to suggest that he is in such demand that he has to limit the number of patients he can see. This is guaranteed to keep him busy.

Another quack, Dr. William Read, began life as a jobbing tailor in Aberdeen.[12] He later moved to Dublin and from there to London, where he settled in rooms in the Strand. His "infallible eye-wash" apparently helped Queen Anne who suffered from chronic eye weakness. She was so grateful that he was knighted in 1705. Another recipient of a knighthood at the same time was Sir William Hannes. The two honours were accepted with some criticism by many, and their knighthoods were celebrated by one cynic in the following verse:

"The Queen, like Heav'n, shines equally on all, Her favours now without distinction fall, Great Read and slender Hannes, both knighted show That none their honours shall to merit owe.'"

Queen Anne had a partiality for "irregular practitioners" as have many members of British Royalty over the years.

Scientists are often initially ridiculed when they describe a new finding. Whenever a new invention is discovered the cynics state that time is needed to show that the invention works. When enough time has elapsed to show that the device works they then say "Yes, it works, but it is no longer new".

Nobel prizes are awarded annually in several fields. They are not awarded to quacks, but they do have some unusual competition. The annual Ig Nobel Prizes, conferred by the Annals of Improbable Research (AIR), are now among the most coveted prizes in science.[13]

They honour "achievements that first make people laugh and then make them think." They do not offer financial rewards or offers of funding. The prizes are often mere plastic mock-ups of humorous items, and they have been awarded to some of the world's quirkiest scientists. Recent winners included a UK-Mexico collaboration, for perfecting a method to collect whale snot using a remote-controlled helicopter. Another was the demonstration by a team from Otago University in New Zealand that people slip and fall less often on icy footpaths in winter if they wear their socks on the outside of their shoes.

Andre Geim from Manchester won the 2000 Ig Nobel Prize in Physics and then went on to win the real 2010 Nobel Physics Prize for his research on graphene. His work, by that time, had come to be regarded more seriously. In 2009, Catherine Douglas and Peter Rowlinson of Newcastle University won an Ig Nobel award for revealing that cows with names give more milk than cows that are nameless.

Sometimes the Ig Nobel prizes drifted into irony. The 2010 economics prize was awarded to the executives and directors of Goldman Sachs, AIG, Lehman Brothers, Bear Stearns, Merrill Lynch, and Magnetar for creating and promoting new ways to invest money - ways that maximised financial gain and minimised financial risk for the world economy or for a portion thereof

One piece of British research was a study called "Courtship Behaviour of Ostriches Towards Humans Under Farming Conditions in Britain" and, amazingly, a 2008 prize was awarded to a University of New Mexico team for discovering that professional lap dancers earn higher tips when they are ovulating. The physiology prize was awarded in September 2011 to Anna Wilkinson of the University of Lincoln in England and her colleagues for investigating if the yawning of red-footed tortoises was social and contagious. The full list of previous years' winners can be found at: http://improbable.[14]

This is not quackery it is scientists having fun. On a much more serious note and completely at the other end of the scale patients had their hopes raised, and then dashed, when a much-hyped cancer "breakthrough" was reported in the HealthWatch newsletter.[15] It was even claimed in this article that cancer would soon be a disease of the past. Sadly, the claims were premature. The theory behind the research was good. It showed that two drugs, endostatin and angiostatin, reduced the blood supply in developing tissues such as cancers resulting in the death of these tissues. It was hoped that the rapidly developing growth of certain cancers would be curtailed. Unfortunately, this work could not be replicated.[16] This was not quackery. Sometimes science gets it wrong. The premature announcement by the media, of hope as opposed to fact, was wrong and harmful.

A magazine advertisement recently promised "You name it; I will make it happen..." A spiritualist by the name of Queenie Lane, described in the headline as a "High Priestess", stated that she could be called upon to undertake such tasks as, "removal of a curse, revenge, confidence, weight loss, weight gain, appearance and job status." This advertisement was quackery. It was the subject of a complaint upheld by the Advertising Standards Authority. They considered that the specific claim included in the advertisement "I will make your dreams come true. Guaranteed …" could not be substantiated by the information submitted to them. The advertiser was asked to remove the claim and amend the advertisement wording accordingly. There the matter ended after the "High Priestess" had made her money. No punishment followed. Some of the public were poorer.

American Dietetic Association, American Institute of Nutrition and American Society of Clinical Nutrition) recently issued a warning of ten red flags.[17] The ten flags advised consumers to avoid recommendations that promised a quick fix, claims that sounded too good to be true, simplistic conclusions drawn from complex studies, recommendations based on a single study, dramatic statements that were refuted by reputable scientific organisations should be avoided, lists of "good" and "bad" foods, recommendations made to help sell a product, recommendations based on studies published without peer review and recommendations from studies that ignored differences among individuals or groups. There were dire warnings of danger from a single product or regimen.

Martin Gardner[18] and Ben Goldacre[19] cover the subject of quackery in great detail and very enterprising style. I thoroughly recommend both of these books to anyone interested in the subject. Gardner's book has the following on the main cover "The curious theories of modern pseudoscientists and the strange, amusing and alarming cults that surround them. A Study in Human Gullibility." Ben Goldacre's book was a *Sunday Times* Top Ten Bestseller.

I could certainly not improve on their coverage of the subject, but I will discuss certain aspects of quackery which pertain to obstetrics and gynaecology and I might stray slightly!

References:

1. Kenneth Walker. (1959). *The Story of Medicine.* Arrow Books. Grey Arrow Edition. London. p 20.
2. Martin Gardner. (1957). *"Fads and Fallacies in the Name of Science".* Dover Edition. Dover Publications. New York. p 241. Fads and Fallacies in the Name of Science - Wikipedia, the..,
http://en.wikipedia.org/wiki/Fads_and_Fallacies_in_the_Name_of_Science (accessed July 20, 2013).
3. Wikileaks. En.wikipedia.org/wiki/Philipp Bozzini. History of Endoscopy: Chapter 06. Bozzini: The Beginning of ..,
http://laparoscopy.blogs.com/endoscopyhistory/chapter_06/ (accessed April 27, 2012).
4. History of Endoscopy: Chapter 6. Bozzini: The Beginning of ..,
http://laparoscopy.blogs.com/endoscopyhistory/2008/05/chapter-6.html (accessed July 20, 2013).
5. Ibid.
6. Kenneth Walker. (1959). *The Story of Medicine.* Arrow Books. Grey Arrow Edition. London. p 301.
7. Ibid. p 301.
8. Ibid p 302.
9. Ibid. Quoted from C. J. S. Thompson. (1928). *The Quacks of Old London.* p 303.

10. Kenneth Walker. (1959). *The Story of Medicine.* Arrow Books. Grey Arrow Edition. London. Ibid. p 304.
11. Ibid. p 307.
12. Ibid. p 308.
13. Victoria Lambert. *The Weekly Telegraph.* September 28th - October 4th, 2011. Ig Nobel awards: the triumph of silly science - Telegraph, http://www.telegraph.co.uk/science/science-news/8775127/Ig-Nobel-awards-the-triumph-of-silly-science.html (accessed April 27, 2012).
14. List of Ig Nobel Prize winners - Wikipedia, the free encyclopedia, http://en.wikipedia.org/wiki/Ig_Nobel_Prize_Winners (accessed July 2013).
15. Dr. Neville W. Goodman. HealthWatch newsletter. Issue 30. July 1998. HealthWatch Newsletter no 26, http://www.healthwatch-uk.org/newsletterarchive/nlett26.html (accessed April 27, 2012.
16. The Observer. *"Cancer drug hopes dashed".* 15th November 1998.
17. HealthWatch newsletter. Issue 26. July 1997.
18. Martin Gardner. (1957). *"Fads and Fallacies in the Name of Science".* Dover Edition. Dover Publications. New York. 19. Ben Goldacre. (2009). *"Bad Science".* Fourth Estate. London.

CHAPTER TWO - QUACKERY - HORMONES

In 2002 Michael Henk,[1] an Honorary Clinical Oncologist Consultant at the Royal Marsden Hospital, London questioned the sensational reporting of the Women's Health Initiative. The reported results of this research caused tremendous alarm. Was it all really necessary?

On 10th July, 2002 *The Times* carried the headline "HRT is linked to breast cancer: US study is halted after health fears rise: patients suffer 41 per cent increase in stroke: 22 per cent increase in risk of heart disease"! Equally sensational headlines appeared in other newspapers. Behind these headlines which caused alarm and despondency to millions of woman was the publication of preliminary results from the large USA randomised controlled trial of hormone replacement therapy (HRT) in post-menopausal women in the Journal of the American Medical Association.[2,3] This study will be discussed in the chapter under evidence based medicine but what did the trial actually show?

The study was stopped after 5.2 years because the excess incidence of breast cancer had just hit the conventional five per cent significance level, while the global index supposedly supported risks exceeding benefits. Coronary artery disease and thrombo-embolic disease, in addition to breast cancer and strokes, were more frequent in the HRT group, while fractures attributable to osteoporosis and colorectal cancer were less frequent. The incidence of all these events was very low, and differences between them small, yet all were deemed to be statistically significant. There was no difference in deaths or in the total number of cancers, between the two groups.

Michael Henk stated that "It is sad that despite the enormous amount of work the investigators put into this study, their paper, and especially the reaction of the media to it, tell us much about the pitfalls of statistics and little new about HRT. Focussing on relative risks when absolute risks are small can make a negligible effect appear huge. For example, only 212 of the 16,000 women in the study actually suffered a stroke, 127 (16 fatal) in the HRT group and 85 (13 fatal) in the placebo group. The percentages are 0.29 and 0.21 respectively. Therefore the "41 per cent increase" in strokes actually represents a 0.08 per cent absolute increase, or put another way, 8 more strokes per 10,000 person-years in those taking the HRT. Someone so minded could have extracted from the above data the contrary claim that HRT confers a 22 per cent improvement in the chance of surviving a stroke, but Henk says that he must have missed that headline! The increased risk of breast cancer also works out to be eight cases per 10,000 person-years. He goes on to explain that "The use of the five per cent probability level, '$p<0.05$', as the index of a 'statistically significant' result has become a ritual in clinical research. All it means is that the probability that the observed result of a trial would occur by chance if there were no real difference is no more than five per cent. In other words, one in twenty 'significant' results are false positives. The five per cent level was chosen arbitrarily by Sir Ronald Fisher many years ago, only because it was mathematically convenient, yet it has become the yardstick for publication of clinical trials. It is something of a quirk of mathematics that the smaller the absolute percentages the smaller the difference between them that will achieve statistical significance, hence the number of reportedly significant risks of HRT. Moreover, the $p<0.05$ figure for breast cancer is based on a calculation of 'nominal confidence intervals', i.e. the variability that would arise from a simple trial with a single outcome. When the investigators applied a more complex adjusted method that takes into account multiple testing over time and outcome categories, only thrombo-embolic disease and fractures attained five per cent significance."

These were already known hazards and benefits respectively of HRT. Some of the other apparent effects that this trial purported to demonstrate could well have occurred by chance and might not be a genuine effect of the treatment. Most British medical statisticians, according to Henk, would say that a probability of 0.01 is the maximum that gives grounds for stopping a clinical trial prematurely. However, the action of the trial group in this respect was understandable; breast cancer is such an emotive subject and "$p<0.05$" is so ingrained in both the scientific and legal mind that the fear of litigation in USA left them with no alternative but to stop the trial. In fact, litigation was already underway. The *Sunday Telegraph* reported that lawyers in America had started a worldwide class action against Wyeth, the leading manufacturer of HRT. British women who suffered strokes or other illness while on HRT joined in, claiming they had been used as guinea pigs. The alternativists also entered the fray. In the weekly "What's the Alternative" page in the *Sunday Times* colour supplement the writer Susan Clark pointed out the results of the trial, of course quoting the relative rather than the absolute risks. Instead of HRT she recommended treating menopausal symptoms with a cocktail of phytochemicals, one of which happened to be an estrogen and another, a progestin! Of course she omitted to mention that there had been no objective assessment of the risks of the therapy she recommended. Presumably as it was derived from plants it must be, by definition, "natural" and therefore considered by the alternative therapy adherents to be perfectly safe.

Henk concluded that there was little in the study that should cause alarm to women who took HRT and whose quality of life was enhanced by this treatment but millions of women did indeed stop taking it. Such, according to Henk, were "the consequences of the misapplication of statistics in medicine and journalism."

"Natural" progesterone

Many ladies purchase "natural" progesterone. It is claimed to be the universal panacea curing everything from premenstrual tension to puerperal depression.

To digress to puerperal depression as I have mentioned it; on *Sky News* on the 3rd of October 2011 there was an item describing this "complex and common syndrome" and saying that thousands of women in the United Kingdom, about 33 per cent of new mothers were too scared to mention their depression for fear of being stigmatised. If indeed it is that common, I certainly never realised it. The commentator said that doctors could and should detect the syndrome more often and even warn their patients about the possibility. They could be more sympathetic when it is diagnosed rather than merely prescribing sedatives and anxiolytics. These are probably very valid points.

One of my patients, a very nice nursing sister who was in hospital for a prolonged period of time with threatened preterm labour suffered very severe puerperal depression and she wrote a very poignant poem titled "Mind to let". I have not seen this patient for many years and do not know how to contact her but I have decided to include her poem in this book in the hope that it may help other mothers who suffer from the same condition. I am sure that the lady will not mind me doing this. I am also glad to relate that when I last saw her she had fully recovered and was leading a full, successful and happy life. Puerperal depression is a truly traumatic condition and very few sufferers have the ability to relate their feelings during their period of illness. She was.

Mind to Let

Mind to let, it's vacant,
The owner's packed and gone,
They don't know how it happened,
They say it won't be long.

But try and make them realise,
That I'm no longer here
This other "Mind" is stronger,
They've put mine "out of gear".

There are words and phrases shouting
And screaming in my mind,
With long- forgotten memories,
Of words that were unkind,

"Snap out of it", they tell me
I'm trying, can't they see?
This strange, bizarre behaviour,
It really isn't me,

A great abyss divides me,
From friends and every day,
How will I find a footbridge,
Nobody knows the way.

Along a long dark tunnel,
With no light at the end,
And only love to help me,
A husband and a friend.

and the rest

Back to "natural" progesterone.

Many patients are dissatisfied with estrogen replacement therapy (ERT) because doctors may not explain this treatment adequately due to time constraints, the patients lack true knowledge of the risks and benefits of the treatment, they fear cancer, they do not want the inconvenience of monthly withdrawal vaginal bleeds, they wish to control their own health and they dislike the thought of taking medication for the rest of their lives. No more than 30 per cent of women comply with their prescribed estrogen regimens. In women prescribed estrogens for the first time 20 to 30 per cent never even have the prescription filled. Moreover, 20 per cent discontinue therapy within the first nine months and another 10 per cent use estrogen therapy in an intermittent fashion. Approximately two-thirds of those who start therapy with an estrogen progestin sequential regimen discontinue the progestin after 12 months. Because of this limited acceptability of prolonged estrogen replacement therapy many patients are looking for substitutes and they are prepared to accept alternative forms of treatment even though these may be untried and unproven but marketed very successfully by misguided well wishers or, being uncharitable, unscrupulous money-makers.

In addition to this, as a result of the publication of the Women's Health Initiative report in July 2002 mentioned above, many more women sought alternative treatment.[4] One alternative that was promoted was a transdermal cream containing bio-identical progesterone. In 1974, Dr. John R. Lee, a Californian general practitioner with a background in pharmacology, had developed this cream. It was intended to deliver 10–12 mg. progesterone daily. In the normal menstrual cycle following ovulation, the secretion of progesterone increases to between 20 to 25 mg. per day.

Lee reported that most patients using the cream experienced an improved sense of well-being. On the basis of these anecdotal responses, he developed and promoted progesterone cream as a commercial product. Pharmaceutical companies in the United States, France, and Australia marketed the progesterone creams.

Clinical information on the benefits and use of this transdermal progesterone cream, without the addition of estrogen, was based on reports mostly from the United States. Many claims were made but the paucity of credible supportive scientific data raised considerable concern regarding the potency of this form of progesterone therapy [5, 6, 7, 8] and peer-reviewed studies have failed to confirm the expectations expounded by proponents of this treatment regimen. Currently, available progesterone creams cannot be recommended for treatment of symptoms associated with menopause.[9]

Lee[10] the most prominent promoter of so called "natural progesterone" in his book stated quite openly that "as with other hormones, any use of progesterone as a therapeutic modality should be undertaken only with consultation with one's physician".

Yet there are today, in Zimbabwe and elsewhere, certain unqualified totally non-medical people openly promoting the sale of "natural progesterone". Everyone has the fundamental right to treat their own body as they wish. They have the right to take whatever medication they wish or they need not take any medication at all if they do not want to. After all some people smoke! What is totally wrong however is that many of these people selling "natural progesterone" are advising patients to stop taking the estrogen and other treatment which has been prescribed by their doctors. By advising patients, who would otherwise live longer and in whom the quality of life would be enhanced by their estrogen treatment, to stop the treatment, these persons are effectively shortening their patients' lives.

Bioharmony, a company registered in South Africa, wrote to me on 15th May, 1997 regarding their product Ultrafemme which they described as an "original formulation of natural progesterone derived from selected Wild Yam (Dioscorea)" and making many extravagant claims for this product. They went on to state that Dr. Beverly Hoffman of Stellenbosch University near Cape Town, and they gave her telephone numbers, "has taken a personal academic interest in the formulation and is currently embarking on a three-year clinical research program on the product together with Tygerberg Hospital to establish its clinical effects on osteoporosis". I have a letter in my possession from Professor Kobie van der Merwe of Tygerberg Hospital, after I requested specific information on Dr Beverly Hoffman's work, in which he states "I spoke to Beverly Hoffman. She said that she has been quoted on something she said informally. She does not do any research on Ultrafemme or any other drug. There is no scientific evidence of Ultrafemme being used in postmenopausal women".

Bioharmony continued their letter saying that the Wild Yam is extracted through an "Alcohol Extraction" process. It works more on a homeopathic basis whereby the Progesterone receptors are stimulated thus ensuring increased production of Progesterone at the body's natural pace of action." What abject nonsense.

In another letter dated 27th June, 1997 written by a Maria Ascencao she states that "The product ('natural progesterone') has been well researched, thoroughly tested and arrived at after many years of intensive research. Thousands of women are currently reaping enormously positive and health-enhancing effects from the use of the product." "The product has been on the market for two years with NO (in capitals) side effects." In the same letter Ms Ascencao states that "The Dioscorea villosa extract (Wild Yam) is Nature's storehouse of natural steroidal saponins and phyto-progesterones". No mention that the Dioscorea villosa is also a precursor of estrogens!

This misconception that wild yam contains hormones or hormonal precursors is largely due to the historical fact that progesterone, androgens, and cortisone were chemically manufactured from Mexican wild yam in the 1960s. Some herbalists even recommend Wild Yam as a natural contraceptive or birth control measure. Herbal roulette!

According to Martindale, the "bible" of the pharmaceutical profession and published by The Royal Pharmaceutical Society, progesterone in its natural state in a double-blind placebo-controlled crossover study involving 168 women in a dose of 400 to 800 mg given daily by the vaginal route did not significantly improve symptoms of the premenstrual syndrome[11]. The results of this trial were questioned by a Katherine Dalton.[12] She suggested that the dose and frequency of administration needed to be individualised and that if the response to treatment was inadequate then the intramuscular route should have been tried. More recent studies have found oral micronized progesterone in an initial dose of 300 mg. four times daily, to be no better than placebo in the management of severe premenstrual syndrome.[13, 14]

Doctors have nothing to gain by prescribing estrogen rather than "natural progesterone". Unlike the purveyors of progesterone creams doctors obtain no monetary reward whatever they prescribe. They prescribe estrogen for treatment of the climacteric and they prescribe progesterone for the conditions for which it is indicated.

This upsurge of interest in "natural" medicines is not confined to Zimbabwe. Patients are looking for alternatives to estrogen for the reasons mentioned previously. "Natural progesterone" is really being promoted sometimes, although misguided, with the best of intentions and sometimes solely for pecuniary reasons. It should be noted that, in addition to progesterone, all the natural estrogens other than conjugated equine estrogen (which is derived from the urine of pregnant mares) are derived from plants, cactus or soya bean. If progesterone is natural then so is estrogen.

As mentioned previously the quack may only be distinguished from the physician by means of their predominant motive and not by the mode of their treatment. If purveyors of "natural" progesterone cream genuinely believe that they are doing good and are not merely selling their products for the purpose of monetary gain then they possibly should not be termed "quacks".

Dr Barbara Gross, Chief Scientist for the Sydney Menopause Centre, wrote an article on progesterone creams for the Australian Menopause Society (Amarant).[15]

According to her more and more women were rejecting synthetic hormones and turning to what they believe are "natural" products. They were purchasing so-called "natural" remedies over-the-counter from pharmacies, health food stores, or from direct sellers. They were often unaware that these preparations are also medicines or pharmaceutical preparations. Unlike most prescribed products, however these preparations or "natural" remedies are often not required to be registered. Legally in Australia and in many other countries claims cannot be made by the sellers of these items that their preparations can have a particular effect on the body even though this message is often conveyed by word of mouth by the sales force. If claims are made, they have to be in accordance with advertising codes. Manufacturers often do not, or cannot, list all the active ingredients. They are not required to show that the products do in fact contain the stated amount of a particular ingredient i.e. there is no required quality control from batch to batch. One has to rely on the integrity of the companies manufacturing and distributing the products. There are obviously many very ethical companies who do have strict quality controls but how can the consumer tell the difference between these products?

More importantly the companies are not required to carry out research to test the effectiveness or the safety of many of these listed preparations. This is in contrast to the requirements of the Australian Drug Regulatory authorities for most pharmaceutical companies which are required to thoroughly research and prove the effectiveness and safety of the preparations they wish to register. This often requires ten or more years of research on animals and humans and thousands to millions of dollars in costs.

A few years ago I attended a New Product Information Seminar in Australia where Bullivant's Natural Health Products were discussed. Amongst their outrageous claims was one for "Hypericum 2000 + L-Tyrosine" a substance which they labelled "natural nutrition". In the key points of description for this substance was the statement: "Specific for the treatment of viral conditions such as influenza, herpes, glandular fever and AIDS". At the bottom of each page of the booklet which they supplied was stated quite clearly: "FOR PROFESSIONAL USE ONLY. NOT FOR ADVERTISING". This statement was obviously made to circumvent illegal advertising.

What, in fact, does "natural" mean? Is it harmless? Many people consider that if the product comes from plants then usually it is natural and therefore it is better than synthetic medicines. Here are examples of some "natural" products that are not good for one. Lead, uranium, radon, arsenic, thallium, strychnine, cyanide (in *Sorghum* and *Prunus* species), stinging nettles, poison ivy, yew, deadly nightshade, castor beans (ricin), tobacco, curare, foxglove, fly agaric, (muscarine), death cap (amanita phalloides).[16] There are many more.

What many people do not realise is that many, if not most, of our medicines do actually originally come from plants. Aspirin for example comes from the bark of the willow tree therefore aspirin could be considered natural. Digitalis, the heart drug, comes from foxglove. As stated previously both estradiol and progesterone come from soy bean or wild yam. One is sold in skin creams and gels, oral capsules, and vaginal gels and the other as creams, tablets or implants. Why is one considered to be "natural" and the other is not unless this is a marketing ploy? It gets worse. As Bioharmony and Maria Ascencao both said, so-called "natural" progesterone is modified or synthesised from Dioscorea villosa. The plant itself does not contain estradiol or progesterone but it does contain a fat or saponin called diosgenin. This fat is extracted from the wild yam root or rhizome and then by a series of steps, progesterone or estradiol, and also cortisone and testosterone can be made in the laboratory. Many of these so-called "natural" hormones are therefore in fact produced in a laboratory by either clinical or enzyme processes. The estradiol and progesterone, produced in the laboratory from soy or wild yam, have exactly the same chemical structure as the hormones produced in human ovaries, the real or biological human hormones.

Do the "natural progesterone" creams contain hormones? If they do they should be subject to the same regulations required for other pharmaceutical products containing hormones. Hormones are potent compounds affecting many body tissues and should be treated with respect for that reason! In Australia, the companies that distribute the creams cannot, by law, use the word "Progesterone" on the label nor state that the creams contain progesterone nor make any claims related to progesterone. There are several creams available, for example, Natra Gest, Endau, Progest, Renewed Balance all of which are believed to contain different amounts of progesterone but they can only be marketed as moisturising or skin creams, Other creams have ingredients labelled "Wild Yam extract". They may or may not have progesterone added to the cream. Still other creams are labelled "Wild Yam Cream". Many have no progesterone at all in them!

A laboratory in California[17] analysed several progesterone and wild yam creams available in the USA and there are many. The amount of progesterone in the creams ranged from none to very high (2,000 mg. per ounce) amounts. They all claimed to have progesterone-like action and benefits! Like most steroids, progesterone can be absorbed through the skin but achieving normal blood levels, e.g. levels seen in the second half of the menstrual cycle (20-25 mg/day) is difficult. After twice daily applications of a high dose (15 mg.) of a progesterone cream a study in the USA reported levels of progesterone equivalent to the low range of the second half of the menstrual cycle. Absorption can be improved by using a carrier (e.g. vitamin E or liposomes) to increase the solubility of progesterone, which is fat soluble. A recent study in the United Kingdom[18], after double the recommended dose of cream was applied twice daily, found low levels of progesterone in the blood.

Progesterone creams are currently being extensively promoted in the writings of Dr Lee[19] and other authors who freely quote him e.g. Sherril Selman, Leslie Kenton, women's magazines, and distributors of progesterone and wild yam creams for use for some of the following conditions: premenstrual symptoms/syndrome, menopause symptoms particularly hot flushes and night sweats, prevention and treatment of osteoporosis and fibrocystic breasts. Dr Gross, in the Amarant article, said that there have been no well-designed prospective clinical trials which prove the effectiveness of the use of transdermal progesterone creams for any of these conditions in the human female, with the possible exception of premenstrual painful breasts.

There have been many reports that women have substituted using progesterone cream for their progestogen tablets, A woman could be putting herself at risk if, while continuing to take or use estrogen and without medical advice, she does this. If a woman still has her uterus and is using an estrogen preparation (tablet, patch, cream, gel, implant or injection) alone, she is at risk of having abnormal changes in the lining of the uterus which could lead to cancer of the uterus. For this reason, women who still have a uterus are prescribed progesterone as well as estrogens for management of their symptoms. Although progesterone in large doses (100 to 200 mg.), taken by mouth (capsules) or administered vaginally (capsules or pessaries), has been shown to protect the uterus, there have been no studies to show that progesterone cream will deliver sufficient, progesterone to protect the lining of the uterus. The most important concern is safety.

Dr. Lee has reported on his clinical observations of the benefit for women of using progesterone cream for treatment of hot flushes but he has not carried out any clinical trials. There is a plethora of anecdotal evidence by women using the same cream who attest to relief of symptoms such as hot flushes. The effectiveness of the use of progesterone-based skin creams needs to be evaluated against placebo creams. The observations and comments contained in books written by Dr. Lee have been used as the basis for numerous companies and authors to promote their creams despite the absence of scientific studies or even clinical observations.

The American College of Obstetrics and Gynecology Task Force [20] issued a review statement concerning topical progesterone, testosterone and other "Natural Hormones" sold in health food stores and via the Internet.

The Task Force stated that no formal studies had been conducted to determine the safety and/or effectiveness of these products.

Many so-called "natural" progesterone creams did not contain substances that the human body can use as progesterone. These products are often derived from wild yam extracts and contain diosgenin that only plants can metabolise into active progesterone.

They also warned that some treatments have the potential to cause drug interactions with other medications. Dietary supplements, including herbal products, were not as strictly regulated as were prescription and over-the-counter drugs.[21] As a result, potency might vary from product to product, or even from batch to batch of the same product. "Natural" did not mean that the remedies were without risks or side effects. They advised taking the same care when using alternative supplements or products as one would when using any prescription medication.

Dr. Gorski an Obstetrician and Gynaecologist in Arlington, Texas, and president of the Greater Dallas-Fort Worth Council Against Health Fraud gave a detailed Medscape interview titled "Wild Yam Cream Threatens Women's Health".[22]

His comments were very much in line with the American College of Obstetrics and Gynecology Task Force statement. He stated that the greatest danger posed by this product and its deceptive promotion was that it would lead many menopausal women to forego or even discontinue appropriate hormone-replacement therapy (HRT) and that the last thing American women needed was another unproven "natural alternative" promoted by a campaign of deceit at the expense of their lives, health, and well-being.

He also pointed out that wild yam cream[23] cost more than Premarin. A month's supply of Wild Yam Cream cost about $US 27 whereas a month's supply of Premarin cost $US 12. Progesterone cream is at present being sold in Harare at $US 34.00 for 50 grams of Progest. It depends how often and in what dose the cream is applied as to how long 50 grams will last. The amount of 50 grams is supposed to be one month's treatment but if a twice daily dose of 15 mg. of Progesterone as mentioned above i.e. 30 mg. per day is used, then 50 grams would last for approximately 16 to 17 days. Double that to make roughly a month's supply and that would cost $US 68.00.

Premarin, the correct treatment for symptoms of the climacteric is being sold for $US 28.00 for one month's treatment. Progesterone cream treatment is not cheap! Not a bad profit for something that is not effective.

Gorski described, what he called, "The most outrageous promotion I have encountered" a "Medical Recall Notice" mailing from "Health Notification Service" of Henderson, Nevada.

The official-looking contents purported to be a recall of all "Prescription Estrogens and Progestins" because of "Severe and Prolonged Life-Threatening Side Effects." According to this mailing, the "Indicated Treatment" to be substituted was a "Natural Progesterone Cream" with "No Harmful Side Effects," with the order form, of course, conveniently enclosed. In September 2000, the United States Food and Drug Administration warned the owners of the company, Roger J. and Debra L. Peeples, that it was illegal to suggest that their "Miracle Wild Yam Cream" was useful in treating or preventing osteoporosis, symptoms of menopause, depression, premenstrual syndrome, breast cancer, postpartum depression, ovarian cysts, fibrocystic mastitis, infertility, or other diseases and conditions.

In February 2002, the Illinois Attorney General charged the company and owners with violating the Consumer Fraud and Deceptive Business Practices Act and the Illinois Food, Drug and Cosmetic Act.

Bio-identical hormones

With the fear of breast cancer generated by the findings of the Women's Health Initiative study, women sought alternatives for their menopausal symptoms. Celebrities can markedly influence the practice of medicine. This has been shown many times over by notables including Steve McQueen, Larry King, Prince Charles, David Beckham, Roger Moore, Tom Cruise and Peter Sellers. Suzanne Somers, an actress, Oprah Winfrey, and others even including some doctors, achieved a certain amount of success in promoting bioidentical hormones.

Somers, the actress, believed that estrogen replacement therapy caused heart disease, blood clots and cancer because they were made by big pharmaceutical companies. If women used natural hormones found in plants or so-called "Natural bioidentical hormones" made by small isolated pharmacies they would avoid these risks.

Paul Offit[24] makes the point "that estrogen is estrogen. Whether it's isolated from soybeans, wild yams, or horse's urine, it's the same molecule; the source is irrelevant. The only thing that matters is the molecular structure of the final product. " Dr Offit quotes Joe Schwarz from McGill University as saying: "When it comes to assessing effectiveness and safety, whether the substance is synthetic or natural is totally irrelevant."

Another point made by Offit is that bioidentical and conventional hormones are primarily all made in the same way. They are synthesized from plants in factories and then sent to small compounding pharmacies and to the major pharmaceutical companies." They therefore carry the same risks. The bioidentical industry claim that their products have all the benefits and carry none of the risks of those produced by the big pharmaceutical companies is simply not true.

Wulf Utian,[25] a professor of obstetrics and gynecology at Case Western University, quoted by Dr Offit, said that if you believe that "you might as well believe in the Tooth Fairy."

Dr Offit says that "The difference between bioidentical and conventional hormones isn't that one is natural and the other isn't. Or that one is safe and the other isn't. It's that one is the product of an unsupervised industry and the other isn't."

In 2001, the FDA analyzed twenty-nine products from twelve compounding pharmacies and found that 34 percent failed standard quality or potency tests. The

American College of Obstetricians and Gynecologists, the American Association of Clinical Endocrinologists, the American Medical Association, the American Cancer Society, the Mayo Clinic, and the FDA have all issued statements asserting that bioidentical hormones are probably as risky as their conventional counterparts.

The following is from an article which appeared on the USA Food and Drug Administration's Consumer Updates page[26], which features the latest on all FDA-regulated products. It was updated on April 8th, 2008.

Sellers of compounded "bio-identical" hormones[27] often claim that their products are identical to hormones made by the body and that these "all-natural" pills, creams, lotions, and gels are without the risks of standard drugs approved by the Food and Drug Administration for menopausal hormone therapy.

"Bio-identical hormone replacement therapy" (BHRT)[28] is a marketing term not recognised by the United States Food and Drug Administration.

They have not approved compounded "BHRT" drugs as they cannot assure their safety or effectiveness. This has not stopped the makers of these "bio-identical" hormones from claiming that their wares are: "A natural, safer alternative to dangerous prescription drugs", "Can slim you down by reducing hormonal imbalances" and "Prevents Alzheimer's disease and senility". These claims are unproven and the Food and Drug Administration is concerned that claims like these mislead women and health care professionals, giving them a false sense of assurance about using potentially dangerous hormone products.

Drugs that are approved by the Food and Drug Administration must undergo the agency's rigorous evaluation process, which scrutinises everything about the drug to ensure its safety and effectiveness from early testing, to the design and results of large clinical trials, to the severity of side effects and to the conditions under which the drug is manufactured. All Food and Drug Administration-approved drugs have undergone this process and all must meet federal standards for approval. No compounded "BHRT" drug has met these standards.

Steve Silverman, Assistant Director of the Office of Compliance in the Food and Drug Administration's Centre for Drug Evaluation and Research said that "Unlike commercial drug manufacturers, pharmacies are not required to report adverse events associated with compounded drugs. One of the big problems is that we just do not know what risks are associated with these so-called 'bio-identicals.' "

On January 9th, 2008 the U.S. Food and Drug Administration issued a news release stating that they had sent letters warning seven pharmacy operations that the claims they had made about the safety and effectiveness of their so-called "bio-identical hormone replacement therapy," products were unsupported by medical evidence, and were considered false and misleading by the agency. The pharmacy operations had improperly claimed that their drugs, which contained hormones such as estrogen and progesterone, were superior to Food and Drug Administration approved menopausal hormone therapy drugs and prevented or treated serious diseases, including Alzheimer's disease, stroke, and various forms of cancer.

Compounded drugs are not reviewed by the Food and Drug Administration for safety and effectiveness, and the Food and Drug Administration encourages patients to use Food and Drug Administration approved drugs whenever possible. The warning letters stated that the pharmacy operations violated federal law by making false and misleading claims about their hormone therapy drugs. The Food and Drug Administration regarded the use of the term "bio-identical" as a marketing term implying a benefit for the drug, for which there was no medical or scientific basis. The pharmacy operations used the terms "bio-identical hormone replacement therapy" to imply that their drugs are natural or identical to the hormones made by the body.

Firms that did not properly address the violations identified in the warning letters risked further enforcement, including injunctions that would prevent additional violations as well as seizure of certain products.

On a visit to Beacon Bay near East London in South Africa in February 2012 I went into a "Health" shop and enquired as to whether they sold "natural" progesterone cream. I was informed by a very pleasant saleslady that the product had been rescheduled and could now only be obtained from pharmacies. She did offer to obtain some for me but I told her that I was only enquiring as I considered it to be "quackery". She then laughingly and quite openly told me that the shop had many other "quackery" products. This was a lovely and very refreshing approach.

References:

1. Michael Henk. HealthWatch. (October 2002). *Damned lies, statistics and HRT.* Newsletter no 47.
2. Fletcher SW, Colditz GA. Failure of estrogen plus progestin therapy for prevention. JAMA 288:366-368, 2002.
3. Writing Group for the Women's Health Initiative Investigators. Risks and benefits of estrogen plus progestin in healthy postmenopausal women: Principal results from the Women's Health Initiative Randomized Controlled Trial. JAMA 288:321-333, 2002.
4. Barry G. Wren. Clinical Update. (2005). *The Medical Journal of Australia. (MJA)* 182: p 237-239.
5. Eagon, P. K., Elm, M. S., Hunter, D. S. et al. (Jun 8-11. 2000). *Medicinal herbs: modulation of estrogen action. Era of Hope* Mtg. Dept Defense; Breast Cancer Res Prog, Atlanta, GA.
6. Freeman, E. W. et al. (1990). *Ineffectiveness of progesterone suppository treatment for premenstrual syndrome.* JAMA; 264: p 349-353.
7. Dalton, K. (1988). *Treating the premenstrual syndrome.* Br. Med. J. 297: p 490.
8. Freeman, E. W. et al. (1995) *A double-blind trial of oral progesterone, alprazolam and placebo in treatment of severe premenstrual syndrome.* JAMA; p 51-57.
9. Barry G. Wren. Clinical Update. (2005). *The Medical Journal of Australia. (MJA)* 182: p 237-239.
10. John R. Lee and Virginia Hopkins (1996) *What your doctor may not tell you about menopause.* Warner Books, New York. USA.
11. Sean C. Sweetman, ed. (2011). *Martindale: The Complete Drug Reference* (37th edition ed.). London: Pharmaceutical Press. ISBN 978-0-85369-933-0.

12. Dalton, K. (1988). *Treating the premenstrual syndrome.* Br Med J.; 297: p 490.
13. Freeman, E. W. et al. (1990). *Ineffectiveness of progesterone suppository treatment for premenstrual syndrome.* JAMA; 264: p 349-353.
14. Freeman, E. W. et al. (1995). *A double-blind trial of oral progesterone, alprazolam and placebo in treatment of severe premenstrual syndrome.* JAMA; 274: p 51-57.
15. Barbara Gross, Dr.. Amarant Newsletter. Sydney Menopause Centre, Royal Hospital for Women, Randwick, New South Wales, Australia.
16. The quack page, http://www.ucl.ac.uk/pharmacology/dc-bits-old/quack4.html (accessed July 20, 2013).
17. USA Study: Dollbaum & Duwe. (1996). *Abstracts of 7th Annual Meeting of North American Menopause Society.*
18. UK study cited Lancet 1997, as reported at the 1997 meeting of the British Menopause Society.
19. John R. Lee and Virginia Hopkins (1996) *What your doctor may not tell you about menopause.* Warner Books, New York. USA.
20. The American College of Obstetrics and Gynecology Task Force Review on *Topical Progesterone, Testosterone and other "natural" hormones.* www. ACOG. Task Force Review.
21. Women's Health Information at Bayside Gynecology, http://baysidegyn.com/health%20information.htm (accessed July 20, 2013).
22. Timothy N. Gorski, M.D. (April 8th, 2008).Greater Dallas-Fort Worth Council Against Health Fraud. Quackwatch Home Page. This article was revised on July 19, 2002.
23. WILD YAM CREAM, http://lesann.tripod.com/wild%20yam%20cream.htm (accessed July 20, 2013).
24. Dr. Paul Offit. Killing Us Softly.The Sense and Nonsense of Alternative Medicine. Fourth Estate. London. ISBN 978-0-00-749172-8. p 116.
25. Ibid. p 117.
26. FDA Consumer Update.
27. When it comes to estrogen and progesterone, what is the .., http://www.everydayhealth.com/health-questions/hormone-replacement-therapy/when-it-comes-to-estrogen-and-progesterone-what-is-the-difference (accessed July 20, 2013).
28. Ibid.

CHAPTER THREE - QUACKERY - COMPLEMENTARY AND ALTERNATIVE MEDICINE (CAM)

What is CAM?

In recent years a wide range of unconventional therapies have been offered as "alternative" or "complementary" to mainstream medicine. These include everything from herbal medicines, homeopathy, and aromatherapy to the use of acupuncture, therapeutic touch, prayer at a distance, faith healing, chelation therapy, "miraculous" cancer cures and others.[1] The charter Members of the Council for Scientific Medicine posted a statement[2] saying that the need for objective, scientific critiques of the claims of "alternative" or non-conventional medicine has never been greater.

They argued that there was a lack of readily available, reliable information about the efficacy of such treatments. This impaired people's free choice and increased risks to their health. The potential harm was incalculable but appeared to be growing. The trend was abetted by those who promoted unproven treatments, especially those who were "naive, greedy, or unscrupulous." They criticised the media for dwelling on controversial and false claims without providing critical examination of them. The public was often subjected to anecdotal testimony of people allegedly cured. Many best-selling books promoted the power of such alleged healings, but they "hardly passed the scrutiny of peer review." The results of proper scientific research were not published enough. Instead several journals devoted exclusively to "alternative" medicine had appeared recently. These merely advocated unconventional treatments and rarely assessed them objectively. The statement, in fairness, pointed out that credible, scientific assessments of many "alternative" medicine claims already existed and that new evaluations based on available information were possible. Both the public and some medical professionals seemed unaware of this. The statement stressed that there was a critical need to test new claims before they were marketed to the public.

The signatories to the statement welcomed the founding of a new journal; *The Scientific Review of Alternative Medicine*,[3] the first peer-reviewed journal dedicated entirely to the scientific, rational evaluation of unconventional health claims. The purpose of the journal was to "apply the best tools of science and reason to determine the validity of hypotheses and the effectiveness of treatments." It would seek to answer two questions: "Is it true?" and "Does this treatment work?" It would call for double-blind controlled trials of "alternative" therapies. It is a prime requisite for any scientist or doctor to know the answers to these questions. They called on physicians, scientists, health practitioners, and citizens everywhere to support the journal in advancing scientific medicine and expanding the benefits of free and informed choice.

Alternative medicine is any healing practice, "that does not fall within the realm of conventional medicine."[4] It is based on historical or cultural traditions, rather than on scientific evidence. It is frequently grouped with complementary medicine under the umbrella term complementary and alternative medicine, or CAM but, unlike mainstream medicine, claims about the efficacy of alternative medicine tend to lack evidence.

The United States National Science Foundation[5] has defined alternative medicine as "all treatments that have not been proven effective using scientific methods". Proponents of evidence-based medicine agree that all treatments, whether "mainstream" or "alternative", ought to be held to the standards of the scientific method.[6] Angell and Kassirer[7] have stated that "healthcare practices should be classified based solely on scientific evidence. It is time for the scientific community to stop giving alternative medicine "a free ride".

There cannot be two kinds of medicine – conventional and alternative. There is only medicine that has been adequately tested and medicine that has not, medicine that works and medicine that may or may not work. There is no alternative to science-based medicine, just as there is no alternative to astronomy or chemistry unless one accepts astrology or alchemy.[8]

Therefore, a middle ground somewhere between science and validity on one hand, and pseudoscience and indeterminacy on the other, cannot logically exist or be acceptable to a rational society. Once a treatment has been tested rigorously and shown beyond doubt to be effective, it no longer matters whether it was considered alternative at the outset.[9] If it is found to be reasonably safe and effective, it will and should be accepted. But assertions, speculation, and testimonials do not substitute for evidence. Once accepted it ceases to be "alternative" and becomes just like any other part of medical knowledge. That means, though, that "alternative medicine" must consist, at present, entirely of unproven treatments. Alternative treatments should be subjected to scientific testing no less rigorous than that required for conventional treatments."[10]

Integrative medicine or integrative health is the combination of practices and methods of alternative medicine with conventional medicine.[11] Some universities and hospitals have departments of integrative medicine but Dr. Arnold Relman, editor in chief emeritus of The New England Journal of Medicine wrote[12]: "There are not two kinds of medicine, one conventional and the other unconventional, that can be practiced jointly in a new kind of 'integrative medicine.' In the best kind of medical practice, all proposed treatments must be tested objectively. In the end, there will only be treatments that pass that test and those that do not, those that are proven worthwhile and those that are not. Can there be any reasonable 'alternative'?" Dr. Marcia Angell, executive editor of The New England Journal of Medicine said, "It's a new name for snake oil."[13]

The legal aspects of alternative medicine vary from state to state in the United States. For example in California naturopaths are licensed. In Tennessee it is illegal and in Arkansas, it is not addressed legally. The FDA has jurisdiction for herbs, nutritional supplements and alternative medical devises sold across state lines.[14] The regulation and prevalence of homeopathy is discussed in the next chapter. It is practised fairly commonly in some countries in Europe while being uncommon in others. Regulations vary depending on the country. In some countries, there are no specific legal regulations concerning the use of homeopathy, while in others, licenses or degrees in conventional medicine from accredited universities are required.

In its December 2nd, 2002 issue, *Newsweek* published a special report on "The Science of Alternative Medicine." Dr. William M. London, a former president of the National Council against Health Fraud, commented on this special report. He referred to the report as "Newsweek's Misleading Report on Alternative Medicine" [15] and wrote a very detailed and well referenced exposé of the article. London emphasised that "the science of alternative medicine" falsely implied that a meaningful category of healthcare called "alternative medicine" existed and was scientifically based but, in common usage, he said that the term "alternative medicine" was "a euphemism used by enthusiasts and profiteers to give the appearance of legitimacy to methods promoted with scientifically implausible, invalidated, or non-validated claims". His article is well worth reading. He discussed the comments in the article on acupuncture, chiropractors, traditional Chinese medicine, herbal products such as ginkgo biloba and the placebo effect amidst others and he concluded that "Instead of attempting a special report on "The Science of Alternative Medicine," *Newsweek* should have served its readers well by providing an exposé of "Pseudoscience Promoted as Alternative Medicine."

Edzard Ernst, the world's first Professor of Complementary Medicine, retired in May, 2011 after 18 years in his post at Exeter University. Despite his title, Dr Ernst was described as "no breathless promoter of snake oil". According to one study he had pioneered the rigorous study of everything from acupuncture and crystal healing to Reiki channelling and herbal remedies. Professor Ernst wrote *The Desktop Guide to Complementary and Alternative Medicine. An evidence-based approach.* [16] This book provided evidence-based information on 69 popular forms of complementary and alternative medicine, and 46 common conditions frequently treated with CAM. It summarised clinical trial data on the effectiveness of CAM for specific conditions and alerted readers to cases where CAM might be risky or inappropriate.

Ernst was also awarded the 2005 HealthWatch Award which he regarded as very courageous on the part of HealthWatch as Ernst was a researcher of the very subject HealthWatch often criticised and also courageous on his part to accept the award as it would be unlikely to result in praise from the proponents of complementary medicine. In receiving the award Ernst spoke[17] on the good and bad points of complementary medicine. He said that when it comes to healthcare, "likes and dislikes should matter far less than evidence."

Healthcare is not a fashion where one might legitimately have this or that opinion, nor should it be confused with religion in which one either believes or doesn't. Medical treatments either demonstrably and reproducibly work or they don't." He quoted the example of the recent (first ever) trial of shark cartilage for cancer[18] showing that this form of treatment had no beneficial effect. Ernst considered this good news all round. Sharks would not die needlessly, cancer patients would not attach false hopes to a bogus treatment and money could be saved for effective treatments.[19] The only people who could possibly perceive this finding as "negative" were those involved in "peddling bogus cancer cures and swindling desperate patients and their families of their savings."[20]

He pointed out that examples of CAM that did work included real acupuncture which was shown to be better than sham acupuncture for a range of pain-related syndromes, e.g. back pain[21] and several systematic reviews of rigorous clinical trials which had demonstrated that certain herbal medicines were efficacious for certain indications.[22] As long as the findings were based on good science, it was good news.

Ernst listed Cochrane systematic reviews that he said "suggested" efficacy of herbal medicines.[23] These included andrographis for upper respiratory tract infection, cranberry for urinary tract infection, devil's claw for osteoarthritis and back pain, ginkgo for intermittent claudication and dementia, ginger for morning sickness, hawthorn for chronic heart failure, horse chestnut for chronic venous insufficiency, lava for anxiety and menopausal symptoms, nettle for benign prostatic hyperplasia, peppermint for abdominal pain, non ulcer dyspepsia and the irritable bowel syndrome, saw palmetto for benign prostatic hyperplasia, St. John's Wort for depression and yohimbe for erectile dysfunction, but Ernst's feelings of "suggested" efficacy were often not shared.

Other authors have concluded that saw palmetto, used by over two million men in the United States, was not effective for benign prostatic hyperplasia."[24] and Ernst himself, in a later publication merely said that there was evidence "suggesting" that St. John's Wort, a herbal remedy, "could help" with mild depression.[25]

In October 1991 the U.S. Congress provided $2 million in funding for the fiscal year 1992 to establish an office within the National Institutes of Health (NIH) to investigate and evaluate promising unconventional medical practices. This was the Office of Alternative Medicine (OAM) which became the National Centre for Complementary and Alternative Medicine (NCCAM) after it was established by the U.S. Congress in October 1998. At the same time its status was elevated from "Office" to "Centre".

Gunnar B. Stickler,[26] Emeritus Professor of Paediatrics at the Mayo Clinic said that according to the NCCAM Web site, 30 centre grants, 67 research grants, 14 co-operative agreements, and four training grants were awarded from 1993 to 1998. By 2001, "remarkably little had been found effective and, surprisingly, there had been few enlightening publications of any kind."

In February 2000 NCCAM provided a complete bibliography of the research it supported. There were 62 entries between 1995 and 1999. They included seven reports of controlled studies in humans. Two were about the use of acupuncture for pain control after tooth extraction[27] and knee pain in patients with osteoarthritis.[28] A small benefit was reported for each but these two studies were repeats of similar earlier investigations by the same authors.[29, 30] In other studies, massage therapy of 14 infants of HIV-positive mothers,[31] and of bone marrow transplant patients[32] found results slightly superior to those in controls. One study on absorption and "imagery instruction" on immunoglobulin A (IgA) levels in saliva, the clinical significance of which is unknown, showed positive effects.[33] In one trial patients in a methadone maintenance program were randomised into two groups. One received dynamic group psychotherapy and another group practiced Hatha yoga weekly for six months.[34] Both groups experienced significantly decreased drug use and decreased criminal activity, but there was no difference between the two groups, nor was there a no treatment control group.

A group in Munich, Germany, found 89 studies with data adequate for meta-analysis.[35] This was done on 185 placebo-controlled trials of homeopathic preparations. The authors reported that they "found insufficient evidence from these studies that homeopathy is clearly efficacious for any clinical condition." The findings were similar to other studies of the same type.[36] Also in the bibliography were 13 surveys of the practice and teaching of complementary medicine, eight uncontrolled treatment trials, eight animal or tissue culture studies, five pilot studies, and three plans for future study.[37] Twelve reports were listed as "in press" or "submitted for publication," one paper was listed twice, and five could not be found using MEDLINE. "None of these contained information useful for medical practice."[38]

While there are many reports of controlled studies about alternative medicine, just two reviews are mentioned.[39] From a meta-analysis of homeopathy it was concluded that "at the moment the evidence of clinical trials is positive but not sufficient to draw definite conclusions because most trials are of low methodological quality and because of the unknown role of publication bias."[40]

In a position paper released in 1988 and published in 1991,[41] the National Council Against Health Fraud concluded that the scientific literature up to that time had provided no evidence that acupuncture performed consistently better than a placebo in pain control, and stated that "acupuncture cures nothing." Efforts should be made to distinguish clearly between food supplements and drugs. For instance, they said that it was difficult to understand why St. John's wort is protected as a food supplement and not required to be tested by the FDA as a drug.

The American Medical Association (H-480.964 Alternative Medicine) said that there was "little evidence" to confirm the safety or efficacy of most alternative therapies. Many have not been shown to be efficacious and they recommended that "well designed, stringently controlled research should be done to evaluate the efficacy of alternative therapies."[42] They also said that physicians should routinely inquire about the use of alternative or unconventional therapy by their patients, and educate themselves and their patients about the state of scientific knowledge with regard to alternative therapy that may be used or contemplated.[43]

Patients who choose alternative therapies should be educated as to the hazards that might result from postponing or stopping conventional medical treatment.[44] It was also resolved that the American Medical Association support the incorporation of complementary and alternative medicine (CAM) in medical education as well as continuing medical education curricula, covering CAM's benefits, risks, and efficacy.

The American Medical Association amended the Alternative Medicine Resolution in June 2006.[45] They added the words "and that the American Medical Association promote awareness among medical students and physicians of the wide use of complementary and alternative medicine, including its benefits, risks and evidence of efficacy or lack thereof". The addition of the words "or lack thereof" is significant.

Stickler, in the paper mentioned above, concluded that there was "insufficient evidence from previous studies or from studies supported by the NCCAM to accept any "alternative" procedures into the realm of scientific medicine."[46] He said that to that point, "the National Centre for Complementary and Alternative Medicine had not sponsored significant research in a responsible manner. Millions of NCCAM dollars have enabled the continuation of ill-conceived research projects. These projects support positions of advocacy in academic medical centres and continuing calls for more and better research because of defective and inconclusive data." He proposed that insurance companies exercise voluntary restraint and insure only for methods backed by scientific evidence rather than insuring for methods demanded by poorly informed consumers.

Professor Ernst, in England, felt that the incessant criticism directed at the work of his unit by enthusiasts of CAM, was based on a profound misunderstanding.[47] His unit sometimes showed that certain forms of CAM "were not effective or safe but this was not in any way negative. It benefited those who, in medicine, mattered most, the patients." His critics, the died-in-the-wool protagonists of CAM failed to see his work in that light. Ernst said that many researchers seem to use science to prove that what they believe is correct but that science is not for proving but for testing. The former approach reveals an unprofessional attitude and is misleading. "Emotions and strong beliefs can lead to bias[48] and bias leads to bad science. Sadly poor science is rife in complementary medicine".

Poor science is bad because it leads to wrong decisions in healthcare. It is detrimental to patients. Ernst described the prevention either directly or indirectly of patients receiving the best available healthcare as "ugly".[49] Many aspects of complementary medicine fell into this category: dishonesty, neglect of medical ethics, exploitation of vulnerable patients and political interventions were some.

Under the administration of unsafe treatments Ernst listed Asian herbal mixtures and upper spinal manipulation.[50] The former were sometimes contaminated with toxic heavy metals and the latter had been repeatedly linked to arterial dissection followed by stroke. Iridology had been frequently tested and not found to be reliable and "Live blood analysis" has been used without evidence that it is valid.

"Millions of web sites, hundreds of books, weekly columns in the print media, and even a UK government-sponsored patient-guide" all failed to provide responsible advice, said Ernst.[51] This was misleading consumers.[52] The scarce research funds allocated by the Department of Health had not been used for studying efficacy and safety as recommended by the "Lord's Report" and despite the lack of reliable data, the "Smallwood Inquiry 2005" had recommended that large sums of money could be saved if more homeopathy was used in the NHS.

Ernst derided the application or promotion of one standard for conventional medicine and another for complimentary or alternative medicine. The proponents of "integrated medicine", according to Ernst,[53] claim that it cares for the individual as a whole rather than "looking at a diagnostic label". He goes on to say that caring for the whole individual has always been and will always be a hallmark of any good medicine[54] and that conventional healthcare professionals who work towards optimising patient care must feel insulted by this statement.[55] He is correct although one practitioner[56] stated that when there is time, he tries to step back and address his patients as a whole and tries to listen to their concerns, but he admitted: "I've been known to refer to a patient as "the pneumonia in Room 5133" or to describe an emotional patient as "a bit squirrelly!"

"Best" medicine should be applied and Ernst described this term as "those treatments that demonstrably and reproducibly do more good than harm" and "this is precisely what evidence based medicine (EBM) is all about."[57] Ernst goes on to say that considering what "integrative medicine" in the United Kingdom currently promotes, this discloses integrative medicine as "an elaborate smoke screen for adopting unproven treatments into routine healthcare"[58] and in the long run, this strategy will be detrimental to everybody, including patients and even complimentary or alternative medicine itself.

Ernst concluded that CAM had much to offer. In the past 12 years, he and others had identified numerous CAM interventions that generated more good than harm.[59] Many more therapies needed scientific testing and some of them would turn out to be useful. The only way to find out was to conduct rigorous research. Poor science will inevitably mislead, double standards were detrimental for everyone. He said that "In a nutshell, good science is good, bad science is bad and increasing the risk of patients not receiving the best available healthcare is ugly."

In one study, Ernst and his colleagues examined fields as diverse as acupuncture, herbal medicine, homeopathy and reflexology. The results of around 95 per cent of the treatments were statistically indistinguishable from those of placebo treatments.[60] In only five per cent of cases was there either a clear benefit above and beyond a placebo "or even just a hint that something interesting was happening to suggest that further research might be warranted". Professor Ernst said that, unlike their conventional counterparts, practitioners of alternative medicine often excelled at harnessing the placebo effect. They offered long, relaxed consultations with their customers and they believed passionately in their treatments, which were often delivered with great and reassuring ceremony. "That alone can be enough to do good, even though the magnets, crystals and ultra-dilute solutions applied to the patients are, by themselves, completely useless" and this from a Professor of alternative medicine!

Despite the power of placebos, many conventional doctors are wary of prescribing them. As mentioned previously they worry that to do so is to deceive their patients. Professor Ernst stated that alternative medicine practitioners provide exactly the sort of "good bedside manner" that "harried" modern doctors struggled to provide. This is a very generalised comment and I would like to see the evidence for it. Did he possibly mean the deception of the patient by "being economical with the truth?"

A good health provider is "a teacher, a coach, a friend and a fan." Many alternative practitioners manage to play those roles, with the result that their patients trust them and have faith in their treatments. Within the constraints of the conventional health-care system in the USA with "its 15-minute office visits, recurrent insurance denials and unnecessary diagnostic tests to avert malpractice suits" a doctor might find it hard to perform all of these important interpersonal tasks.[61]

Practitioners of alternative medicine became increasingly reluctant to co-operate with Professor Ernst's group as the negative results of research piled up. He had an argument in 2005 with an alternative-medicine lobby group founded by Prince Charles. Conservative MP Jacob Rees-Mogg tweeted that "for his latest attack on Prince Charles, Ernst should be locked up in the Tower of London." At a press conference to mark his retirement Ernst agreed with a *Daily Mail* reporter's suggestion that the Prince of Wales was a "snake-oil salesman". Ernst said that "He owns a firm that sells this stuff and I have no qualms at all defending the notion that a tincture of dandelion and artichoke (Duchy Herbals detox remedy) doesn't do anything to detoxify your body and therefore it is a snake oil."[62]

Although traditional medical-research bodies saw investigations into things like Ayurvedic healing as a waste of time and money, Professor Ernst believed his work helped to address a serious public-health problem. He pointed out that conventional medicines must be shown to be both safe and efficacious before they could be licensed for sale. That was rarely true of alternative treatments. Despite the lack of evidence, and despite the possibility that some alternative practitioners might be harming patients, either directly, or by convincing them to forego more conventional treatments for their ailments, Professor Ernst believed that conventional doctors could usefully learn the therapeutic value of the placebo effect from chiropractors and homeopaths.

For the past few years, Ernst has been on the frontline of a battle between practitioners of complementary medicine and their supporters on the one hand, and a small group of scientists and free speech campaigners on the other.[63] "I have enemies," he said, "there's no question about it."[64] He was the author, with journalist Simon Singh, of a book that led, via an article in the Guardian, to the latter being sued by the British Chiropractic Association for libel.[65] The case was abandoned after Singh won in the court of appeal, but not before both men had spent two years defending it. It became a cause celebre. Ernst believed the chiropractors would have targeted him if they could have, and that Singh was attacked as a result of their association.[66] Chiropractors had been complaining about Ernst for years, particularly after he questioned the safety of spinal manipulation.

Politics and costs of CAM

When asked how to tell the difference between homeopaths and witch doctors one wag answered that "witch doctors were not publicly funded within the National Health Service, not so far, anyway!" However The Islington Tribune of 11th May 2007 revealed that spiritual healers were being paid by the National

Health Service. The National Secular Society commented: "Spiritual healers using up scarce NHS resources.[67] The University College London Hospital is to spend £80,000 on testing whether 'spiritual healers' can have an effect on cancer". Martin Lerner the Divisional Manager of Cancer Services agreed that "University College London Hospital does employ the staff and provide some of the budget (about £90,000 this year) towards the cost of this service, with a similar amount raised through charitable fundraising.[68] By making these complementary therapy services an integral part of the clinical service, we show that we take responsibility for the whole of the patient's wellbeing" he said.

As long ago as 2002 E. Marshall[69] criticised the politics of alternative medicine in the USA. In discussing the resignation of the head of the USA's National Institute of Health's Office of Alternative Medicine (NIH's OAM), Joseph Jacobs, Marshall described how one powerful senator, Tom Harkin, a democrat from Iowa and advocates of unconventional therapies were shaping the OAM's research agenda. He stated that: "Devising a plan to study unconventional medicine, says one observer on Capitol Hill, is like 'orchestrating a roomful of cats or setting the agenda for a convention of anarchists'. The field is a smorgasbord of therapies ranging from meditation and prayer to acupuncture, homeopathy, shark cartilage enemas for cancer, biofeedback, massage, dosing with bee pollen to stop allergies and many, many more. Each school is confident that its methods are the best. All distrust 'the medical establishment'. And most are not skilled in collecting data." On resigning, Jacobs, in an interview with *Science,* blasted politicians especially Senator Harkin and some advocates of alternative medicine for pressuring his office, promoting certain therapies and, he said, attempting "an end run around objective science." Jacobs, allegedly resigned under Harkin's pressure having objected to Harkin's OAM Council nominees who represented cancer scams such as Laetrile and Tijuana cancer clinics.[70]

In the United States concerns about the cost-effectiveness of CAM are supported by negative results. After ten years of existence and over $US 200 million in expenditures the National Centre for Complementary and Alternative Medicine (NCCAM) in the United States has not proved effective for any "alternative" method of treatment.[71]

This research has largely not demonstrated the efficacy of alternative treatments.[72,73,74] The NCCAM budget has been criticised[75] because there have been exactly zero effective CAM treatments supported by scientific evidence to date.[76] Despite this, the National Centre for Complementary and Alternative Medicine budget has been on a sharp sustained rise to support complementary medicine. In fact, the whole CAM field has been called by critics "the SCAM". Perhaps more important, NCCAM has not declared any method to be ineffective, thus keeping open continuing congressional appropriations. NCCAM is ridden with potential and actual conflicts of interest. Ten individuals account for 20 per cent of NCCAM awards. None of them has produced a definitively positive or negative report. Most recipients have produced no report at all. Two individuals originally on the Advisory Council that approves NCCAM policy were awarded over $US 4 million and $US 5 million in repeated awards.

Scientists look at facts.[77] Looking at the most popularly promoted methods, acupuncture, after thirty years, over 400 clinical trials, and 33 comprehensive literature reviews of those trials, only two specific conditions were found affected by acupuncture more than sham procedures. But even those effects are minimal; they are not superior to standard medical methods, and they remain implausible and unpredictable. They will probably not be confirmed because their results are best explained by biased experimental errors.[78]

After 100 years and many trials, chiropractic manipulation has not been proven to influence the course of any disease and has not been proven effective for treating back pain.[79] As for homeopathy, after 200 years and hundreds of studies, researchers cannot prove an effect for any homeopathic remedy for any condition. Some products have been adulterated with common pharmaceutical drugs that account for their apparent effects.[80]

NCCAM Director, Steven Straus, M.D., a career National Institute of Health physician now oversees the $US 113 million annual budget. He wants more funding for more NCCAM trials![81] They recently announced research on "chelation therapy" for heart disease, a method already disproved and potentially dangerous.[82] And $US10 million is planned for research into herbs with their uncontrollable contents and unreliable results.[83]

Similarly troubling is NCCAM's awards of over $US1million into psychic healing, and $US1.5 million for homeopathy.[84] Both are highly implausible, being not only repeated failures, but promoted falsely as well. NCCAM recently awarded $US15 million to nine medical schools to develop teaching of these subjects, all by advocates of CAM.[85] It gave no funds to the five medical school courses with curricula already developed that teach about the subject rationally. In other words, NCCAM's research agenda fits its congressional supporters' ideological vision and finds unproductive ways to use up its ballooning appropriations.

Wallace I. Sampson is the Editor in Chief of *The Scientific Review of Alternative Medicine and Aberrant Medical Practices*.[86] This is the only peer-reviewed journal devoted exclusively to objectively analysing the claims of "alternative medicine." Its purpose is to apply the best tools of science and reason to determine whether hypotheses are valid and treatments are effective.[87] It seeks answers to two questions: "Is it true?" and "Does this treatment work?"[88] Its publication has been endorsed by the Council for Scientific Medicine, a panel that includes 50 prominent physicians and scientists and five Nobel Prize winners. This is in comparison with other publications that focus on unconventional therapies, merely advocate them and rarely assess them objectively.

Sampson wrote an article titled: "Why the National Centre for Complementary and Alternative Medicine (NCCAM) Should Be Defunded."[89] It describes clearly what is wrong with NCCAM. This organisation had government funding of $US122.7 million in 2006. Since its foundation (as the Office of Alternative Medicine), it has received not much short of a billion dollars ($US 842 million). What has the US taxpayer had for this money? NCCAM was called "a disgrace to science". Sampson wrote "… it has not proved effectiveness for any 'alternative' method. It has added evidence of ineffectiveness of some methods that we knew did not work before NCCAM was formed". NCCAM's major accomplishment, according to Sampson, has been "to ensure the positions of medical school faculty who might become otherwise employed in more productive pursuits." "NCCAM could be dissolved, its functions returned to other NIH centers, with no loss of knowledge, and an economic gain. Funds could be invested into studies of how such misadventures into "alternative" medicine can be avoided, and on studying the warping of human perceptions and beliefs that led to the present situation."

An article appeared in the *Washington Post*[90] encouraging scientists to show their concern that the National Institute of Health (NIH) was funding pseudoscience. Steven Salzberg, from the Centre for Integrative Medicine (CIM) in the University of Maryland School of Medicine suggested that NCCAM be defunded. "Now is the time for scientists to start speaking up about issues that concern us"[91] Steven Salzberg, a genome researcher and computational biologist at the University of Maryland, said. "One of our concerns is that NIH is funding pseudoscience." This proposal was posted on an electronic bulletin board that the Obama transition team had set up to solicit ideas after the President's election. The proposal generated 218 comments, most of them in favour, before the bulletin board closed.[92]

According to the Washington Post writer, many scientists have "been rankled" that "the world's best-known medical research agency sponsors studies of homeopathy, acupuncture, therapeutic touch and herbal medicine."[93] With the lack of effectiveness of NCCAM Steven Novella,[94] a neurologist at Yale School of Medicine and editor of the Web site *Science-Based Medicine* complained that "the very fact NIH is supporting a study is used to market alternative medicine. It is used to lend an appearance of legitimacy to treatments that are not legitimate."

Even Senator Harkin was disappointed.[95] He said that one of the purposes when legislation was drafted in 1992 was to investigate and validate alternative approaches. "Quite frankly, I must say it's fallen short," he told the committee. Most of NCCAM's results have been negative or inconclusive, not positive and encouraging.[96] A randomised controlled trial of the botanical echinacea published in 2003 found it was ineffective in treating upper respiratory infections.[97] Neither the Japanese "palm healing" therapy known as reiki, nor sham reiki, reduced the symptoms of fibromyalgia, a chronic pain syndrome.[98] A study comparing real and sham acupuncture in 162 cancer patients who had undergone surgery found no difference in their levels of pain. At the same time, it is difficult to determine the clinical implications of some of the positive studies.[99] For example, reiki blunted the rise in heart rate, but not the rise in blood pressure, in rats put under stress by loud noise. Therapeutic touch, a different modality, increased the growth of normal bone cells in culture dishes, but decreased the growth of bone cancer cells.

In the United States and in Britain too! The following letter dated 19th May 2006 was sent to the chief executives of 476 National Health Service Trusts.[100]

It was the main headline in *The Times,* and the lead item on the BBC's *Today* Program. From Professor Michael Baum and others it read:[101]

"Dear …

Re: Use of 'alternative' medicine in the NHS

We are a group of physicians and scientists who are concerned about ways in which unproven or disproved treatments are being encouraged for general use in the NHS. We would ask you to review practices in your own trust, and to join us in representing our concerns to the Department of Health because we want patients to benefit from the best treatments available.

There are two particular developments to which we would like to draw your attention. First, there is now overt promotion of homeopathy in parts of the NHS (including the *NHS Direct* website). It is an implausible treatment for which over a dozen systematic reviews have failed to produce convincing evidence of effectiveness. Despite this, a recently-published patient guide, promoting use of homeopathy without making the lack of proven efficacy clear to patients, is being made available through government funding. Further suggestions about benefits of homeopathy in the treatment of asthma have been made in the 'Smallwood Report' and in another publication by the Department of Health designed to give primary care groups "a basic source of reference on complementary and alternative therapies." A Cochrane review of all relevant studies, however, failed to confirm any benefits for asthma treatment.

Secondly, as you may know, there has been a concerted campaign to promote complementary and alternative medicine as a component of healthcare provision. Treatments covered by this definition include some which have not been tested as pharmaceutical products, but which are known to cause adverse effects, and others that have no demonstrable benefits. While medical practice must remain open to new discoveries for which there is convincing evidence, including any branded as 'alternative', it would be highly irresponsible to embrace any medicine as though it were a matter of principle.

At a time when the NHS is under intense pressure, patients, the public and the NHS are best served by using the available funds for treatments that are based on solid evidence. Furthermore, as someone in a position of accountability for resource distribution, you will be familiar with just how publicly emotive the decisions concerning which therapies to provide under the NHS can be; our ability to explain and justify to patients the selection of treatments, and to account for expenditure on them more widely, is compromised if we abandon our reference to evidence. We are sensitive to the needs of patients for complementary care to enhance well-being and for spiritual support to deal with the fear of death at a time of critical illness, all of which can be supported through services already available within the NHS without resorting to false claims.

These are not trivial matters. We urge you to take an early opportunity to review practice in your own trust with a view to ensuring that patients do not receive misleading information about the effectiveness of alternative medicines. We would also ask you to write to the Department of Health requesting evidence-based information for trusts and for patients with respect to alternative medicine.

Yours sincerely

The signatories to this letter were Professor Michael Baum, Emeritus Professor of Surgery, University College London, Professor Frances Ashcroft FRS, University Laboratory of Physiology, Oxford, Professor Sir Colin Berry, Emeritus Professor of Pathology, Queen Mary, London, Professor Gustav Born FRS, Emeritus Professor of Pharmacology, Kings College London, Professor Sir James Black FRS, Kings College London, Professor David Colquhoun FRS, University College London, Professor Peter Dawson, Clinical Director of Imaging, University College London, Professor Edzard Ernst, Peninsula Medical School, Exeter, Professor John Garrow, Emeritus Professor of Human Nutrition, London, Professor Sir Keith Peters FRS, President, The Academy of Medical Sciences, Mr Leslie Rose, Consultant Clinical Scientist, Professor Raymond Tallis, Emeritus Professor of Geriatric Medicine, University of Manchester, and Professor Lewis Wolpert CBE FRS, University College London.[102]

The letter was discussed in *The Times* of 23rd May 2006 by the Science Editor, Mark Henderson under the title "NHS told to abandon alternative medicine". He considered that the appeal of these 13 learned gentlemen, including "some of the most eminent names in British medicine" was a direct challenge to the Prince of Wales's outspoken campaign to widen access to complementary therapies.[103]

The scientists demanded that only evidence-based therapies were provided free to patients. The letter's signatories included Sir James Black,[104] who won the Nobel Prize for Medicine in 1988, and Sir Keith Peters, President of the Academy of Medical Science, which represents Britain's leading clinical researchers. It was organised by Michael Baum, Emeritus Professor of Surgery at University College London, and other supporters included six Fellows of the Royal Society, Britain's national academy of science and even Professor Edzard Ernst.

Professor Baum, a cancer specialist, said that he had organised the letter because of his "utter despair" at growing National Health Service acceptance of alternative treatments while drugs of proven effectiveness are being withheld.[105] "At a time when we are struggling to gain access for our patients to Herceptin, which is absolutely proven to extend survival in breast cancer, I find it appalling that the NHS should be funding a therapy like homoeopathy that is utterly bogus," he said.

He said that he was happy for the NHS to offer the treatments once research has proven them effective but that very few had reached the required standards.[106] "If people want to spend their own money on it, fine, but it shouldn't be NHS money" he said.

Alternative medicine is big business. Since it is largely unregulated, reliable statistics are hard to come by and the United Kingdom Department of Health apparently does not keep figures on the total NHS spending on alternative medicine. Britain's total market is estimated at between £210 million and £1.6 billion with one in five adults thought to be consumers, and some treatments, notably homeopathy, being available on the National Health Service. Around the world, according to an estimate made in 2008, the industry's value is about US $60 billion. All this money is a real waste in the UK, in the USA and almost certainly in a great many other countries all round the world. It could be very much better spent.

The letter by Professor Baum and others had been sent as the Prince was preparing a controversial speech to the World Health Organisation assembly in Geneva asking them to embrace alternative therapies in the fight against serious disease.[107] His views have outraged clinicians and researchers, who claim that many of the therapies that he advocates have been shown to be ineffective in trials or have never been properly tested. The letter criticised two of the Prince's flagship initiatives on complementary medicine: a government-funded patient guide prepared by his Foundation for Integrated Medicine, and the Smallwood report, which he had commissioned to make a financial case for increasing NHS provision.[108]

Prince Charles commissioned the Smallwood report on *The Role of Complementary and Alternative Medicine in the NHS*.[109] The report was published on 9 August 2005. The report stated that the evidence that CAM works was slim, and simply passed the buck. Their principal recommendation being that "the Health Ministers should invite the National Institute for Health and Clinical Excellence (NICE) to carry out a full assessment of the cost effectiveness of the therapies which we have identified and their potential role within the NHS in particular with a view to the closing of 'effectiveness gaps'."[110] Contrary to widespread misreporting of its conclusions, therefore, the report, did not recommend that more CAM be made available on the NHS. That judgement was passed on to NICE.

The report, written by an economist Christopher Smallwood, did not address the central dilemma of whether CAM works or not. It did confirm the well-known views of its sponsor. It discussed evidence, and the lack thereof, using so-called "expert advice". Which "experts" provided this advice? Strange to say the list of interview summaries did not contain a single pharmacologist (clinical or otherwise), nor did it contain any statistician. Eight of the 10 names were deeply committed to CAM or made their living from it. The only exceptions were Professor Peter Littlejohns (National Institute for Clinical Excellence - NICE) and Dr John Appleby (Chief economist of the Kings Fund).[111] The report has been strongly criticised for the lack of "respectable" scientists among the experts involved. Despite the views of his sponsor[112] and despite the very unbalanced group of people from whom he took evidence, Smallwood nevertheless concluded that not enough was known about benefits to do a cost-benefit analysis.[113] The buck was again simply passed to NICE.

The Medicine and Healthcare products Regulators Agency (MHRA) is an executive agency of the Department of Health. It is roughly the UK equivalent of the Food and Drugs Administration (FDA) in the USA. It was founded in 2003 by merging the Medicines Control Agency (MCA) and the Medical Devices Agency (MDA). The MCA was created by the UK Medicines Act 1968, in the wake of the thalidomide disaster.

The MHRA recently betrayed the trust placed in it by the public by allowing untrue claims to be put on the labels of homeopathic and herbal treatments. Homeopathic medicines on the market before 1968 were given Product Licences of Right (PLR), which has now allowed them to make claims about health benefits.[114] Hitherto they were not allowed to make such claims. Once the United Kingdom entered the European Union in the 1970's this delayed new products coming on to the market, because the nature of homeopathic medicines meant there was not the clinical evidence to support licensing regulations.[115] A simplified version was introduced in 1992, which allowed homeopathic medicines to be licensed, but prevented them from making health claims. Now over 3,000 homeopathic medicines have licenses, most of them PLRs. Previously a homeopathic remedy in a high street chemist would have been labelled "6c dilution of Gelsemium sempervirens", or something similarly obscure. It can now be sold, quite legally, as 'NoCold-Max cold and flu remedy ... homeopathic'.[116] To make such a claim, the manufacturers need only show that the product has been used to treat those particular conditions within the homeopathic industry.[117]

No scientific basis. No clinical trials. No evidence of effectiveness. Decisions of this kind should be made on the basis of scientific and medical evidence, not anecdotes. A press release dated November 8th 2006 was the first example of the MHRA decision to allow totally misleading labels to be put on over-the-counter treatments. They granted the first United Kingdom product registration under the European Directive on traditional herbal medicinal products. Nobody knows exactly what caused them to take this action but it is clear that they were under pressure from both the Department of Health and from the Prince of Wales. Homeopathic remedies have not been able to make health claims since 1968 but the MHRA suddenly decided to introduce rules to allow remedies to advertise and specify the ailments for which they can be used. They will be allowed to indicate what sort of symptoms they can relieve, although this will be limited to minor ailments such as colds, coughs and hay fever.[118]

Manufacturers did not have to provide evidence of efficacy from clinical trials and needed only to show that the product had been used to treat those particular conditions within the homeopathic industry.[119]

The MHRA argued that failure to introduce the new system would inhibit the homeopathic industry's expansion. They said its key motivations were "protecting consumers and promoting choice" rather than boosting the industry.[120] Professor Michael Baum said he was perplexed by the new system as the MHRA was giving approval to products that had not been rigorously tested.[121] This would boost the homeopathic industry but would not benefit anyone else. It could put patients at risk. Dr. Evan Harris, science spokesman for the Liberal Democrats, said: "It is wrong that this country's medicines regulatory arrangements which need to be scientific and rigorous, are being diluted and polluted by processes which allow ineffective products to be licensed as medicines without having to provide any scientific evidence of effectiveness.[122] There are very tight standards for proper medicines for very good reasons, the need to protect vulnerable consumers from exploitation."

The MHRA admitted to having received at least seven letters from the Prince of Wales, and an MHRA member had met the Prince at Clarence House at least once. All the contents and discussions were kept secret from the public. The Chairman of the MHRA Agency Board, Professor Alasdair Breckenridge, and chairman of their Herbal Medicines committee, Professor Philip Routledge, both admitted to being under pressure from the Prince of Wales. Neither would give any details, despite having been condemned by their own professional organisation, the British Pharmacological Society.

Max Hastings in the Guardian was not so reticent. He said that "To make good use of evidence, it is essential to possess not only intelligence, but a capacity for disciplined analysis. The prince has considerable virtues, a good heart notable among them. But he has always lacked discipline in his life and in his treatment of issues. Again and again, he gets himself into trouble by seeking to address matters that are, frankly, beyond his intellectual reach."

It was also reported by some papers[123] that Tony Blair spoke to European Union leaders, to oppose the very sensible and modest European Food Supplements Directive. This directive is a small move to prevent the most fraudulent claims for *"food supplements"* and to prevent sale of those that are actually dangerous.[124] It would, for example, prevent the sale of Viridian Trace Mineral Complex, which contains Manganese, Selenium, Boron, Copper, Vanadium, Chromium and Molybdenum. Why would Tony Blair oppose this?

Margaret Thatcher was a devotee of mystical "electric baths" and Ayurveda therapy.[125] Cherie Blair expressed an interest in New Age spirituality, [126] inviting a feng-shui expert to rearrange the furniture at No 10 and wearing a "magic pendant" known as a BioElectric Shield,[127] which has "a matrix of specially cut quartz crystals" that surround the wearer with "a cocoon of energy" to ward off evil forces. She has also dabbled in other forms of unorthodox ventures. She employed a "lifestyle guru" and also had her swollen ankles treated by swinging a crystal pendulum over the affected area and eating strawberry leaves grown within the "electro-magnetic field" of a neolithic circle. [128] Both Tony and Cherie Blair had a "rebirthing experience" under the supervision of a Nancy Aguilar while holidaying on the Mexican Riviera in the summer of 2001.

Some of Cherie Blair's other peculiar obsessions have already been adopted as official policy.[129] In January 1999 the government recruited a feng-shui consultant, Renuka Wickmaratne, for advice on how to improve inner-city council estates. "Red and orange flowers would reduce crime," she concluded, "and introducing a water feature would reduce poverty. I was brought up with this ancient knowledge." Two years later, the government announced that, for the first time since the creation of the National Health Service, remedies such as acupuncture and Indian ayurvedic medicine could be granted the same status as conventional treatments.[130] According to the *Sunday Times,* "The inclusion of Indian ayurvedic medicine, a preventative approach to healing using diet, yoga and meditation, is thought to have been influenced by Cherie Blair's interest in alternative therapy." An all too believable suggestion, since Cherie was a client of the ayurvedic guru Bharti Vyas and officiated at the opening ceremony for her holistic therapy centre in London. The Queen apparently carries homeopathic remedies with her at all times. Princess Diana was a devotee of reflexology and Prince Charles has been a prominent champion of CAM.

With regard to feng shui, Thomas Sutcliffe wrote in the *The Independent* of 20 Feb, 2007, "It's never easy being a world leader in any field.[131] You're always liable to be demoted by some upstart. So it must be good news for Los Angelos that their city has cemented its reputation as the global epicentre of New Age dim-wittedness by hiring a feng shui expert to advise on the construction of a monkey enclosure at Los Angeles Zoo. Simona Mainini was reportedly paid $4,500 for feng shui-ing a new home for three Chinese golden monkeys. She has advised that the angle of the monkey house be rotated a few degrees to "transform the energy distribution" and that a water feature be added.[132] The zoo hasn't revealed whether the monkeys will also receive high colonics, botox and reiki massages - but anything less would surely count as cruel neglect."

The MHRA was condemned by just about every professional organisation in Britain including The Royal Society, the Medical Research Council, the Academy of Medical Sciences, the Royal College of Pathologists, the Biosciences Federation, the Physiological Society and the British Pharmacological Society. In contrast, the main medical organisations were silent. Nothing was heard from the British Medical Association. Nothing either from the Royal College of General Practitioners or from the Royal Society of Medicine although the BBC reported on 26th October 2006 that hundreds of doctors and scientists had signed a statement opposing the rules that allowed homeopathic medicines to make medical claims. The Royal College of Pathologists said it was "deeply alarmed" that the regulation of medicine had "moved away from science and clear information for the public."[133] The Medical Research Council said claims should not be made about efficacy of products without "rigorous and objective evidence", and the BioSciences Federation claimed that the MHRA had "bowed to industry pressure". The chairman of the campaign group Sense about Science, Lord Dick Taverne, said: "As many of the medical specialists contacting us have pointed out, evidence-based medicine has been a major public gain of the twentieth century. This is the first time, since the thalidomide tragedy and the 1968 Medicines Act that the regulation of medicines has moved away from the science rather than towards it."[134]

Which? health policy expert Frances Blunden[135] warned: "This approach gives homeopathic products the veneer of efficacy. Claims for any homeopathic products ought to be based on independently verified and reliable evidence of their efficacy. Without this there's a danger that consumers are being misled and ultimately ripped off. Consumers shouldn't be fooled that despite homeopathic medicines being 'alternative', there is still a significant profit-making industry behind them.

The Physiological Society stated in a newsletter[136] that it was concerned with the scientific investigation of how the body works. It was their view that "alternative medicine" had, with very few exceptions, no scientific foundation, either empirical or theoretical. As an extreme example, many homeopathic medicines contained no molecules of their ingredient, so they could have no effect (beyond that of a placebo).[137] To claim otherwise it would be necessary to abandon the entire molecular basis of chemistry. The Society believes that any claim made for a medicine must be based on evidence, and that it was a duty of the regulatory authorities to ensure that this was done." Austin Elliott, the writer of the newsletter continued as the web site of the European Council for Classical Homeopathy puts it: "To make such a claim, the manufacturers need only show that the product has been used to treat those particular conditions within the homeopathic industry." No scientific basis was needed. No clinical trials. No evidence of effectiveness.[138,139]

The homeopaths, and the companies that produce over-the-counter homeopathic remedies were understandably delighted. To allow labeling like this is wrong. The MHRA is supposed to "enhance and safeguard the health of the public by ensuring that medicines and medical devices work and are acceptably safe."[140] Decisions of this kind should be made on the basis of scientific and medical evidence not under pressure from other interested parties without the requisite scientific knowledge.

Nevertheless the MHRA granted the first United Kingdom product registration under the European Directive on traditional herbal medicinal products.[141] Professor Kent Woods, Chief Executive of the MHRA said "This first product registration is an important landmark. We hope that Atrogel Gel[142] will be the first of many products to receive a traditional herbal registration. Our aim is to enable those consumers who wish to take herbal medicines to make an informed choice from a wide range of products which have been made to assured standards of safety, quality and patient information."

David Colquhoun asked what evidence there was that Arnica Gel was the slightest good for the conditions that would appear on the label? The answer was essentially none. Of the papers he could find in Medline, the first showed no detectable effect of arnica gel compared with vehicle alone.[143] The second paper claimed a positive effect, but it was worthless because it was an open trial with no proper controls.[144] The last author on this paper, incidentally, gave his address as Bioforce AG. Atrogel was not yet on the market in Britain but the application for registration was from Bioforce(UK).

Another paper in the Journal of the Royal Society of Medicine concluded that arnica "had no effect on postoperative recovery". This trial, by researchers at the University of Southampton, examined the effects of arnica C30 on pain and post-operative recovery in 73 women following total abdominal hysterectomy at Southampton's Princess Anne Hospital. The trial was double-blind, placebo-controlled and randomised. The paper concluded, "In terms of pain, analgesia, infection and operative severity, this study revealed no significant differences between the arnica and placebo groups."[145]

Professor Woods is correct the MHRA's press release was indeed a landmark. It was the first time that they allowed a medicine to be labelled with a therapeutic claim when there was no reason to believe it to be true and this is the government agency that is responsible for ensuring that medicines and medical devices work.[146]

The MHRA decision was based on European Directive 2004/24/EC paragraph 6 of which contains the following statement. "The long tradition of the medicinal product makes it possible to reduce the need for clinical trials, in so far as the efficacy of the medicinal product is plausible on the basis of long-standing use and experience.[147] Pre-clinical tests do not seem necessary, where the medicinal product on the basis of the information on its traditional use proves not to be harmful in specified conditions of use." Evidently the MHRA acceded to the European Directive.

The new rules outlined that homeopathic products would receive a licence if data could be provided proving the treatment was safe. The makers would not have to produce evidence of efficacy from clinical trials. To make such a claim, the manufacturers needed only to show that the product had been used to treat those particular conditions within the homeopathic industry.[148] Critics argued that, as the products did not need to undergo the clinical trials orthodox drugs do, the treatments would not be rigorously tested. A licence would be obtained without this testing. Critics were also angered by suggestions that the decisions of the MHRA had been partly motivated by a desire to boost the homeopathic industry. They felt that patients would be put at risk by the new regulatory system.

To claim that "It helps relieve symptoms including …" will now be quite legal and totally nonsensical even if the proviso that evidence for this statement is "based exclusively on long-standing use." On *BBC News* "Michael Baum said: "This is like licensing a witches' brew as a medicine so long as the bat wings are sterile."

The Executive Board of the MHRA who made this momentous decision consisted of the Chief Executive Officer, Professor Kent Woods who qualified in medicine from Cambridge in 1972 and is now a Professor in therapeutics at Leicester University, Professor Sir Alasdair Breckenridge, CBE, most recently Professor of Clinical Pharmacology at the University of Liverpool, Professor Angus Mackay, OBE, is Mental Health Service Director / Consultant Psychiatrist at the Argyll and Bute Hospital, Michael Fox, Chief Executive of the Prince of Wales' Foundation for Integrated Health since 1998, Shelley Dolan, Nurse Consultant Cancer and Critical Care at the Royal Marsden NHS Trust, Charles Kernahan, Chief executive of the National Kidney Research Fund with over 25 years experience in healthcare products and service provision, Garry Watts, a Chartered Accountant and Chief Executive of SSL International plc, an international healthcare company and Lisa Arnold, currently involved on a voluntary basis with RAFT, a medical research charity, both as a Trustee and on a consultancy basis.

According to David Colquhoun, the group that was responsible for the MHRA decision on whether or not Arnica works had, as its members, apart from the Chief Executive Officer, one pharmacologist, one psychiatrist, a representative of an organisation "devoted to crackpot medicine",[149] a nurse and three accountants/bankers/marketers with strong industry connections which he detailed on his website. Perhaps that, according to Colquhoun, accounted for their bizarre decision. He could only assume that the one pharmacologist was outvoted and that the MHRA now seemed to regard its role as promotion of the "homeopathic industry." He said "The new government regulations allow claims to be made that sugar pills can treat illnesses when there isn't a fragment of reason to believe the claims are true. This is simply government-endorsed lying." Even Professor Edzard Ernst, said that "This makes a mockery out of evidence-based medicine."

The regulations that allowed unjustified claims to be made for homeopathic pills were the subject of an annulment debate in the House of Lords on 26 October 2006 where the MHRA were censured.[150] The regulations were introduced as a statutory instrument. This is a form of legislation which allow the provisions of an Act of Parliament to be subsequently brought into force or altered without Parliament having to pass a new Act.[151] In other words a minister just decides to do it without any debate or parliamentary approval. The instrument is laid after making, subject to annulment if a motion to annul is passed within 40 days.

In the House of Lords, Lord Taverne moved: "That an humble Address be presented to Her Majesty praying that the regulations, laid before the House on 21 July, be annulled (S.I. 2006/1952). 44th Report from the Merits Committee."[152]

He argued that "There is one very important, absolutely fundamental objection to this regulation. For the first time in the history of the regulation of medical products, it allows claims of efficacy to be made without scientific evidence. It is an abandonment of science and the evidence-based approach. Under this new regulation, the sole basis on which claims of efficacy can be made for homeopathic products quite legally is "homeopathic provings". There is no need for clinical or scientific tests. Homeopathy is not based on science and is not a science in any sense whatever."[153] He read a comment stating that "The British Pharmacological Society believes that any claim for a medicine must be based on evidence, and that it is the duty of the regulatory authorities, in particular the MHRA, to ensure that no claims can be made for the efficacy of any form of medicine unless there is good evidence that the claim is true. Despite many years of investigation, we have no convincing scientific evidence that homeopathic remedies work any better than placebo. What it has done is to promote what is in effect the selling of snake oil. This statutory instrument should be withdrawn, it is a disgrace. I beg to move."[154]

Lord Rees of Ludlow said: " My Lords, the Royal Society, of which I have the honour to be president, believes that all complementary and alternative medicines should be subject to careful evaluation of their efficacy and their safety.[155] All treatments so labelled should be properly tested and patients should not receive misleading information. There are no great concerns about the safety of homeopathic treatments. What is at issue is their effectiveness. Obviously placebo effects can be powerful, nobody denies that. It is, however, quite different to assert that homeopathic treatments offer benefits beyond a placebo. Indeed, if medicines can really work even when so diluted that barely a single molecule is left, this would entail some fundamentally new scientific principle with amazingly broad ramifications. It would mean that materials like water carry imprints of their past and can remember their history, as it were, in some quite novel and mysterious way. If that were the case, it would have fundamental implications for precise experiments over the whole of science. So it seems to me that the burden of proof on homeopathic remedies should actually be higher, not lower, than for conventional ones. Extraordinary claims demand extraordinary evidence. To put it mildly, so-called "homeopathic provings" seem to fall far short of that. That is why I wholeheartedly support what the noble Lord, Lord Taverne, is saying on this issue."

The 30th Countess of Mar, a hereditary peer and organic farmer and Lord Colwyn, CBE, a Conservative peer opposed the annulment. The 30th Countess of Mar quoted Professor Madeleine Ennis whose research showed that high dilutions of the active ingredients in homeopathic solutions worked, whether the active ingredient was present in the water or not. The Countess, according to David Colquhoun, omitted to mention that the first author on both of Ennis's papers was Philippe Belon. who is a director of the huge French homeopathic company, Boiron. Boiron makes profits from homeopathy of about 20 million Euros a year. It is big business. Small wonder that all Belon's papers seem to favour homeopathy. Lord Colwyn quite forgot to declare his interests. He is vice-president of the Blackie Foundation Trust. This trust was founded by Dr Margery Blackie in 1971, at that time homoeopathic physician to Her Majesty, the Queen. He also forgot to mention that he is a patron of the National Federation of Spiritual Healers.

The MHRA by their action have made it legal to advertise items such as "Nelsons Coldenza is a homeopathic remedy specifically designed to bring fast, effective relief for the symptoms of cold and flu."[156] "Active ingredients: 6c homeopathic potency of Gelsemium sempervirens." "Precautions: Keep out of the reach of children.[157] If symptoms persist or worsen, consult your doctor or homeopath." These "Coldenza" tablets can in no way influence the course of a cold or flu. This is not "information" for the patient. As Colquhoun says: "It is misinformation. It is lies, endorsed by the MHRA." He also says that the MHRA were acting under instructions from the Department of Health, and the Executive Board failed to resist bad instructions. The idea that the decision of the MHRA had been required by European legislation was apparently not true. Colquhoun says that it was a decision of the MHRA by itself or perhaps as a result of pressure from ministers.

On 1st October 2006 Colquhoun had a reply from Sue Harris the Assessment Team Manager, Licensing Division at the MHRA in response to a question about how the decision was made. The answer stated: "The decision to implement the National Rules Scheme was agreed by the Executive Board in response to the ministerial request and not by the Agency Board as the Agency Board does not have executive responsibility. The Chair and non-executive board members were not involved in the decision making process and the final decision was taken by the Minister. " The Minister of State's views on CAM were abundantly clear and are discussed later under "The Department of Health view on homeopathy".

Colquhoun felt that "this certainly suggests that the MHRA made their bizarre decision on instructions from above. It does not explain why the MHRA knuckled under and implemented a policy that is in direct contradiction to their mission."

The editor of the British Medical Journal, Fiona Godlee wrote "Drug regulators too seem unequal to their task. Critics focus on their close relationship with industry; their lack of transparency; and an emphasis on efficacy over patient safety, which favours industry"[158]

Which? magazine[159] quoted the MHRA as saying: "our role is not to protect industry interests. We have a responsibility to ensure that regulation is designed to enable rather than hinder the development of new products that would improve health." But this claim stands in stark contrast with the MHRA's "Explanatory Memorandum". This memorandum states "Although the development of national rules by Member States under Directive 2001/83/EC is optional, failing to introduce the scheme would inhibit the expansion of the homeopathic industry by the prevention of the development of new products with indications."[160]

The discussion document issued by the MHRA said that: "The industry as a whole will benefit from the opportunity to gain indications for products for which use within the homeopathic tradition can be demonstrated, but cannot currently carry indications." "Legislation enabling the products to be labeled with indications is also considered to be of significant benefit to patients." "Reviewing the Product Licences of Right will provide an opportunity to rectify any cases where products are being marketed with inappropriate indications." Colquhoun questioned whether it was part of the MHRA's brief to promote any industries? He asked how lying to patients benefited them and who would decide what indications were "appropriate" for pills that contain nothing whatsoever?

The MHRA is responsible for the regulation of medicines and medical devices and equipment used in healthcare, and the investigation of harmful incidents.[161] The MHRA also looks after blood and blood products, working with United Kingdom blood services, healthcare providers, and other relevant organisations to improve blood quality and safety. Whether it is a medicine you buy, or one prescribed for you as part of a course of treatment, it should be reassuring to know that all medicines available in the UK are subject to rigorous scrutiny by the MHRA before they can be used by patients.[162] This ensures that medicines meet acceptable standards on safety, quality and efficacy. They do this for medicines but what is, and is not, a medicine?[163]

The law in Britain defines a medicine as something used in disease, whether it is used to prevent, treat or diagnose it, in anaesthesia, investigating conditions or interfering with the normal operation of the body.[164] It does not include such things as contact lens fluids, food supplements and cosmetics. Many factors are considered in deciding whether a product is actually a medicine such as what it contains, what it is advertised or used for,[165] the way it will be used, any particular targeting of the marketing information and what the promotional literature says.

Claims that a product "supports" health or a healthy lifestyle is not usually considered as medicinal. Control of medicines starts as soon as they are first discovered and tested in healthy volunteers, all the way through to when a company wants to change the conditions its products are approved for, such as changing the colour of the tablet or what it is used for.

Francis Wheen, writing in the London Evening Standard of May 16th 2006 in a piece titled "There's no remedy for the Prince of Quacks" questioned why Prince Charles had been asked to deliver the keynote speech at the annual assembly of the World Health Organisation.[166] He said that: "The WHO describes Charles as the president of the Prince's Foundation for Integrated Health and 'patron of a number of health charities'.[167] It omits to add that his views on medicine are barmy - and pernicious.[168] WHO delegates from 192 nations have plenty to discuss during their five-day meeting - HIV/Aids, sickle-cell anaemia, preparations for a flu pandemic, the eradication of polio and smallpox. Why waste precious time listening to the heir to the British throne, who has spent more than 20 years displaying his ignorance of medical science?" "The prince has never met a snake oil vendor he didn't like. A couple of years ago he urged doctors to prescribe coffee enemas to cancer patients, a suggestion which provoked this rebuke from Professor Michael Baum of University College London: 'The power of my authority comes with a knowledge built on 40 years of study and 25 years of active involvement in cancer research. Your power and authority rest on an accident of birth'."[169]

The Prince's Foundation for Integrated Health publishes *Complementary Healthcare: a guide for patients*. It tells the unfortunate patient that: "Homeopathy is most often used to treat chronic conditions such as asthma; eczema; arthritis; fatigue disorders like ME; headache and migraine; menstrual and menopausal problems; irritable bowel syndrome; Crohn's disease; allergies; repeated ear, nose, throat and chest infections or urine infections; depression and anxiety" but it says nothing at all about whether or not it works.[170] That is just irresponsible and to describe pills that contain no trace of the substance on the label as "very diluted" is dishonest.[171]

Edzard Ernst, having been sent a draft of the Smallwood report, described the initial findings as "outrageous and deeply flawed". He added that it was based on such poor science, that it was just "hair-raising" and that the Prince "also seems to have overstepped his constitutional role". As a result Ernst was subjected to a very prolonged disciplinary procedure. A letter alleging a breach of confidence by Ernst was sent from Clarence House to the vice-chancellor of Exeter University, Steve Smith. For a year it was not obvious whether Ernst would keep his chair. For a Prince, in a constitutional monarchy, to put pressure on a university to silence a conspicuously honest academic should not be acceptable. Professor Smith, instead of supporting his staff and supporting academic freedom, appeared to cower before the Clarence House letterhead. After keeping Prof Ernst on tenterhooks for an entire year he eventually deigned not to fire him.

Peter Hain, the Minister for Northern Ireland, said "I would certainly never advocate the squandering of public money on so called treatments that have no proven benefits and which take money away from existing therapies that are shown to work." In the same speech he said: "I am certain, as a user of complementary medicine myself, that this has the potential to improve health substantially." He was "delighted that Northern Ireland is leading the way in integrating complementary and alternative therapies into the National Health Service". GetwellUK a company in Northern Ireland was due to receive £200,000 of taxpayers' money. General Practitioners in two areas would now for the first time be able to refer patients for therapies like acupuncture, homeopathy and massage. But these treatments have "no proven benefits." How inconsistent can one get?

Who are GetwellUK? They are a private company financed largely by taxpayers' money supported by Prince Charles. This is done partly through yet another of the Prince's lobby groups, "GP Associates". "GP Associates" was the forerunner of "Integrated Health Associates" the inaugural meeting of which was sponsored by Solgar Vitamins, a drug company and a purveyor of "supplements".

In a commentary by Elizabeth Wager titled "Authors, Ghosts, Damned Lies and Statisticians", the author concludes "perhaps we should now admit that there are four types of lie: lies, damned lies, statistics, and the authorship lists of scientific papers, and that statisticians may be able to help prevent both the third and fourth types."[172]

Cancer researcher Andrew J. Vickers has stated: The label "unproven" is inappropriate for many therapies; it is time to assert that many alternative cancer therapies have been "disproven."[173]

Dangers of CAM

Some "alternative" medicine providers reach beyond their expertise and provide potential for disaster. A woman in her 30s with a prosthetic heart valve who had done well for years on blood-thinning medicine was told by her faith healer that she was "cured." She discontinued her lifesaving medication and within weeks a blood clot had formed near her heart valve. She died in the operating room.[174]

In Australia 39 separate incidents were reported to the Paediatric Surveillance Unit between 2001 and 2003.[175] Four children died because their parents chose ineffective naturopathic, homeopathic, or other alternative medicines and diets rather than conventional therapies. In all, 17 instances occurred in which children were significantly harmed by a failure to use conventional medicine. The children ranged from babies to 16 year olds. Parents sometimes think CAM remedies are "more natural" with fewer side effects than conventional drugs but in nearly two thirds of the cases the side effects were rated as severe. In 30 cases, the issues were "probably or definitely" related to complementary medicine, and in 17 the patient was regarded as being harmed by a failure to use conventional medicine. The report says that all four deaths resulted from a failure to use conventional medicine. One death involved an eight-month-old baby admitted to hospital "with malnutrition and septic shock following naturopathic treatment with a rice milk diet from the age of three months for 'congestion'". Edzard Ernst said that inert remedies like homeopathy, even though they in themselves may be harmless, can be life threatening when they replace effective treatments."

Another death involved a 10-month-old infant who presented with septic shock following treatment with homeopathic medicines and dietary restriction for chronic eczema.[176] One child had multiple seizures after complementary and alternative medicines were used instead of anti-seizure drugs due to concerns about potential side effects.[177] The fourth death was of a child who needed blood-clotting drugs but was given complementary medicine instead. The study found that parents used alternative therapies to treat anything from constipation to clotting disorders, and diabetes to cerebral palsy.

The authors of the report from the Royal Children's Hospital in Melbourne, said: "Many of the adverse events associated with failure to use conventional medicine resulted from the family's belief in complementary and alternative medicine and determination to use it despite medical advice."[178]

Dr William Van't Hoff, a consultant paediatrician and a spokesman for the Royal College of Paediatrics and Child Health, described the study as being an important and well constructed study that demonstrated "a high and unacceptable rate of adverse events" associated with the use of complementary and alternative medicine (CAM).[179] The four deaths related to the failure of the families to use conventional medicine. Probably the most important risk is that families abandon or delay the use of conventional medicine and rely on CAMs.[180] The second concern was that CAMs can interact with other medicines or have toxic effects.[181]

There is a presumption that natural remedies must be harmless. Families may not appreciate this and may even attribute the toxic effect to the conventional therapy.

Neck manipulation can maim and kill and it has no proven benefit for any disease. The chiropractor's defence when adverse events occur is that standard medicine also has its victims.[182] Medications are dangerous, so are surgery and anaesthesia, immunisation and antibiotics. It is true, medical treatments can cause great harm, but each of them can be judged on a benefit-risk ratio so that the benefit will be less harmful than the disease for which it is applied.[183] Medicine is also a science that tracks adverse events while chiropractic "is a self-serving guild that denies its dangers and covers up its adverse effects."[184]

Chiropractic is a false health care practice that has flourished basically unchallenged over the past century. A survey of 27 American Medical College deans concluded that there is no scientific validity to the "ill-defined" chiropractic theory of "a vertebral body subluxation pressing on a nerve and interfering with the passage of energy down that nerve to various organs of the body thereby causing disease and that such disease can be treated by chiropractic adjustments of these subluxations or that chiropractic can cure disease or promote wellness in any way."[185]

Edzard Ernst, said that it was well known that alternative therapies could have side effects, especially in vulnerable groups like children. Parents could be "misguided by the 50 million alternative medicine websites."[186] The children are victims of lots of nonsense and false claims. All of these treatments can have side effects but there's also a risk of alternative therapies replacing effective treatments.[187] "So inert remedies like homeopathy, even though they in themselves are harmless, can be life-threatening when they replace effective treatments."

Popularity of CAM

More than a third of American adults use alternative therapies and almost all of those patients also see conventional doctors.[188]

The popularity of complementary therapies in Britain is currently at its peak. Authors have speculated on the reasons for the appeal of alternative medicines being used *in lieu* of conventional medicine. Among these reasons is the vigorous marketing[189] of extravagant claims by the alternative medical community combined with inadequate media scrutiny and attacks on critics.[190,191]

There is also an increase in conspiracy theories toward conventional medicine[192] and pharmaceutical companies, mistrust of traditional authority figures, such as physicians, and a dislike of the current delivery methods of scientific biomedicine, all of which have led patients to seek out alternative medicine.[193] Many patients also lack access to contemporary medicine,[194] due to a lack of private or public health insurance, which leads them to seek out lower-cost alternatives.[195] Medical doctors are also aggressively marketing alternative medicine to profit from this market.[196]

Is CAM effective?

The popularity of CAM may be related to other factors.[197] In an interview with Edzard Ernst, *The Independent* wrote: Why is it so popular, then? Ernst blames the providers, customers and the doctors whose neglect, he says, has created the opening into which alternative therapists have stepped. "People are told lies. There are 40 million websites and 39.9 million tell lies, sometimes outrageous lies. They mislead cancer patients, who are encouraged not only to pay their last penny but to be treated with something that shortens their lives. At the same time, people are gullible. It needs gullibility for the industry to succeed. It doesn't make me popular with the public, but it's the truth."[198]

Ernst published a study in the Annals of Oncology which concluded that nearly 50 per cent of the 32 most popular websites on Complementary and Alternative Medicine for cancer were not of good quality.[199] Ernst said that the study should raise patients' awareness on the variability of the quality of websites on CAM for specific diseases. "The cancer cures discussed on these websites are not supported by good scientific evidence," according to the study. Even worse, three websites were qualified as "outright dangerous". These three sites had applied, but were rejected, by Health On the Net Foundation for HON code certification.[200] HON counts more than 5,000 certified Websites in some 72 countries worldwide that bear the HON code seal.

Professor Antoine Geissbühler, President of the HON Foundation and Director of the Service of Medical informatics of the Geneva University Hospitals said that HON can today implement an action plan in order to protect and guide citizens to safer and better quality online information. On the positive side, "four websites stand out" from the rest for the exemplary quality of their information and treatments. They included quackwatch.org, ebandolier.com, cis.nci.nih.gov and rosenthal.hs.columbia.edu.

Despite the increase in popularity, chiropractic and osteopathy are currently the only two complementary and alternative medical professions that are subject to statutory regulation in Britain. The United Kingdom Department of Health has been examining proposed extensions of regulations to include herbal medicine and acupuncture.

To enhance any placebo effect it should be accompanied by as much impressive "mumbo jumbo" as possible or to lie to the patient as much as possible[201] and certainly to disguise from them the fact that, for example, their homeopathic pill contains nothing but lactose. Therein lies a problem. The whole trend in medicine has been to be more transparent with the patient and to tell them the truth.[202] To maximise the benefit of alternative medicine, it is necessary to lie to the patient as much as possible.[203]

In addition, who trains CAM practitioners? Are the trainers expected to tell their students the same lies? Certain Universities in the United Kingdom offer courses in various aspects of alternative medicine.

BBC2 TV showed a much-advertised and heavily criticised series on alternative medicine in early 2006. It was billed as "the deepest investigation into the efficacy of alternative medicine ever attempted on TV".[204] Presented by Kathy Sykes it was claimed to investigate "why science is starting to respond to these centuries-old remedies" but Simon Singh who writes in the Daily Telegraph (14th Feb., 2006) asked: "Did we really witness the 'amazing power' of acupuncture?" He said that the series was devoid of scepticism and rigour. "Although the second program was indeed a rational look at the placebo effect,[205] the other two episodes were little more than rose-tinted adverts for the alternative medicine industry." "For example, the scene showing a patient punctured with needles and undergoing open heart surgery left viewers with the strong impression that acupuncture was providing immense pain relief. In fact, in addition to acupuncture, the patient had a combination of three very powerful sedatives (Midazolam, Droperidol, Fentanyl) and large volumes of local anaesthetic injected into the tissues on the front of the chest.[206] With such a cocktail of chemicals, the acupuncture needles were apparently cosmetic. In short, this memorable bit of telly was emotionally powerful, but scientifically meaningless in building a case for acupuncture. This TV series pretended to be scientific and had the chance to set the record straight, but instead it chickened out of confronting the widespread failure of alternative medicine."

Among the many criticisms was one from Ernst, the main consultant for the series. He felt that the BBC had abused him.[207] "It was as if they had instructions from higher up that this had to be a happy story about complementary medicine without any complexity, and they used me to give a veneer of respectability" he is quoted as saying.

A letter, unequivocal in its defence of the BBC was published by *The Guardian* on April 1st, 2006, a very appropriate day. The letter had ten signatories but was actually written by the BBC who also compiled the signatories.[208] The letter had not even been seen by some of the people whose names appeared as signatories. *The* Guardian later published a correction. How far can quackery go?

The *British Medical Journal*[209] had a debate on whether or not CAM should be referred for evaluation to the National Institute for Clinical Excellence (NICE). Two of the comments that followed the debate were as follows:[210] John R King, a Consultant Psychiatrist, commented that there was a very large and ever expanding array of alternative treatments, some more bizarre than others, which could tie up the resources of NICE for an indefinite period but, he stated that, if people wanted to believe in them or in fairies or leprechauns, they should be left in peace to do so.[211] It was no concern of scientific medicine.

David Colquhoun, replied that "Nobody is proposing to ban fairies or leprechauns.[212] It would be both undesirable and impossible. There does seem to be a case, though, for not providing leprechauns at the tax payers' expense. And really all leprechauns that are sold to the public should have labels that don't make false claims for their powers."

The Royal Society, the United Kingdom's national academy of science, put a statement about alternative medicine on its "science issues" web site. It stated that the Royal Society believes that complementary and alternative medicines, like conventional medicines, should be subject to careful evaluation of their effectiveness and safety. It is important that treatments labelled as complementary and alternative medicines are properly tested and that patients do not receive misleading information about the effectiveness of complementary medicine.

Furthermore, National Health Service provision for complementary and alternative medicines, as for conventional medicines, should be confined to treatments that are supported by adequate diagnosis together with evidence of both effectiveness and safety. Note the statement that patients do not receive misleading information about the efficacy of the alternative medicine.

Convenient slogans such as "integrated therapy", "alternative medicine" or even the favourite of creationists "intelligent design" are all convenient slogans that permit the credulous to con the gullible.[213]

In 1834, Dr. Oliver Wendell Holmes, poet, essayist, and Professor-to-be of Anatomy at the Harvard Medical School, returned to Boston from study in Paris with microscope in hand. He was convinced that French quantitative science would find a new home in the city, which he christened "the Hub" of the universe. But Boston in 1834 had permitted curious forms of the healing art to flower[214] and Holmes was appalled. By 1842, he had had enough and wrote the definitive critique of the practice: *Homeopathy and its Kindred Delusions*.[215] He found that homeopathy was "lucrative, and so long as it continues to be will surely survive, as surely as astrology, palmistry and other methods of getting a living out of the weakness and credulity of mankind and womankind."

Holmes also said that "Some of you will probably be more or less troubled by that parody of medieval theology which finds its dogma in the doctrine of homeopathy, its miracle of transubstantiation in the mystery of its dilutions, its church in the people who have mistaken their century, and its priests in those who have mistaken their calling."[216]

CAM and the Cochrane Collaboration

In their efforts to put "alternative" medicine on to a more scientific basis and much to their credit a Cochrane CAM Field was set up in 1996. This is an international group of individuals dedicated to facilitating the production of systematic reviews of randomised clinical trials in areas such as acupuncture, massage, chiropractic, herbal medicine, homeopathy and mind-body therapy.[217] It was founded and coordinated by the University of Maryland Centre for Integrative Medicine and is a member entity of the *Cochrane Collaboration*. They are actively involved in the preparation of systematic reviews. Over the last five years Cochrane CAM Field staff have published more than ten systematic reviews, for both *The Cochrane Library* and for print journals.[218]

In May 2007, the Cochrane CAM Field was awarded a five-year 2.1 million dollar research grant from NCCAM to support and extend the work of the Field.[219] They identify published clinical trials of alternative therapies, prepare systematic reviews, train systematic reviewers, disseminate systematic reviews to the general public and healthcare providers, and conduct research to improve systematic review methodology. Symposia and workshops on research methodology, study design, and systematic reviews have been organized in San Francisco, Baltimore, Barcelona, Ottawa, Melbourne, Dublin, Hong Kong and Israel. All of these symposia and workshops have focused on or highlighted the work of the *Cochrane Collaboration*.[220] The CAM-related Cochrane, Issue 12.

2011, reviews and protocols, organised by CAM topics are available in *The Cochrane Library* at: http://www.cochrane.org/reviews/ en/subtopics/22.html.[221]

The reviews are also linked to summaries and abstracts free of charge.

Cochrane CAM Field staff published a paper in the January 2004 issue of *Complementary Therapies in Medicine,* that outlined the many projects the CAM Field was undertaking on behalf of the *Cochrane Collaboration.*[222] In the journal *Explore,* a regular column called "Cochrane for CAM Providers", was launched by the CAM Field[223] to promote the awareness of the *Cochrane Collaboration* and to improve the understanding of randomised controlled trials and systematic review methodology among the CAM community. A series has been launched in the *Journal of Alternative and Complementary Medicine*,[224] to provide an overview of the Cochrane CAM-related reviews.[225] A book titled *Complementary Therapies on the Internet* has been written to facilitate both professionals and consumers' acquisition of reliable information on CAM therapies and research.[226]

Another core function of the CAM Field is maintaining the register of CAM trials.[227] The entire contents of the CAM Field register is submitted regularly to the US Cochrane Centre for publication in The Cochrane Library's *CENTRAL Register of Controlled Trials*, the most comprehensive register of trials in the world. As well as maintaining the register of CAM trials,[228] the CAM Field has compiled a register of *CAM-related systematic reviews,* which currently numbers 340 non-*Cochrane CAM-related systematic reviews* and over 150 *Cochrane systematic reviews.*

Universities and CAM

Much of alternative medicine is positively anti-science, yet three-year BSc degrees are now being awarded in this subject by 16 British Universities.[229] Is it honest to award Bachelor of Science degrees for these courses?

David Colquhoun said he was "appalled". "These courses are basically anti science. Universities that run them should be ashamed of themselves"[230] he said. He argued that awarding a Bachelor of Science degree for an alternative medicine course is a failing in quality assurance. Not only were some of the doctrines of CAM incompatible with science or common sense, but they are often also incompatible with each other.[231] Homeopaths subscribe to the bizarre doctrine that the less you give the bigger the effect, but herbalists do not. They want to give a sensible dose, but do not know what it is.[232] Nutritional therapists go to the opposite extreme and want to give huge and sometimes toxic doses. Students of reflexology, according to Colquhoun, are taught that a small area on the big toe is connected with the pituitary gland.[233] Not only is this incompatible with physiology, but it is also incompatible with homeopathy, herbal medicine and nutritional therapy. Brian Isbell the head of the department of complementary therapies at Westminster University stated that homeopathy had a conflict as, "although there is scientific evidence for its efficacy, current theory cannot explain how the intervention works".

Edzard Ernst weighed in saying that most complementary medicine degrees were "scandalously unacademic". Peter Fisher, the clinical director of the Royal

London Homeopathic Hospital, admitted that much more work needed to be done to establish a scientific basis for homeopathy.

The National Health Service Centre for Reviews and Dissemination from the University of York said that "There is currently insufficient evidence of effectiveness either to recommend homeopathy as a treatment for any specific condition". [234]

In a BBC London News (BBC1 TV) program Riz Lateef the presenter asked Dr. Peter Fisher if he could ever see homeopathy as a science degree in the future.[235] Fisher responded: "I would hope so. I wouldn't deny that a lot of scientific research needs to be done, and I would hope that in the future it would have a scientific basis. I have to say that at the moment that basis isn't comprehensive. To that extent I would agree with Professor Colquhoun." Comments in the newspapers following this program included:

"Faith-based degree damages science" - *The Times*. "Homeopathy science degrees 'gobbledygook' ". the *Guardian*. "Alternative medicine degrees 'anti-scientific'". *The Daily Telegraph*.[236]

"Universities 'are duping students with homeopathy science degrees' " *The Independent*. "Less than complementary?" *The Glasgow Herald*.[237] "Alternative therapy degree attack" "UK universities are teaching "gobbledygook" following the explosion in science degrees in complementary medicine, a leading expert says." *BBC News* web site. "University homoeopathy degrees 'gobbledygook', claims Professor". *Daily Mail*. "British health expert brands homeopathy 'gobbledygook'". Daily India.com.[238] "Homeopathic Degree in Britain Puts Scientific Gloss on Nonscientific Dross, Critics Say". *The Chronicle of Higher Education* (USA).

One comment, from *The Guardian*'s "Comment is Free" asked "So why not homeopathy alongside medicine?" Colquhoun answered: "Right. Why not Levitation alongside Aeronautical Engineering?"

Colquhoun also said that the new universities had been much-mocked for offering degrees in subjects like Golf Course Management (e.g. Bournemouth, Lincoln).[239] While it was true that there is little relationship between the intellectual content of such courses and that of a B.Sc. in Physics, Golf Course Management was not dishonest.[240] It is useful for some people. A B.Sc. in plumbing, would be just as intellectual, and a lot more useful than golf. He said that "What is truly disgraceful is not so much that degrees are being offered in subjects with little intellectual content, but that degrees are being offered in subjects that have negative intellectual content. Degrees in subjects where the words have no discernable meaning at all, but are pure mumbo jumbo".[241]

The sceptic might say that degrees in theology may not be based on scientific fact but no university has ever offered a Bachelor of Science degree in theology.[242] Nobody, according to Colquhoun, pretends that religion is a subject that is amenable to the methods of science yet, incredibly, it is possible to find places that offer B.Sc. degrees in subjects like homeopathy which bears no relationship whatsoever to science.[243] The University of Westminster, for example, boasts proudly that "The School has developed the widest range of complementary therapy courses in Europe.[244] The BSc (Hons.) Health Sciences degrees in herbal medicine, homeopathy, nutritional therapy and therapeutic bodywork and the Traditional Chinese Medicine: Acupuncture course were the first named degrees of their kind in the UK. They have recently been supplemented by a new pathway in naturopathy." In similar vein the University of Lincoln advertises: "Complementary Medicine BSc (Hons.). This exciting and innovative degree programme will give you an appreciation of the orthodox western model of health and illness as a foundation to your complementary medicine studies in either western herbal medicine or traditional Chinese acupuncture."[245] Another institution at the forefront of promoting gobbledygook in the name of science, is Thames Valley University,[246] whose brochure offers aromatherapy, reflexology and shiatsu massage as though they were science (B.Sc (Hons)). Colquhoun advised that if a B.Sc. was too much for one, Thames Valley University also offered a short course in homeopathy,[247] which was described thus. "Would you like to know how to treat your relatives and friends for colds and flu, injuries, travel illnesses, pre-exam stress and acute emotional difficulties? These are just some of the conditions that can be treated with Homeopathy medicine and which will be covered in the course." The suggestion that homeopathy can cure colds and flu is false and irresponsible.

The University of Salford also offers Complementary Medicine and Health Sciences, BSc (Hons).[248] They state that "If you complete all of the homeopathy modules in the degree you will be able to apply for entry into year two of the four-year part-time homeopathy professional training programme at the North West College of Homeopathy in Manchester. You will also receive a certificate in Homeopathic First Aid."[249]

Colquhoun enquires what will be offered next? "B.Sc. degrees in Black Magic and the Casting of Spells? Astrology? Why not? They would be little different from things on offer already. There would be no objection to teaching homeopathy etc. as part of the history of ideas, or as a sociological phenomenon. What is deeply objectionable, if not downright fraudulent, is to label them as science".[250]

The University of Maryland Medical Centre in the USA had a good reputation in medicine. They now have a website with a whole section devoted to "Alternative/Complementary Medicine". This is a serious indication of how far universities have acquiesced in delusional thinking.[251] In fact it is worse, because the bad advice comes from what seems like an authoritative source.[252] In 1991 Brian Berman, M.D founded the Centre for Integrative Medicine (CIM) within the University of Maryland School of Medicine. The CIM is a National Institutes of Health (NIH) Centre of Excellence for research, patient care, education and training in integrative medicine. It emphasizes an approach to healing that values mind, body, and spirit. The Centre is "committed to evaluating the scientific foundation of complementary medicine, educating health professionals and the public; and integrating evidence-based complementary therapies into clinical care to help people achieve and maintain optimal health and well-being."[253] Dr Stephen Barrett of *Quackwatch* searched the Maryland site with Google and found articles that promoted homeopathy for about 300 health problems.[254]

The University of Pennsylvania, America's first School of Medicine has entered into a collaboration agreement with the Tai Sophia Institute of Applied Healing Arts. The University press release reads: "The University of

Pennsylvania School of Medicine and the Tai Sophia Institute for the Applied Healing Arts of Laurel, Maryland,[255] have signed an affiliation agreement to collaborate on education, research and clinical activities in complementary and alternative medicine." Another real medical school decided to forego science and throw in its lot with the delusional age. The initiatives will include[256] the creation of a Master's Degree in Complementary and Alternative Medicine, to be offered by the Tai Sophia Institute and developed in collaboration with Pennsylvania School of Medicine faculty.[257] "This degree program is one of the first of its kind in the nation," stated Alfred P. Fishman, MD, Senior Associate Dean for Program Development at Penn's School of Medicine and co-director of the collaboration.[258] The Tai Sophia "institutional values" include: "All members of Tai Sophia Institute''s community – faculty, staff, administration, and students will operate from a Declaration of Oneness, a unity with all creation and they will use nature and the rhythms of the earth as a guide in teaching our students and each other."[259] The values go on "Continue our learning in the presence of each other, acting not as truth-tellers but as guides for self-discovery."[260]

Gerald Weissmann wrote a very entertaining and delightfully titled article about homeopathy published in the *Federation of American Societies for Experimental Biology Journal*[261] in which he mentions Dana Ullman. Weissman's article is well worth reading. Dana Ullman is an ardent practitioner of homeopathy in the United States.[262] He has written six major texts on the subject and he serves on the Advisory Council of the Alternative Medicine Centre at Columbia University's College of Physicians and Surgeons. He is also a consultant to Harvard Medical School's Centre to Assess Alternative Therapy for Chronic Illness,[263] During an anthrax outbreak in October 2001, Mr. Ullman advised use of the homeopathic medicine *Anthracinum* for the prevention and treatment of anthrax. This agent, obtained from infected pigs, is called a nosode and its producers reassure the public that they are "diluted to a point where no molecules of the disease product remain."[264]

The Alternative Medicine Centre at Columbia University's College of Physicians and Surgeons is one of the Centers Ullman has advised.[265] Columbia University's Rosenthal Centre offers[266] "integrative medicine" for children with cancer provided by staff "experienced in *Shiatsu*, reflexology, aromatherapy, *Reiki*, Flow Alignment and Connection, *So Tai*, and *Tui Na*."[267] Harvard Medical School's Osher Institute where Ullman is also a consultant offers clinical fellowships, funded by NCCAM, to study remedies that meet Prince Charles's criteria of being[268] "rooted in ancient traditions acupuncture, herbal therapies, chiropractic, relaxation techniques, therapeutic massage, and other proto-scientific measures that sidestep the laws of chemistry and physics.[269] When Columbia's Rosenthal Centre celebrated its 10th anniversary among the awardees of honour was Prince Charles.[270]

Florida State University, allegedly under political pressure, was also proposing to set up a school of Chiropractic. One of the University professors, Albert Stiegman, predicted the future campus map including buildings for chiropractice medicine, Yeti Foundation, School of Astrology, Institute of Telekinesia, Department of ESP studies, College of Homeopathic Medicine, Bigfoot Institute, Faith Healing, Foundation for Prayer Healing Studies, School of

UFO Abduction Studies, School of Channelling and Remote Sensing, Creationism Foundation, Tarot Studies, Palmistry, College of Dowsing, Past Life Studies, Crop Circle Simulation Studies. In the end, reason won. The Florida Board of Governors voted 10-3 to deny Florida State University's request to build a chiropractic school.

Elsevier the publishers have introduced a new "scientific" journal. Titled *Explore: The Journal of Science & Healing*[271] and advertised as "an interdisciplinary journal that explores the healing arts, consciousness, spirituality, eco-environmental issues, and basic science as all these fields relate to health." Its contents include:[272] Acupuncture/Acupressure, Ayurveda, Biofeedback, Botanical or Herbal Medicine, Chiropractic, Consciousness, Creative Therapies, Diet/Nutrition/Nutritional Supplements, Environmental Medicine, Holistic Medicine/Nursing, Homeopathy, Indigenous Medical Practices, Manual Therapies, Mind-Body Therapies, Naturopathy, Osteopathic Medicine, Qigong/Tai Chi, Touch Therapies, Spiritual/Transpersonal Healing/Prayer, Tibetan Medicine, Traditional Chinese Medicine and Yoga. But how much science despite the word being used in the title?

A CAM teaching program was advertised in the Bulletin of the British Pharmacological Society in 2001. The cost of the program was £25.00 for "UK HE" and £350.00 for others! The teaching document starts with the statement "Please note that many of the statements/ claims made concerning the therapies in this program are those of the practitioners of the therapies.[273] The claims may or may not have a factual basis, and are not necessarily the views of the authors". In the program there is no attempt whatsoever to assess the truth of any of the statements and claims that are made.[274]

To that extent, the program is not about science at all. David Colquhoun considered pharmacology to be the science concerned with what drugs do and how they do it and science to be concerned with distinguishing truth from fiction.[275] By those criteria, he commented that this program was concerned with neither pharmacology nor science and that it was "a disgrace to both". Alternative-medicine providers have been looked on in the same light as good used car salesmen; that is, with little scientific proof for their treatments, they find many willing customers.[276]

<u>Why do people accept CAM?</u>

Barry Beyerstein[277], a biopsychologist at Simon Fraser University in Burnaby, British Columbia, Canada, proposed several reasons why so many otherwise intelligent patients and therapists pay considerable sums of money for products and therapies of alternative medicine when they know that most of them are useless or dangerous or have not been subjected to rigorous scientific testing? He said that there were social and cultural reasons e.g., many citizens' inability to make an informed choice about a health care product; anti-scientific attitudes meshed with New Age mysticism; vigorous marketing and extravagant claims; dislike of the delivery of scientific biomedicine and belief in the superiority of natural products. There were psychological reasons e.g., the will to believe;[278]

logical errors of judgment; wishful thinking, and demand characteristics and there was the illusion that an ineffective therapy works,[279] when actually other factors were at work e.g., the natural course or cyclic nature of the disease; the placebo effect; spontaneous remission or misdiagnosis.

The extravagant claims of the CAM advocates and the oft promised certain cure are both attractive but Beyerstein cautioned potential clients to be suspicious if those treatments were not supported by reliable scientific research, or, among other things, if the promises of cures sounded too good to be true.

The belief in alternative medicine by fools can be accepted. The belief in alternative medicine when all scientific and proven methods of treatment have been exhausted and found to be ineffective can be understood. Many people who use CAM are neither foolish, ill-educated nor desperate. Some intelligent people accept complementary or alternative medicine. Personal experience causes different people to think differently. This is especially true if emotions, doctrines or monetary factors are involved. Controlled observations and formal logic, according to Beyerstein, are far superior to anecdotes and surmises that "can so easily lead us astray."

The providers of any form of treatment have the obligation to prove that their products are safe and effective.[280] The latter is often difficult to prove. Proof of effectiveness is provided by proper scientific evidence such as randomised clinical trials. This is evidence-based medicine and without such evidence it is questionable to offer that treatment to the public. Subjective testimonials as provided by advocates of CAM are not proof of effectiveness and there are many subtle ways that patients and health care providers can be led into thinking that a useless treatment has produced a cure.

Why do intelligent people use CAM? They do so even if the alternative therapy is implausible, lacks scientifically acceptable rationale of its own,[281] has insufficient supporting evidence derived from adequately controlled double-blind, randomised, placebo-controlled clinical trials, has failed in well-controlled clinical studies done by impartial evaluators and should seem improbable, even to the lay person, on "commonsense" grounds.[282] Beyerstein believes that they do so because of vigorous marketing of unsubstantiated claims by "alternative" healers,[283] the poor level of scientific knowledge in the public at large,[284] and the "will to believe."[285,286] He explains these reasons in great detail.

Many diseases are self-limiting and some are cyclical.[287] Arthritis, multiple sclerosis, allergies, and gastrointestinal complaints are examples of diseases that normally "have their ups and downs." Sufferers naturally, tend to seek therapy during the downturn of any given cycle.[288] In this way, a bogus treatment will have repeated opportunities to coincide with upturns that would have happened anyway. "Spontaneous remissions" even of some cancers can occur. They are rare but possible and are often reported anecdotally. Alternative therapies may receive unearned acclaim for remissions of this sort because many desperate patients turn to them when they feel that they have nothing left to lose.[289] Statistical evidence that the "cure rates" exceed the known spontaneous remission rate and the placebo response rate is needed for the treatment to be regarded as successful.[290]

The placebo effect provides a major reason why bogus remedies are credited with subjective, and occasionally objective, improvements.[291, 292]

Some allegedly cured symptoms may be psychosomatic to begin with and these may have been alleviated merely by support and reassurance. This may quite easily be extended to subtle criticism of conventional medicine and its practitioners. Beyerstein states that a large portion of those diagnosed with "chronic fatigue," "environmental sensitivity syndrome," various stress disorders and interestingly enough those affected by the allegedly harmful effects of silicone breast implants, very much the topic of the news in January 2012.[293, 294, 295] may fall into this category.

Support in similar cases may even be in the form of pseudoscientific diagnostic devices provided by the CAM advocate. This may explain the reported success of various devices which throughout history have been claimed to "cure" various illnesses.

When CAM has been shown to be ineffective in a particular case it might be too psychologically disconcerting for a patient to admit that it has been a waste of time and money and there might be a strong psychological pressure to find some redeeming value in the treatment.[296] This is a self-serving bias to help maintain self-esteem and smooth social functioning.[297] Because core beliefs tend to be vigorously defended by warping perception and memory, patients and practitioners of CAM may misinterpret cues and remember things as they wish they had happened.[298] They may be selective in what they recall. They may overestimate their apparent successes while ignoring, downplaying, or explaining away their failures.

Dean and colleagues[299] showed that without sophisticated statistical aids, human cognitive abilities are simply not up to the task of sifting valid relationships out of masses of interacting data. Similar difficulties would have confronted the pioneers of pre-scientific medicine and their followers, and for that reason, their anecdotal reports cannot be accepted as support for their assertions.

Beyerstein concluded that individual testimonials counted for very little in evaluating therapies. Any putative treatment should be tested under conditions that control for placebo responses, compliance effects, and judgmental errors.[300]

Before anyone agrees to undergo any kind of treatment, he or she should be confident that it has been validated in properly controlled clinical trials. Supporting evidence should be published in peer-reviewed scientific journals. Potential clients should be wary if the "evidence" consists merely of testimonials, self-published pamphlets or books, or items from the popular media.[301] Finally, because any single positive outcome, even from a carefully done experiment published in a reputable journal, could always be a fluke, replication by independent research groups is the ultimate standard of proof. [302] He stresses that if the practitioner "claims persecution, is ignorant of or openly hostile to mainstream science, cannot supply a reasonable scientific rationale for his or her methods, and promises results that go well beyond those claimed by orthodox biomedicine, there is strong reason to suspect that one is dealing with a quack."[303]

False hope easily supplants common sense. Patients in a vulnerable state need hard-nosed appraisal of proposed treatment. Normally "savvy" consumers, felled by disease,[304] "often insist upon less evidence to support the claims of alternative healers than they would previously have demanded from someone hawking a used car."

Prayer and CAM

In a discussion on the golf course practice range one day a family practitioner, who I knew very well, claimed that prayer helped to cure certain illnesses. I had, incidentally, taken this doctor for his final examinations in Obstetrics and Gynaecology when he qualified a few years previously and I had given him a very good pass. I knew him to be very bright. I expressed doubt at the supposed effects of prayer but, as my friend was adamant, I decided to research prayer and its effects on illnesses.

Francis Galton, the famous English scientist argued that regardless of how it worked the efficacy of prayer was a "perfectly appropriate and legitimate subject of scientific inquiry" because it could be tested statistically.[305] He reasoned that clergy should be the longest lived of all since they prayed the most and were also among the most prayed for but when he compared the longevity of eminent clergy with eminent doctors and lawyers, the clergy were the shortest lived of the three groups.[306] He then considered royalty who he felt, when compared to other members of the aristocracy, were much prayed for. Galton concluded that "Sovereigns are literally the shortest lived of all who have the advantage of affluence." It is of interest that when Diana and Charles divorced, Queen Elizabeth had Diana's name removed from the list of beneficiaries of the public prayer. Galton looked at the premiums that the insurance companies charged to insure ships. He reasoned, that missionaries and pilgrims prayed a great deal and ships that carried missionaries and pilgrims should therefore have provided a great deal of prayer for the safety of the ship. Therefore the insurance premiums should be lower for such ships.[307] But apparently the insurance premiums were exactly the same. Insurance companies had found that ships carrying pilgrims and missionaries sank just as often as did other ships.[308] Apparently the prayers did not help.

Rupert Sheldrake, a Cambridge trained plant biologist examined the effects of prayer in India. Most people there preferred having a son, and a tremendous amount of praying is used in the effort to produce one.[309] Sheldrake examined statistics of live male births in India and used data from England as a control where the preference for sons was less strong. He found that in both England and India there were 106 males to 100 females, just as in every other country. He stated, "If this enormous amount of psychic effort and praying of holy men were working, you would expect on average the percentage of live male births to be higher."[310]

Although these statistical studies from the nineteenth century strongly suggest that prayer is not effective,[311] they do not meet the "gold standard," of a completely valid scientific study. Actually, there are only three studies that meet the "gold standard." For a finding to be considered statistically significant the P or probability value must be 0.05 or less, which means the probability that it could be due to chance is five in 100 or less. The figure of 0.05 is the one usually accepted for "ordinary" scientific studies but what criterion should be applied in proving a supernatural finding? [312]

The James Randi Educational Foundation, mentioned later, has a standing offer of one million dollars to anyone who can demonstrate any supernatural event under carefully controlled scientific conditions.[313] The members of the foundation think that a study that would prove a claim of the supernatural should eliminate any possibility that the result could be by chance. They think a test should be devised where the possibility of a supernatural event happening would be in the range of 1 in 10,000,000, a far cry from five in 100. Extraordinary claims should require extraordinary proof and this requirement should especially apply to claims of the supernatural.[314]

Dr. Randolph Byrd's paper in 1988[315] was the first to purport to establish the positive effects of intercessory prayer (prayer by one or more persons on behalf of another), without the recipients' knowledge,[316] on the hospital course of patients.

Using twenty-six indicators in patients admitted to a coronary care unit (CCU),[317] he had found no statistically significant differences between prayed-for and control patients. He did report a significant decrease in certain medical complications[318] in the prayed-for group: less congestive heart failure, pneumonia, and cardiopulmonary arrest; less need for diuretic therapy, antibiotics, and respiratory intubation and/or ventilation. Byrd also devised a scoring system to rate the overall hospital course as "Good," "Intermediate," or "Bad," and reported a statistically significant decrease in the number of "Bad" outcomes among the prayed-for patients. Byrd's study found no statistically significant differences in length of CCU stay, total days hospitalised, or number of deaths but despite its procedural and statistical shortcomings,[319] the 1988 Byrd study has been frequently quoted as showing positive effects of prayer.[320, 321, 322, 323]

When Irwin Tessman, professor of biological sciences at Perdue University, requested of Dr. Byrd that he be allowed to review the raw data that went into the study, he was refused.[324] Since Dr. Byrd's claim was one of the supernatural, it would seem appropriate that all aspects of the study be reviewed by independent investigators.[325] In addition the degree of religiosity communicated by Dr. Byrd raised doubts that he could be completely objective on a scientific investigation of prayer, something that he deeply believed was effective. At the end of his paper he acknowledges; "... and Mrs. Janet Greene for her dedication to this study. In addition, I thank God for responding to the many prayers made on behalf of the patients."[326]

A study by Harris and others[327] attempted to replicate Byrd's findings by testing the hypothesis that patients who are unknowingly and remotely prayed for by blinded intercessors[328] would experience fewer complications and have a shorter hospital stay than patients not receiving such prayer. Harris's study showed that in a comparison of two groups in a coronary care unit, although the lengths of coronary care unit and hospital stays were not different in the two groups, intercessory prayer was associated with more favourable outcomes. The authors stated: "Our findings support Byrd's conclusions despite the fact that we could not document an effect of prayer using his scoring method"[329] and they suggested that prayer might be an effective adjunct to standard medical care. Their findings not only do not support Byrd's conclusions but they directly refute them. Nevertheless the editorial board that agreed to publish this article allowed this statement to stand.[330]

Harris's study caused significant publicity when it was first published but it has been thoroughly discredited since. There were many valid criticisms of both Byrd's and Harris's papers.[331] Carl Sagan said "extraordinary claims require extraordinary proof." Byrd's and Harris's claims were certainly extraordinary. If their findings were true they would suggest the existence, if not scientific proof, of a supernatural power. That is an extraordinary claim and would require extraordinary proof. This was not the case.

In 1988, there had only been three controlled examinations of the effects of prayer by third parties on people who were unaware of the prayers.[332] The article by Byrd has been described.[333] This claimed benefit but was poorly designed, whereas the other two were well designed but found no benefit.[334, 335]

Since 1988 four more studies have been published,[336] two showing no benefit and two claiming a positive result. In another study improvement occurred in anxiety, depression, and self-esteem in all of the 406 subjects who received intercessory prayer or no prayer but there were no differences between the two groups.[337] A study of the effects of intercessory prayer on 40 recovering alcoholics also showed no benefit.[338]

Mayo Clinic researchers, in 2001, concluded that "intercessory prayer had no significant effect on medical outcomes after hospitalization in a coronary care unit." Not one difference in medical outcomes showed up between the control group and the prayed-for group in more than 750 patients who were followed for 6 months after discharge from the hospital coronary care unit.[339]

Stephen Barrett[340] feels that intercessory prayer studies accomplish nothing. "Believers" will not change their view if further studies are negative, and nonbelievers will not change theirs if additional studies appear positive.

The statistical studies from the nineteenth century and the three coronary care unit studies on prayer are quite consistent with the fact that humanity is wasting a huge amount of time on a procedure that simply does not work.[341]

Nonetheless, faith in prayer is so pervasive and deeply rooted, believers will continue to devise future studies in a desperate effort to confirm their beliefs.[342] At least, now that I have the scientific information, I can challenge my family practitioner colleague on proper scientific grounds.

Psychic healers

Many "psychics" and "healers" offer help through the mail or by telephone.[343] Some call themselves Sister, Madame, Reverend, Doctor, Father, Prophet, Madame Queen, Reverent Mother, or Reverend Sister. The purported benefits may include better health, better luck or financial benefit. Many people respond and may send a specific sum of money. Rest assured a further letter would arrive indicating that the problem was worse than was initially thought and requesting further cash.

Very few, if any, "faith healers" ever request the medical records of a client. Do they ever enquire as to the health of their client at any later stage? Do they ever keep statistics? On the other hand, many cases have been documented in which people with serious disease have died as a result of abandoning effective medical care after being "healed."[344]

A number of religious sects favor prayer over medical care.[345] Christian Science is probably the best known of these groups in the USA and it is the only form of faith healing that is deductible as a medical expense for federal income tax purposes.[346] Followers of the sect contend that illness is an illusion caused by faulty beliefs [347] and that prayer heals by replacing bad thoughts with good ones. Barrett says that Christian Science practitioners work by trying to argue the sick thoughts out of the person's mind. Consultations can take place in person, by telephone, or even by mail.[348] Individuals may also be able to attain correct beliefs by themselves through prayer or mental concentration. *You can Heal*, a pamphlet of the Christian Science Publishing Society, states that "every student of Christian Science has the God-given ability to heal the sick." Two weeks of class instruction are required to become a practitioner. The weekly magazine *Christian Science Sentinel* publishes several "testimonies" in each issue. Believers have claimed that prayer has brought about recovery from anemia,[349] arthritis, blood poisoning, corns, deafness, defective speech, multiple sclerosis, skin rashes, total body paralysis, visual difficulties, and various injuries but most of these accounts contain little detail, and many of the diagnoses were made without medical consultation.[350]

Rita and Douglas Swan, whose 16-month-old son Matthew died of meningitis under the care of two Christian Science practitioners in 1977, are not surprised by these statistics.[351] Rita and a colleague collected and reviewed the cases of 172 children who died between 1975 and 1995 when parents withheld medical care because of reliance on religious rituals.[352] They concluded that 140 of the deaths were from medical conditions for which survival rates with medical care would have exceeded 90 per cent.[353] These included 22 cases of pneumonia in infants under two years of age,[354] 15 cases of meningitis, and 12 cases of insulin-dependent diabetes. 18 more children had expected survival rates greater than 50 per cent and all but three of the remainder would probably have had some benefit from clinical help.[355]

A 1996 poll of 1,000 adults in the USA found that 79 per cent believed that spiritual faith could help people recover from disease.[356]

This idea is also popular among physicians. Although many studies have found associations between religious belief and health, no well-designed study has demonstrated that religious beliefs or prayer actually benefit health.[357]

One well-designed study found just the opposite.[358] The study involved patients whose progress was followed for nine months after discharge from a British hospital. They evaluated the outpatient records and the responses of 189 patients to questionnaires. The researchers concluded that the health status of patients with stronger spiritual beliefs were more than twice as likely to be unimproved or worse.[359]

The thought that prayer, divine intervention or the ministrations of an individual healer can cure illness has been popular throughout history.[360] Many miraculous recoveries have been attributed to "faith healing."

Louis Rose, a British psychiatrist, investigated hundreds of alleged faith-healing cures. He received communications from healers and patients throughout the world.[361] He sent each correspondent a questionnaire and sought corroborating information from physicians. He concluded, "I have been unsuccessful. After nearly twenty years of work I have yet to find one 'miracle cure'; and without that (or, alternatively, massive statistics which others must provide) I cannot be convinced of the efficacy of what is commonly termed faith healing."[362]

During the early 1970s, Minnesota surgeon William Nolen, M.D., attended a service conducted by Katherine Kuhlman, the leading USA evangelical healer of that period. He noted the names of 25 people who had been "miraculously healed."[363] He contacted and followed up these people with interviews and examinations. He discovered that one woman who had been announced as cured of "lung cancer" actually had Hodgkin's disease.[364] Another woman with cancer of the spine, on Ms. Kuhlman's enthusiastic command, had discarded her brace and run across the stage.[365] The following day her backbone collapsed and four months later she died. Overall, Nolen could not find one person with organic disease who had been helped.[366]

In 1987 C. Eugene Emery, Jr., a science writer for the *Providence Journal*, attended one of the Reverend Ralph DiOrio's, services.[367] DiOrio, a Roman Catholic priest,[368] whose healing services attract people by the thousands, had blessed nine people during the service and nine others had been proclaimed cured. DiOrio's organisation provided ten more cases[369] that supposedly provided irrefutable proof of the priest's ability to cure. During a six-month investigation, Emery found no evidence that any of these 28 individuals had been helped.[370]

James Randi[371] has described how many of the leading evangelistic healers have enriched. themselves with the help of deception and fraud. Randi's most noteworthy experience was the unmasking of Peter Popoff[372] and he also exposed the fraudulent techniques used by evangelists W.V. Grant and Ernest Angley.[373]

Although believers do not see faith healing as a problem, according to Barrett, a few things might help lower faith healing's toll on society:[374] Laws to protect children from medical neglect[375] in the name of healing should be passed and enforced. In states that allow religious exemptions from medical neglect, these exemptions should be revoked. Maybe the practice of faith healing on minors should be illegal. Faith healing should no longer be deductible as a medical expense. Reporters should be encouraged to do follow-up studies of people claimed to have been "healed" and "Healers" who use trickery to raise large sums of money should be prosecuted for grand larceny.

In conclusion of this chapter, I recently operated on a young female doctor from England. She had a large endometriotic ovarian cyst. I removed the cyst and discussed further medical treatment for the endometriosis which will recur if not treated in this way. She preferred meditation and opted for this rather than, in my opinion, the "correct" form of drug therapy. She had that right but I expect her to see someone in England about the endometriosis in the not too distant future. Sad, but her choice.

References:

1. The Scientific Review of Alternative Medicine, http://www.sram.org/info/about (accessed July 20, 2013).
2. A Statement in Defense of Scientific Medicine from the Council for Scientific Medicine. September 1997 Winter 2001 (Volume 5, Number 1). Quackwatch. Posted on May 2, 2006.
3. About | The Scientific Review of Alternative Medicine, http://www.sram.org/info/about (accessed July 20, 2013).
4. Bratman, MD, Steven (1997). *The Alternative Medicine Sourcebook*. Lowell House. p. 7. ISBN 978-1-56565-626-0. What are positive and negative things about alternative .., http://www.chacha.com/question/what-are-positive-and-negative-things-about-alternative-medicine (accessed July 20, 2013).
5. National Science Foundation survey: Science and Technology: *Public Attitudes and Public Understanding. Science Fiction and Pseudoscience.* Alternative_medicine : definition of Alternative_medicine and .., http://dictionary.sensagent.com/Alternative_medicine/en-en/ (accessed July 20, 2013).
6. Alternative_medicine: definition of Alternative_medicine and .., http://dictionary.sensagent.com/Alternative_medicine/en-en/ (accessed July 20, 2013).
7. Angell M., Kassirer J. P. (September 1998). *"Alternative medicine-the risks of untested and unregulated remedies"*. The New England Journal of Medicine . 1998. 339 (12): 839–41. doi:10.1056/NEJM199809173391210. PMID 9738094. http://kitsrus.com/pdf/nejm_998.pdf
8. "Alternative" Medicine: A Review of Studies Supported by .., http://www.sram.org/article/alternative_medicine_a_review_of_studies_supported_by_grants_awarded_by_the (accessed July 20, 2013).
9. Alternative_medicine: definition of Alternative_medicine and .., http://dictionary.sensagent.com/Alternative_medicine/en-en/ (accessed July 20, 2013).
10. Angell M., Kassirer J. P. (September 1998). *"Alternative medicine-the risks of untested and unregulated remedies"*. The New England Journal of Medicine . 1998. 339 (12): 839–41. doi:10.1056/NEJM199809173391210. PMID 9738094. http://kitsrus.com/pdf/nejm_998.pdf Alternative_medicine : definition of Alternative_medicine and .., http://dictionary.sensagent.com/Alternative_medicine/en-en/ (accessed July 20, 2013).
11. Integrative medicine - Wikipedia, the free encyclopedia, http://en.wikipedia.org/wiki/Integrative_medicine (accessed July 20, 2013).
12. Arnold S. Relman. A trip to Stonesville. Some Notes on Andrew Weil (1998). Quackwatch. The New Republic. Dec 14, 1998. Integrative medicine - Wikipedia, the free encyclopedia, http://en.wikipedia.org/wiki/Integrative_medicine (accessed July 20, 2013).
13. Alternative_medicine : definition of Alternative_medicine and .., http://dictionary.sensagent.com/Alternative_medicine/en-en/ (accessed July 20, 2013).
14. http://wiki.answers.com/Q/Who_governs_alternative_medicine#ixzz1i8kkGS005. health topic about Regulation and prevalence of homeopathy ..,

http://healcon.com/health-book/health-topic/Regulation-and-prevalence-of-homeopathy_AzV2MTWzMJZ4KmRjBQpk.htm (accessed July 20, 2013).
15. Dr. William M. London, Newsweek's Misleading Report on "Alternative Medicine." 2 Dec 2002.
www.quackwatch.com/04ConsumerEducation/newsweek.html. National Council against Health Fraud Newsletter .
16. Ernst E, Boddy K, Pittler MH, Wider B. (2006). *The desk top guide to complementary and alternative medicine.* 2nd Edition. Edinburgh; Mosby.
17. Ernst E. *"Complementary medicine: the good the bad and the ugly".* http://www.healthwatch-uk.org/awardwinners/edzardernst.html. Healthwatch Award 2005: Edzard Ernst, http://www.healthwatch-uk.org/awardwinners/edzardernst.html (accessed July 20, 2013).
18. Loprinzi CL, Levitt R, Barton DL, Sloan JA, Ahterton PJ, Smith DJ et al. *Evaluation of shark cartilage in patients with advanced cancer.* Cancer 2005; 104: 176 – 82.
19. Healthwatch Award 2005: Edzard Ernst, http://www.healthwatch-uk.org/awardwinners/edzardernst.html (accessed July 20, 2013).
20. Ibid.
21. Manheimer E, White A, Berman B, Forys K, Ernst E. *Meta-analysis: acupuncture for low back pain.* Ann Intern Med 2004; 142: 651-63.
22. Ernst E, Boddy K, Pittler MH, Wider B. (2006). *The desk top guide to complementary and alternative medicine.* 2nd Edition. Edinburgh; Mosby.
23. Gunnar B. Stickler "Alternative" medicine: a review of studies supported by grants awarded by the national centre for complementary and alternative medicine. The Scientific Review of Alternative Medicine Vol. 5, No. 4 (Fall 2001).
24. Stephen Bent, Christopher Kane, Katsuto Shinohara, John Neuhaus, Esther S. Hudes, Harley Goldberg, and Andrew L. Avins. *"Saw Palmetto for Benign Prostatic Hyperplasia".* New England Journal of Medicine. February 9th 2006. 354, p 557 – 566.
25. Edzard Ernst. *Alternative medical treatments rarely work. But the placebo effect they induce sometimes does.* Economics All Science & technology May 19th 2011 from the print edition Saturday June 4th 2011.
26. Gunnar B. Stickler "Alternative" medicine: a review of studies supported by grants awarded by the national centre for complementary and alternative medicine. The Scientific Review of Alternative Medicine Vol. 5, No. 4 (Fall 2001).
27. Lao L, Bergman S, Hamilton GR, Langenberg P, Bergman B. Evaluation of acupuncture for pain control after oral surgery: a placebo-controlled trial. *Arch Otolaryngol Head Neck Surg.* 1999;125:567–572.
28. Bergman BM, Singh BB, Lao L, et al. A randomized trial of acupuncture as an adjunctive therapy in osteoarthritis of the knee. *Rheumatology.* 1999;38:346–354.
29. Bergman BM, Lao L, Greene M, et al. Efficacy of traditional Chinese acupuncture in the treatment of symptomatic knee osteoarthritis: a pilot study. *Osteoarthritis Cartilage.* 1995;3:139–142.
30. Lao L, Bergman S, Langenberg P, Wong RH, Bergman BM. Efficacy of Chinese acupuncture on postoperative oral surgery pain. *Oral Surg Oral Med Oral Pathol Oral Radiol Endod.* 1995;79:423–428.
31. Scafidi F, Field T. Massage therapy improves behaviour in neonates born to HIV-positive mothers. *J Pediatr Psychol.* 1996;21:889–897.
32. Ahles TA, Tope DM, Pinkson B, et al. Massage therapy for patients undergoing autologous bone marrow transplantation. *J Pain Symptom Manage.* 1999;18: 157–

163.13. *"Cochrane CAM Field: Integrative Medicine".* University of Maryland Centre for Integrative Medicine (CIM). http://www.compmed.umm.edu/cochrane.asp.
33. Gregerson MB, Roberts IM, Amiri MM. Absorption and imagery locate immune responses in the body. *Biofeedback Self Regul.* 1996;21:149–165.
34. Shaffer HJ, LaSalvia TA, Stein JP. Comparing Hatha yoga with dynamic group psychotherapy for enhancing methadone maintenance treatment: a randomized clinical trial. *Alt Ther Health Med.* 1997,3:57–66.
35. Linde K, Clausius N, Ramirez G, et al. Are the clinical effects of homeopathy placebo effects? A meta-analysis of placebo-controlled trials. *Lancet.* 1997 350:834–843.
36. Kleijnen J, Knipschild P, ter Riet G. Clinical trials of homeopathy. *BMJ.* 1991;302:316–323.
37. "alternative " medicine review of studies supported by .., http://www.sram.org/media/documents/uploads/article_pdfs/5-4-05.Stickler.pdf (accessed July 20, 2013).
38. Gunnar B. Stickler "Alternative" medicine: a review of studies supported by grants awarded by the national centre for complementary and alternative medicine. The Scientific Review of Alternative Medicine Vol. 5, No. 4 (Fall 2001).
39. "ALTERNATIVE " MEDICINE REVIEW OF STUDIES SUPPORTED BY .., http://www.sram.org/media/documents/uploads/article_pdfs/5-4-05.Stickler.pdf (accessed July 20, 2013).
40. Kleijnen J, Knipschild P, ter Riet G. Clinical trials of homeopathy. *BMJ.* 1991;302:316–323. "A LTERNATIVE " MEDICINE REVIEW OF STUDIES SUPPORTED BY .., http://www.sram.org/media/documents/uploads/article_pdfs/5-4-05.Stickler.pdf (accessed July 20, 2013).
41. Sampson W. National Council against Health Fraud position paper on acupuncture. *Clin J Pain.* 1991;7(2): 162–166. "A LTERNATIVE " MEDICINE REVIEW OF STUDIES SUPPORTED BY .., http://www.sram.org/media/documents/uploads/article_pdfs/5-4-05.Stickler.pdf (accessed July 20, 2013).
42. East-West Natural Healing Centre, http://ewnaturalhealingacupuncture.com/index.php?r=news&id=11 (accessed July 20, 2013).
43. Like Curing Like: Homeopathy for Fibromyalgia and More, http://www.prohealth.com/library/showarticle.cfm?libid=11204 (accessed July 20, 2013).
44. "Increasing Awareness of the Benefits and Risks Associated with Complementary and Alternative Medicine." AMA House of Delegates. Michael C Cohen. CAMLAW: Complementary and Alternative Medicine Law Blog. The Integrator Blog. News, Reports and Networking for the .., http://theintegratorblog.com/site/index.php?option=com_content&task=view&id=119 & Itemid=173 (accessed July 20, 2013).
45. Increasing Awareness of the Benefits and Risks Associated with Complementary and Alternative Medicine. June 2006. AMA House of Delegates Resolution #306. Michael C The Integrator Blog. News, Reports and Networking for the .., http://theintegratorblog.com/site/index.php?option=com_content&task=view&id=119 &Itemid=173 (accessed July 20, 2013).

46. Gunnar B. Stickler "Alternative" medicine: a review of studies supported by grants awarded by the National Centre for Complementary and Alternative Medicine. The Scientific Review of Alternative Medicine Vol. 5, No. 4 (Fall 2001).
47. Healthwatch Award 2005: Edzard Ernst, http://www.healthwatch-uk.org/awardwinners/edzardernst.html (accessed July 20, 2013).
48. Ernst E, Canter PH. *Investigator bias and false positive findings in medical research.* Trends in Pharmacological Sci 2003; 24: 219-21. Healthwatch Award 2005: Edzard Ernst, http://www.healthwatch-uk.org/awardwinners/edzardernst.html (accessed July 20, 2013).
49. Healthwatch Award 2005: Edzard Ernst, http://www.healthwatch-uk.org/awardwinners/edzardernst.html (accessed July 20, 2013). 50. Ibid. 51. Ibid. 52. Ibid. 53. Ibid. 54. Calman K. *The profession of medicine.* BMJ 1994; 309: 1140-3.
50. Healthwatch Award 2005: Edzard Ernst, http://www.healthwatch-uk.org/awardwinners/edzardernst.html (accessed July 20, 2013).
55. Healthwatch Award 2005: Edzard Ernst, http://www.healthwatch-uk.org/awardwinners/edzardernst.html (accessed July 20, 2013).
56. Manoj Jain. Even "Snake Oil" Can Help Patients Heal. Special to The Washington Post
Tuesday, March 17, 2009; Page HE01. Even 'Snake Oil' Can Help Patients Heal - Washington Post, http://articles.washingtonpost.com/2009-03-17/news/36798688_1_alternative-medicine-heart-valve-patient (accessed July 27, 2013).
57. The Prince of Wales's Foundation for Integrated Health: *Complementary Healthcare: a guide for patients.* 2005. Healthwatch Award 2005: Edzard Ernst, http://www.healthwatch-uk.org/awardwinners/edzardernst.html (accessed July 27, 2013).
58. Smallwood C (led by). *The Role of Complementary and Alternative Medicine in the NHS. An investigation into the potential contribution of mainstream complementary therapies toHealthcare in the UK.* 2005. Healthwatch Award 2005: Edzard Ernst, http://www.healthwatch-uk.org/awardwinners/edzardernst.html (accessed July 27, 2013).
59. Ernst E, Boddy K, Pittler M H, Wider B. *The desk top guide to complementary and alternative medicine.* 2nd Edition. Edinburgh; Mosby. 2006. Healthwatch Award 2005: Edzard Ernst, http://www.healthwatch-uk.org/awardwinners/edzardernst.html (accessed July 27, 2013).
60. Edzard Ernst. *Alternative medical treatments rarely work. But the placebo effect they induce sometimes does.* Economics All Science & technology May 19th 2011 from the print edition Saturday June 4th 2011. quoteflections: Think into Health, http://quoteflections.blogspot.com/2011/05/think-into-health.html (accessed July 27, 2013).
61. Manoj Jain. Even "Snake Oil" Can Help Patients Heal. Special to The Washington Post
Tuesday, March 17, 2009; Page HE01. http://articles.washingtonpost.com/2009-03-17/news/36798688_1_alternative-medicine-heart-valve-patient (accessed July 27, 2013).
62. Chiro.Org – Providing Chiropractic Information for .., http://www.chiro.org/wordpress/?p=7182 (accessed July 27, 2013).
63. Ibid.
64. Ibid.
65. Ibid.

66. Ibid.
67. DC's Improbable Science page, http://dcscience.net/improbable.html (accessed July 27, 2013).
68. Ibid.
69. Marshall E. *The politics of alternative medicine.* Science. Vol. 265 No. 5181. 30 September, 1994. P 2000-2002. *DOI: 10.1126/science.8091220.* Posted on December 10, 2002.
70. Wallace I. Sampson, M.D. *Why the National Centre for Complementary and Alternative Medicine (NCCAM) Should Be Defunded.* Editor of the Scientific Review of Alternative Medicine and Emeritus Clinical Professor of Medicine at Stanford University. nccamwatch.org/index.html Why the National Centre for Complementary and Alternative ..,
http://www.quackwatch.com/01QuackeryRelatedTopics/nccam.html (accessed July 27, 2013).
71. Green, S. *Stated goals and grants of the Office of Alternative Medicine/National Centre for Complementary and Alternative Medicine Policy.* 2001SRAM 5:205-207.
72. *"$2.5 billion spent, no alternative cures found – Alternative medicine-msnbc.com".* MSNBC. June 10, 2009. http://www.msnbc.msn.com/id/31190909/ Why the National Centre for Complementary and Alternative ..,
http://www.quackwatch.com/01QuackeryRelatedTopics/nccam.html (accessed July 27, 2013).
73. *"NCCAM Funding: Appropriations History".* NCCAM. 2008-01-09. Archived from the original on 2009-06-11.
http://nccam.nih.gov/about/budget/appropriations.htm. Retrieved 2008-04-02.
74. Atwood, Kimball C. (2003-09*). "The Ongoing Problem with the National Centre for Complementary and Alternative Medicine". Skeptical Inquirer.*
http://www.csicop.org/si/ show/ongoing problem with the national centre. Retrieved 2009-11-18.
75. *Scientists Speak Out Against Federal Funds for Research on Alternative Medicine* – washingtonpost.com
76. Wallace I. Sampson, M.D. *Why the National Centre for Complementary and Alternative Medicine (NCCAM) Should Be Defunded.* Editor of the Scientific Review of Alternative Medicine and Emeritus Clinical Professor of Medicine at Stanford University. nccamwatch.org/index.html
77. Why the National Centre for Complementary and Alternative ..,
http://www.quackwatch.com/01QuackeryRelatedTopics/nccam.html (accessed July 27, 2013).
78. Ibid.
79. Koes, B. W. and others. *Spinal manipulation for low back pain: An updated systematic review of randomized clinical trials.* Spine 1996. 21:2860-2873.
80.Why the National Centre for Complementary and Alternative ..,
http://www.quackwatch.com/01QuackeryRelatedTopics/nccam.html (accessed July 27, 2013).
81. Ibid.
82. Ibid.
83. Ibid.
84. Ibid.
85. Ibid.

86. A Statement in Defense of Scientific Medicine from the .., http://www.quackwatch.org/04ConsumerEducation/sram.html (accessed July 27, 2013).
87. Ibid.
88. Ibid.
89. Wallace I. Sampson, M.D. *Why the National Centre for Complementary and Alternative Medicine (NCCAM) Should Be Defunded.* Editor of the Scientific Review of Alternative Medicine and Emeritus Clinical Professor of Medicine at Stanford University. nccamwatch.org/index.html
90. David Brown. Washington Post Staff Writer. Scientists Speak Out Against Federal Funds for Research on Alternative Medicine. Critics Object to 'Pseudoscience' Centre washingtonpost.com > Health Tuesday, March 17, 2009
91 Genomics, Medicine, and Pseudoscience: Washington Post shines .., http://genome.fieldofscience.com/2009/03/washington-post-shines-light-on-waste.html (accessed July 27, 2013).
92. Genomics, Medicine, and Pseudoscience: Washington Post shines .., http://genome.fieldofscience.com/2009/03/washington-post-shines-light-on-waste.html (accessed July 27, 2013).
93. Ibid.
94. Steven Novella, Yale School of Medicine. Editor of the Web site Science-Based Medicine (http://www.sciencebasedmedicine.org) ACHS.edu Holistic Health Education, http://achsedu-natural-health-education.blogspot.com/ (accessed July 27, 2013).
95. ACHS.edu Holistic Health Education, http://achsedu-natural-health-education.blogspot.com/ (accessed July 27, 2013).
96. Ibid.
97. Ibid.
98. Ibid.
99. Ibid.
100. The quack page, http://www.ucl.ac.uk/pharmacology/dc-bits-old/quack4.html (accessed July 27, 2013).
101. Letter from Professor Baum and other scientists to NHS Trusts .., http://www.senseaboutscience.org/pages/letter-from-professor-baum-and-other-scientists-to-nhs-trusts.html (accessed July 27, 2013).
102. British Professors Attack Homeopathy - Homeowatch, http://www.homeowatch.org/news/baum.html (accessed July 27, 2013).
103. Skeptical News - North Texas Skeptics | Helping people make .., http://www.ntskeptics.org/news/news2006-05-26.htm (accessed July 27, 2013).
104. SOCIALIZED MEDICINE: May 2006, http://socglory.blogspot.com/2006_05_01_archive.html (accessed July 27, 2013).
105. Skeptical News - North Texas Skeptics | Helping people make .., http://www.ntskeptics.org/news/news2006-05-26.htm (accessed July 27, 2013).
106. Ibid.
107. Ibid.
108. Ibid.
109. The quack page, http://www.ucl.ac.uk/pharmacology/dc-bits-old/quack4.html (accessed July 27, 2013).
110. Ibid.
111. Ibid.
112. Ibid.

113. Ibid.
114. BBC NEWS | Health | Fears over homeopathy regulation, http://news.bbc.co.uk/2/hi/health/5303080.stm (accessed July 27, 2013).
115. Ibid.
116. Austin Elliott. *Physiology News.* Editorial No. 65. PN 3. Winter 2006. www.physoc.org
117. BBC NEWS | Health | Fears over homeopathy regulation, http://news.bbc.co.uk/2/hi/health/5303080.stm (accessed July 27, 2013).
118. Ibid.
119. Ibid.
120. Ibid.
121. Ibid.
122. Ibid.
123. The Independent, 30 June, 2005. The quack page - UCL - London's Global University, http://www.ucl.ac.uk/pharmacology/dc-bits-old/quack-01-06-07.html (accessed July 27, 2013).
124. The quack page - UCL - London's Global University, http://www.ucl.ac.uk/pharmacology/dc-bits-old/quack-01-06-07.html (accessed July 27, 2013).
125. Ibid.
126. Ibid.
127. Ibid.
128. Ibid.
129. Ibid.
130. Ibid.
131. Thomas Sutcliffe: Respect is not a right: it has to be earned .., http://www.independent.co.uk/voices/columnists/thomas-sutcliffe/thomas-sutcliffe-respect-is-not-a-right-it-has-to-be-earned-437121.html (accessed July 27, 2013).
132. Ibid.
133. BBC NEWS | Health | Scientists attack homeopathy move, http://news.bbc.co.uk/2/hi/health/6085242.stm (accessed July 27, 2013).
134. Ibid.
135. Frances Blunden. *Drugs watchdog fails public.* Which? October 2006. pages 24-25. ebm-first - MHRA licensing, http://www.ebm-first.com/homeopathy/mhra-licensing.html (accessed July 27, 2013).
136. Austin Elliott. *"Homeopathic mumbo-jumbo".* The Physiological Society's Newsletter for December 2006. ebm-first - MHRA licensing, http://www.ebm-first.com/homeopathy/mhra-licensing.html (accessed July 27, 2013).
137. ebm-first - MHRA licensing, http://www.ebm-first.com/homeopathy/mhra-licensing.html (accessed July 27, 2013).
138. BBC NEWS | Health | Scientists attack homeopathy move, http://news.bbc.co.uk/2/hi/health/6085242.stm (accessed July 27, 2013).
139. ebm-first - MHRA licensing, http://www.ebm-first.com/homeopathy/mhra-licensing.html (accessed July 27, 2013).
140. Position homeopathic regulation - Healthwatch - for treatment .., http://www.healthwatch-uk.org/Position%20homeopathic%20regulation.pdf (accessed July 27, 2013). 141. The quack page - UCL - London's Global University, http://www.ucl.ac.uk/pharmacology/dc-bits-old/quack-01-06-07.html (accessed July 27, 2013).
142. Ibid.

143. Alonso D, Lazarus MC, Baumann L., *Effects of topical arnica gel on post-laser treatment bruises. Dermatol Surg.* 2002 Aug;28(8):686-8. The quack page - UCL - London's Global University, http://www.ucl.ac.uk/pharmacology/dc-bits-old/quack-01-06-07.html (accessed July 27, 2013).
144. Knuesel O, Weber M, Suter A. *Arnica montana gel in osteoarthritis of the knee: an open, multicenter clinical trial. Adv Ther.* 2002 Sep-Oct;19(5):209-18.) The quack page - UCL - London's Global University, http://www.ucl.ac.uk/pharmacology/dc-bits-old/quack-01-06-07.html (accessed July 27, 2013).
145. Hart O, Mullee MA, Lewith G, Miller J. Double-blind, placebo-controlled, randomized clinical trial of homeopathic arnica C30 for pain and infection after total abdominal hysterectomy. *Journal of the Royal Society of Medicine* 1997; 90: 73-78.
146. The quack page - UCL - London's Global University, http://www.ucl.ac.uk/pharmacology/dc-bits-old/quack-01-06-07.html (accessed July 27, 2013).
147. Ibid.
148. BBC NEWS | Health | Scientists attack homeopathy move, http://news.bbc.co.uk/2/hi/health/6085242.stm (accessed July 27, 2013).
149. ebm-first - MHRA licensing, http://www.ebm-first.com/homeopathy/mhra-licensing.html (accessed July 27, 2013).
150. The quack page - UCL - London's Global University, http://www.ucl.ac.uk/pharmacology/dc-bits-old/quack-01-06-07.html (accessed July 27, 2013).
151. Ibid.
152. Medicines for Human Use (National Rules for Homeopathic .., http://www.theyworkforyou.com/lords/?id=2006-10-26b.1327.3 (accessed July 27, 2013).
153. Ibid.
154. Ibid.
155. Ibid.
156. Nelsons Coldenza™ - Nelsons UK, http://www.nelsonsnaturalworld.com/uk/our-brands/nelsons-homeopathy/nelsons-combination-remedies/coldenza/ (accessed July 27, 2013).
157. Ibid.
158. BBC Expose of GlaxoSmithKline's Marketing of Seroxat (Paxil .., http://www.yoism.org/?q=node/293 (accessed July 27, 2013).
159. *Drugs watchdog fails public.* Which? (October 2006, pages 24-25). GM Rice Contamination How Regulators Tried to Sidestep the Law, http://www.i-sis.org.uk/GMRiceContaminationUK.php (accessed July 27, 2013).
160. Medicines for Human Use (National Rules for Homeopathic .., http://www.theyworkforyou.com/lords/?id=2006-10-26b.1327.3 (accessed July 27, 2013).
161. What we regulate: MHRA - Medicines and Healthcare products .., http://www.mhra.gov.uk/Aboutus/Whatweregulate/index.htm (accessed July 27, 2013).
162. Ibid.
163. Ibid.
164. Ibid.
165. Tuesday1st Correspondence with the MHRA .Patient .., http://tuesday1st-mhra-ppes-correspondence.blogspot.com/ (accessed July 27, 2013).

166. The quack page - UCL - London's Global University, http://www.ucl.ac.uk/pharmacology/dc-bits-old/quack-01-06-07.html (accessed July 27, 2013).
167. Ibid.
168. Ibid.
169. Ibid.
170. Ibid.
171. Ibid.
172. Wager E (2007) Authors, *Ghosts*, Damned Lies, and Statisticians. PLoS Med 4(1): e34. doi:10.1371/journal.pmed.
173. Andrew Vickers PhD (2004). *"Alternative Cancer Cures: "Unproven" or "Disproven"?" CA Cancer J Clin* 54 (2): 110–118. doi:10.3322/canjclin.54.2.110. PMID 15061600. http://caonline.amcancersoc.org/cgi/content/full/54/2/110.
174. Manoj Jain. Alternative Medicine Even 'Snake Oil' Can Help Patients Heal. Health in the News -- And Your Life. Special to The Washington Post. washingtonpost.com > HealthTuesday, March 17, 2009; Page HE01.
175. Dominic Hughes (23 December 2010*). "Alternative remedies 'dangerous' for kids says report"*. BBC News. http://www.bbc.co.uk/news/health-12060507. BBC News - Alternative remedies 'dangerous' for kids says report, http://www.bbc.co.uk/news/health-12060507 (accessed July 27, 2013).
176. BBC News - Alternative remedies "dangerous" for kids says report, http://www.bbc.co.uk/news/health-12060507 (accessed July 27, 2013).
177. Ibid.
178. Ibid.
179. Ibid.
180. Ibid.
181. Ibid.
182. Chiropractic: The Greatest Hoax of the Century? http://www.chirobase.org/05RB/hoax.html (accessed July 27, 2013).
183. Ibid.
184. L.A. Chotkowski. Chiropractic the greatest hoax of the Century? New England Novelty Books (1998-12-31). ISBN: 0965785513 ISBN-13: 9780965785518
185. Ibid.
186. BBC News - Alternative remedies 'dangerous' for kids says report, http://www.bbc.co.uk/news/health-12060507 (accessed July 27, 2013).
187. Ibid.
188. Manoj Jain. Alternative Medicine Even 'Snake Oil' Can Help Patients Heal. Health in the News -- And Your Life. Special to The Washington Post. washingtonpost.com > HealthTuesday, March 17, 2009; Page HE01
189. Weber DO (1998). *"Complementary and alternative medicine. Considering the alternatives". Physician Executive* 24 (6): 6–14. PMID 10351720. Alternative medicine - Wikipedia, the free encyclopedia, http://en.wikipedia.org/?search=NATURAL%20REMEDIES (accessed July 27, 2013).
190. Beyerstein BL (1999). *"Psychology and 'Alternative Medicine' Social and Judgmental Biases That Make Inert Treatments Seem to Work". The Scientific Review of Alternative Medicine* 3 (2).
191. Beyerstein BL (March 2001). *"Alternative medicine and common errors of reasoning". Academic Medicine* 76 (3): 230–7. doi:10.1097/00001888-200103000-00009. PMID 11242572

192. Alternative medicine - Wikipedia, the free encyclopedia, http://en.wikipedia.org/?search=NATURAL%20REMEDIES (accessed July 27, 2013).
193. Beyerstein B. L. (March 2001). Ibid. Alternative medicine - Wikipedia, the free encyclopedia, http://en.wikipedia.org/?search=NATURAL%20REMEDIES (accessed July 27, 2013).
194. Alternative medicine - Wikipedia, the free encyclopedia, http://en.wikipedia.org/?search=NATURAL%20REMEDIES (accessed July 27, 2013).
195. Barnes P. M., Powell-Griner E., McFann K., Nahin R. L. (May 2004). *"Complementary and alternative medicine use among adults: United States, 2002". Advance Data* (343): 1–19. PMID 15188733.
http://www.cdc.gov/nchs/data/ad/ad343.pdf.
196. Weber DO (1998). *"Complementary and alternative medicine. Considering the alternatives". Physician Executive* 24 (6): 6–14. PMID 10351720
197. Complementary and alternative medicine - The Full Wiki, http://www.thefullwiki.org/Complementary_and_alternative_medicine (accessed July 27, 2013).
198. *"Complementary therapies: The big con? – The Independent"*. London. 2008-04-22. http://www.independent.co.uk/life-style/health-and-wellbeing/features/complementary-therapies-the-big-con-813248.html. Retrieved 2010-04-23.
199. "K. Schmidt and E. Ernst. *Assessing websites on complementary and alternative medicine for cancer."* Annals of Oncology number 15, pp 733-742, 2004, http://annonc.oupjournals.org/cgi/content/full/15/5/733
200. Health On the Net Foundation. University Hospital in Geneva. 24 Micheli-du-Crest. 1211 Geneva 14. Switzerland. Email:honsecretariat@healthonnet.org
201. The quack page - UCL - London's Global University, http://www.ucl.ac.uk/Pharmacology/dc-bits/quack4.html (accessed July 27, 2013).
202. Ibid.
203. David Colquhoun, Professor of Pharmacology at University College London. http://dcscience.net/.
204. The quack page - UCL - London's Global University, http://www.ucl.ac.uk/Pharmacology/dc-bits/quack4.html (accessed July 27, 2013).
205. Ibid.
206. Ibid.
207. Ibid.
208. David Colquhoun, Professor of Pharmacology at University College London. http://dcscience.net/.
209. British Medical Journal (2007), 337, 508 – 509. The quack page - UCL - London's Global University, http://www.ucl.ac.uk/Pharmacology/dc-bits/quack4.html (accessed July 27, 2013).210. The quack page - UCL - London's Global University, http://www.ucl.ac.uk/Pharmacology/dc-bits/quack4.html (accessed July 27, 2013).211. Ibid.
212. Ibid.
213. Gerald Weissmann, Editor-in-chief. Feder ation of American Societies for Experimental Biology (FASEB) journal. *The FASEB Journal* 2006;20:1755-1758.
214. Homeopathy deconstructed in the FASEB Journal – Respectful .., http://scienceblogs.com/insolence/2009/10/15/homeopathy-deconstructed-in-the-faseb-jo-1/ (accessed July 27, 2013).

215. Holmes, O. W. (1892) Preface to "Homeopathy and its Kindred Delusions." *Medical Essays, vol. X of The Standard Edition of The Works of Oliver Wendell Holmes* ,xiii Houghton Mifflin Boston.
216. Holmes, Medical Essays ,319 Quoted by Gerald Weissmann. "Homeopathy: Holmes, Hogwarts, and the Prince of Wales". Editor-in-Chief. *The FASEB Journal.* 2006;20:1755-1758. The quack page - UCL - London's Global University, http://www.ucl.ac.uk/pharmacology/dc-bits-old/quack-01-06-07.html (accessed July 27, 2013).
217. About - Cochrane CAM Field: Integrative Medicine: University .., http://www.compmed.umm.edu/cochrane_about.asp (accessed July 27, 2013).
218. Ibid.
219. Ibid.
220. Ibid.
221. Topic list for Cochrane Complementary Medicine Field related .., http://www.cochrane.org/news/blog/topic-list-cochrane-complementary-medicine-field-related-reviews-cochraneorg (accessed July 27, 2013).
222. About - Cochrane CAM Field: Integrative Medicine: University .., http://www.compmed.umm.edu/cochrane_about.asp (accessed July 27, 2013).
223. Ibid.
224. Ibid.
225. Ibid.
226. Ibid.
227. Ibid.
228. Ibid.
229. Times Higher Education Supplement 6th April 2007 Credible endeavour or pseudoscience? David Colquhoun and Brian Isbell. Published: 06 April 2007.
230. DC's Improbable Science page, http://dcscience.net/improbable.html (accessed July 27, 2013).
231. The quack page - UCL – London's Global University, http://www.ucl.ac.uk/pharmacology/dc-bits-old/quack-01-06-07.html (accessed July 27, 2013).
232. Ibid.
233. Ibid.
234. Ibid.
235. Ibid.
236. Ibid.
237. Ibid.
238. Ibid.
239. Ibid.
240. Ibid.
241. Ibid.
242. Ibid.
243. Ibid.
244. Ibid.
245. Ibid.
246. Ibid.
247. Ibid.
248. Ibid.
249. Ibid.
250. Ibid.

251. Ibid.
252. Ibid.
253. University of Maryland – Centre for Integrative Medicine, http://www.greencareersguide.com/university-of-maryland-centre-forintegrative-medicine.html (accessed July 27, 2013).
254. The quack page - UCL - London's Global University, http://www.ucl.ac.uk/pharmacology/dc-bits-old/quack-01-06-07.html (accessed July 27, 2013).
255. Ibid.
256. Ibid.
257. Ibid.
258. Ibid.
259. Ibid.
260. Ibid.
261. Gerald Weissmann. "Homeopathy: Holmes, Hogwarts, and the Prince of Wales". Editor-in-Chief. *The FASEB Journal.* 2006;20:1755-1758. Homeopathy: Holmes, Hogwarts, and the Prince of Wales, http://www.fasebj.org/content/20/11/1755.full (accessed July 27, 2013).
262. Lewis, E. (2005) *Dana Ullman: Treating Children with Homeopathic Medicines* Hpathy Ezinehttp://www.hpathy.com/interviews/danaullman.asp. Accessed July 2006.
263. Penguin Group USA () *About Dana Ullman* http://us.penguingroup.com/nf/Author/AuthorPage/0,,1000040566,00.html. Accessed July 2006. Homeopathy: Holmes, Hogwarts, and the Prince of Wales, http://www.fasebj.org/content/20/11/1755.full (accessed July 27, 2013).
264. Garsombe, K. (Posted October 29, 2001) *Alternative Remedies for Anthrax* Alternet.org. http://www.alternet.org/envirohealth/11814. Accessed July 2006. Homeopathy: Holmes, Hogwarts, and the Prince of Wales, http://www.fasebj.org/content/20/11/1755.full (accessed July 27, 2013).
265. Homeopathy: Holmes, Hogwarts, and the Prince of Wales, http://www.fasebj.org/content/20/11/1755.full (accessed July 27, 2013).
266. Ibid.
267. Integrative Therapies Program for Children with Cancer () About Us. http://www.integrativetherapiesprogram.org/about/staff.php. Accessed July 2006
268. Homeopathy: Holmes, Hogwarts, and the Prince of Wales, http://www.fasebj.org/content/20/11/1755.full (accessed July 27, 2013).
269. Harvard Medical School Osher Institute () http://www.osher.hms.harvard.edu/. Accessed July 2006
270. Rosenthal Centre for Complementary and Alternative Medicine (2003) http://www.rosenthal.hs.columbia.edu/Anniversary_awards.html. Accessed July 2006
271. The quack page - UCL - London's Global University, http://www.ucl.ac.uk/pharmacology/dc-bits-old/quack-01-06-07.html (accessed July 27, 2013).
272. Ibid.
273. Ibid.
274. Ibid.
275. Ibid.
276. Dr. Manoj Jain: Alternative care isn't safe as a substitute .., http://www.commercialappeal.com/news/2009/jun/22/alternative-care-isnt-safe-as-a-substitute/ (accessed July 27, 2013).

277. Barry L. Beyerstein. Alternative Medicine and Common Errors of Reasoning. Social and Judgmental Biases That Make Inert Treatments Seem to Work. Academic Medicine: March 2001 - Volume 76 - Issue 3 - p 230-237. Alternative medicine and common errors of reasoning, http://www.ncbi.nlm.nih.gov/pubmed/11242572 (accessed July 27, 2013).
278. Alternative medicine and common errors of reasoning, http://www.ncbi.nlm.nih.gov/pubmed/11242572 (accessed July 27, 2013).
279. Ibid.
280. Barry L. Beyerstein Why Bogus Therapies Seem to Work. Quackwatch. Committee for Scientific Investigation of Claims of the Paranormal's Skeptical Enquirer. Volume 21.5, September / October 1997. Posted on July 24, 2003.
281. Why Bogus Therapies Seem to Work - CSI, http://www.csicop.org/si/show/why_bogus_therapies_seem_to_work/ (accessed July 27, 2013).
282. Ibid.
283. Beyerstein, B., and W. Sampson. 1996. Traditional medicine and pseudoscience in China. Skeptical Inquirer 20(4): 18-26.
284. Kiernan, V. 1995. Survey plumbs the depths of international ignorance. The New Scientist (April 29): 7.
285. Basil, R., ed. 1988. Not Necessarily the New Age. Amherst, N.Y.: Prometheus Books.
286. Gross, P., and N. Levitt. 1994. Higher Superstition. Baltimore: Johns Hopkins University Press.
287. Why Bogus Therapies Seem to Work - CSI, http://www.csicop.org/si/show/why_bogus_therapies_seem_to_work/ (accessed July 27, 2013).
288. Ibid.
289. Ibid.
290. Ibid.
291. Roberts, A., D. Kewman, and L. Hovell. 1993. The power of nonspecific effects in healing: Implications for psychosocial and biological treatments. Clinical Psychology Review 13: 375-91.
292. Ulett, G. A. 1996. Alternative Medicine or Magical Healing. St. Louis: Warren H. Green.
293. Stewart, D. 1990. Emotional disorders misdiagnosed as physical illness: Environmental hypersensitivity, candidiasis hypersensitivity, and chronic fatigue syndrome. Int. J. Mental Health 19(3): 56-68.
294. Huber, P. 1991. Galileo's Revenge: Junk Science in the Courtroom. New York: Basic Books.
295. Rosenbaum, J. T. 1997. Lessons from litigation over silicone breast implants: A call for activism by scientists. Science 276 (June 6, 1997): 1524-5.
296. Why Bogus Therapies Seem to Work - CSI, http://www.csicop.org/si/show/why_bogus_therapies_seem_to_work/ (accessed July 27, 2013).
297. Beyerstein, B., and P. Hadaway. 1991. On avoiding folly. Journal of Drug Issues 20(4): 689-700.
298. Why Bogus Therapies Seem to Work - CSI, http://www.csicop.org/si/show/why_bogus_therapies_seem_to_work/ (accessed July 27, 2013).

299. Dean, G., I. Kelly, D. Saklofske, and A. Furnham. 1992. Graphology and human judgement. In The Write Stuff, edited by B. and D. Beyerstein. Amherst, N.Y.: Prometheus Books, 342-96.
300. Why Bogus Therapies Seem to Work - CSI, http://www.csicop.org/si/show/why_bogus_therapies_seem_to_work/ (accessed July 27, 2013).
301. Ibid.
302. Ibid.
303. Ibid.
304. Ibid.
305. James Williamson. Scientific Conclusion: Prayer Doesn't Work – Part 1 Orlando Freethinkers & Humanists. www.floridafreethinkers.com/.../scientific-conclusion-prayer-doesnt- How about a prayer? - Yahoo! Answers, http://answers.yahoo.com/question/index?qid=1006022204397 (accessed July 27, 2013).
306. How about a prayer? - Yahoo! Answers, http://answers.yahoo.com/question/index?qid=1006022204397 (accessed July 27, 2013).
307. commonsenseatheism.com, http://commonsenseatheism.com/wp-content/uploads/2010/02/Tessman-vs.-Harris.doc (accessed July 27, 2013).
308. Ibid.
309. How about a prayer? - Yahoo! Answers, http://answers.yahoo.com/question/index?qid=1006022204397 (accessed July 27, 2013).
310. James Williamson. Scientific Conclusion: Prayer Doesn't Work – Part 1. Orlando Freethinkers & Humanists. www.floridafreethinkers.com/.../scientific-conclusion-prayer-doesnt-. How about a prayer? - Yahoo! Answers, http://answers.yahoo.com/question/index?qid=1006022204397 (accessed July 27, 2013).
311. How about a prayer? - Yahoo! Answers, http://answers.yahoo.com/question/index?qid=1006022204397 (accessed July 27, 2013).
312. Ibid.
313. Ibid.
314. Ibid.
315. Randolph Byrd. "Positive Therapeutic Effects of Intercessory Prayer in a Coronary Care Unit Population." Southern Medical Journal. 1988 Jul; 81(7): 826-9. Webglimpse Search Results, http://www.quackwatch.com/search/webglimpse.cgi?ID=1&query=prayer (accessed July 27, 2013).
316. Harris Prayer Study - Gary Posner's Home Page, http://www.gpposner.com/Harris_study.html (accessed July 27, 2013).
317. Ibid.
318. Ibid.
319. Ibid.
320. Posner GP. God in the CCU? *Free Inquiry*. 1990;10 (2):44–45.
321. Witmer J, Zimmerman M. Intercessory prayer as medical treatment? An inquiry. *Skeptical Inquirer*. 1991;15(2): 177–180.
322. Sloan RP, Bagiella E, Powell T. Religion, spirituality, and medicine. *Lancet*. 1999;353:664–667.

323. Tessman I, Tessman J. Efficacy of prayer. *Skeptical Inquirer*. 2000;24(2): 31–33.
324. How about a prayer? - Yahoo! Answers, http://answers.yahoo.com/question/index?qid=1006022204397 (accessed July 27, 2013).
325. Ibid.
326. Positive Therapeutic Effects of Intercessory Prayer in a .., http://www.godandscience.org/apologetics/smj4.html (accessed July 27, 2013).
327. William S. Harris, Manohar Gowda, Jerry W. Kolb, Christopher P. Strychacz, James L. Vacek, Philip G.Jones, Alan Forker, James H. O'Keefe, Ben D. McCallister. A Randomized, Controlled Trial of the Effects of Remote, Intercessory Prayer on Outcomes in Patients Admitted to the Coronary Care Unit. Archives of Internal Medicine. 1999. 159 p 2273-2278. JAMA Network | JAMA Internal Medicine | A Randomized .., http://archinte.jamanetwork.com/article.aspx?articleid=485161 (accessed July 27, 2013).
328. Stai Essay Examples by Mightystudents.com, http://www.mightystudents.com/tag/stai (accessed July 27, 2013).
329. JAMA Network | JAMA Internal Medicine | A Randomized .., http://archinte.jamanetwork.com/article.aspx?articleid=485161 (accessed July 27, 2013).
330. Ibid.
331. http://www.csicop.org/articles/20010810-prayer/ Transcript of the March 13th, 2001, Debate Between William Harris, PhD, Saint Luke's Hospital, Kansas City, MO, and Irwin Tessman, PhD, Purdue University, West Lafayette.
332. Witmer J, Zimmerman M. Intercessory prayer as medical treatment? An inquiry. Skeptical Inquirer 15:177-180, 1991. Webglimpse Search Results, http://www.quackwatch.com/search/webglimpse.cgi?ID=1&query=prayer (accessed July 27, 2013).
333. Randolph Byrd. "Positive Therapeutic Effects of Intercessory Prayer in a Coronary Care Unit Population." Southern Medical Journal. 1988 Jul; 81(7): 826-9
334. Tessman I, Tessman J. Efficacy of prayer. *Skeptical Inquirer*. 2000;24(2): 31–33.
335. Dossey L. *Healing Words*. New York, NY: Harper-Collins; 1993: xv.
336. Webglimpse Search Results, http://www.quackwatch.com/search/webglimpse.cgi?ID=1&query=prayer (accessed July 27, 2013).
337. O'Laoire S. An experimental study of the effects of distant, intercessory prayer on self-esteem, anxiety, and depression. Alternative Therapies in Health & Medicine 3(6):38-53, 1997.
338. Walker SR and others. Intercessory prayer in the treatment of alcohol abuse and dependence: A pilot intervention. Alternative Therapies in Health & Medicine 3(6):79-86, 1997.
339. Aviles JM and others. Intercessory prayer and cardiovascular disease progression in a coronary care unit population: A randomized controlled trial. Mayo Clinic Proceedings 26:1192-19198, 2001.
340. Stephen Barrett. Quackwatch. Some Thoughts about Faith Healing. Revised on December 27, 2009. www.quackwatch.com/01QuackeryRelatedTopics/faith.html
341. Passover in pictures – CNN Belief Blog - CNN.com Blogs, http://religion.blogs.cnn.com/2012/04/06/passover-in-pictures/ (accessed July 27, 2013).

342. James Williamson. Scientific Conclusion: Prayer Doesn't Work – Part 2 Orlando Freethinkers & Humanists. www.floridafreethinkers.com/.../scientific-conclusion-prayer-doesnt-
343. Faith Healing - Quackwatch, http://www.quackwatch.org/dantest/faith.html (accessed July 27, 2013).
344. Some Thoughts about 'Faith Healing' - The Skeptic Tank .., http://www.skeptictank.org/heal1.htm (accessed July 27, 2013).
345. Webglimpse Search Results, http://www.quackwatch.com/search/webglimpse.cgi?ID=1&query=prayer (accessed July 27, 2013).
346. Ibid.
347. Ibid.
348. Ibid.
349. Ibid.
350. Ibid.
351. Some Thoughts about 'Faith Healing' - The Skeptic Tank .., http://www.skeptictank.org/heal1.htm (accessed July 27, 2013).
352. Faith Healing - Quackwatch, http://www.quackwatch.org/dantest/faith.html (accessed July 27, 2013).
353. Some Thoughts about Faith Healing -- Stephen Barrett, M.D, http://www.skeptictank.org/fhealrp.htm (accessed July 27, 2013).
354. Some Thoughts about Faith Healing -- Stephen Barrett, M.D, http://www.skeptictank.org/fhealrp.htm (accessed July 27, 2013).
355. Asser S, Swan R. Child fatalities from religion-motivated medical neglect. Pediatrics 101:625-629, 1998.
356. McNichol T. The new faith in medicine. USA Today, April 7, 1996, p 4.
357. Sloan RP, Bagiella E, Powell T. Religion, spirituality and medicine. Lancet 353:664-667, 1999. Webglimpse Search Results, http://www.quackwatch.com/search/webglimpse.cgi?ID=1&query=prayer (accessed July 27, 2013)..
358. Ibid.
359. King M, Speck P, Thomas A. The effect of spiritual beliefs on outcome from illness. Social Science & Medicine 48:1291-1299, 1999. Webglimpse Search Results, http://www.quackwatch.com/search/webglimpse.cgi?ID=1&query=prayer (accessed July 27, 2013).
360. Stephen Barrett. Quackwatch. Some Thoughts about Faith Healing. Revised on December 27, 2009. This article was revised on December 27, 2009. www.quackwatch.com/01QuackeryRelatedTopics/faith.html. Webglimpse Search Results, http://www.quackwatch.com/search/webglimpse.cgi?ID=1&query=prayer (accessed July 27, 2013).
361. Some Thoughts about Faith Healing -- Stephen Barrett, M.D, http://www.skeptictank.org/fhealrp.htm (accessed July 27, 2013).
362. Rose L. Faith Healing. Baltimore: Penguin Books, 1971. Some Thoughts about Faith Healing -- Stephen Barrett, M.D, http://www.skeptictank.org/fhealrp.htm (accessed July 27, 2013).
363. Some Thoughts about 'Faith Healing' - The Skeptic Tank .., http://www.skeptictank.org/heal1.htm (accessed July 27, 2013).
364. Ibid.
365. Ibid.

366. Nolen W. Healing: A Doctor in Search of a Miracle. New York, 1974, Random House Inc.
367. Some Thoughts about `Faith Healing' - The Skeptic Tank .., http://www.skeptictank.org/heal1.htm (accessed July 27, 2013).
368. Ibid.
369. Ibid.
370. Emery CE. Are they really cured? Providence Sunday Journal Magazine, Jan 15, 1989.. Some Thoughts about `Faith Healing' - The Skeptic Tank .., http://www.skeptictank.org/heal1.htm (accessed July 27, 2013). 371. Randi J. The Faith Healers. Amherst, N.Y.: Prometheus Books,1987.
372. Some Thoughts about `Faith Healing' - The Skeptic Tank .., http://www.skeptictank.org/heal1.htm (accessed July 27, 2013).
373. "A Profitable Prophet". Inside Edition. February 27, 2007. http://www.insideedition.com/ourstories/reports/story.aspx?storyid=639. Retrieved May 7, 2007.
374. Some Thoughts about `Faith Healing' - The Skeptic Tank .., http://www.skeptictank.org/heal1.htm (accessed July 27, 2013).
375 Some Thoughts about Faith Healing -- Stephen Barrett, M.D, http://www.skeptictank.org/fhealrp.htm (accessed July 27, 2013).

CHAPTER FOUR - QUACKERY - HOMEOPATHY

The same David Colquhoun,[1] mentioned previously, published the following lines originally from Bishop William Croswell Doane (1832–1913), first Episcopal bishop of Albany (NY).

> Stir the mixture well
> Lest it prove inferior,
> Then put half a drop
> Into Lake Superior.
>
> Every other day
> Take a drop in water,
> You'll be better soon
> Or at least you oughter!

"Exaggerated claims for the efficacy of a medicament are very seldom the consequence of any intention to deceive; they are usually the outcome of a kindly conspiracy in which everybody has the very best intentions. The patient wants to get well, his physician wants to have made him better, and the pharmaceutical company would have liked to have put it into the physician's power to have made him so. The controlled clinical trial is an attempt to avoid being taken in by this conspiracy of good will."[2]

Homeopathy may be effective because of "regression to the mean". Ben Goldacre[3] explains this beautifully. Many illnesses have what is called a "natural history": they are bad, and then they get better. He quotes Voltaire as saying "'the art of medicine consists in amusing the patient while nature cures the disease." When one recovers from an illness one naturally assumes that whatever treatment one took must be the reason for one's recovery. Credit may be given to a homeopathic remedy, antibiotics, change of circumstances or a number of things whereas it is really due to "regression to the mean".

<u>History of homeopathy</u>

Samuel Hahnemann a German physician was the founder of homeopathy. He published his first paper in 1796. The basic doctrine of homeopathy is that "like cures like." The correct medicine for any disease would therefore be the one capable of producing similar symptoms to those of the disease itself. The efficacy of the substance, according to Hahnemann's theory, also depended on its concentration being reduced to an infinitesimal degree by means of multiple dilutions.

Oliver Wendell Holmes[4] described Hahnemann's method of dilution in detail but it is of interest and a fact not very well known that "sugar of milk", presumably lactose, and alcohol were both used in the original preparations. The dilution of the substance is accompanied by shaking in a very precise manner. According to Hahnemann's own words "A long experience and multiplied observations upon the sick lead me within the last few years to prefer giving only two shakes to medicinal liquids, whereas I formerly used to give ten."

The dilution of the original millionth of a grain of the substance is carried successively to the billionth, trillionth, quadrillionth, quintillionth, and very often much higher fractional divisions. At every successive dilution of the fluid ninety-nine hundredths is cast aside. After all these dilutions it is no wonder that no trace of the actual original substance can be found. Indeed, homeopathy is sometimes described as "the medicine that contains no medicine".

Selling pills that contain nothing whatsoever but sugar as medicines is not just delusional, it's fraud. Most homeopathic solutions contain nothing at all. They are diluted sometimes several million times. Oscillococcinum, a homeopathic product "for the relief of colds and flu-like symptoms," involves dilutions that are even more far-fetched. Its "active ingredient" is prepared by incubating small amounts of a freshly killed duck's liver and heart for 40 days.[5]

Were a single molecule of the duck's heart or liver to survive the dilution, its concentration would be 100^{200}. This huge number, which has 400 zeroes, is vastly greater than the estimated number of molecules in the universe (about one googol, which is a 1 followed by 100 zeroes!). Quackwatch quotes the February 17, 1997, issue of *U.S. News & World Report* as reporting that only one duck per year is needed to manufacture the product, which had total sales of $20 million in 1996. The magazine dubbed that unlucky bird "the $20-million duck."[6]

One of the homeopathic recommendations for travel sickness is cocculus. That is a plant that contains the poisonous alkaloid, picrotoxin. Luckily, the label on the bottle is usually untrue and the pills contain none. Travel sickness is known to be influenced by expectations. That makes it a good candidate for placebo effects and also good for the income of charlatans. The placebo effect is not new, and a fool and his money are soon parted.

Homeopathy, according to Hahnemann, had several other principles. He attributed very little success to the curative powers of nature. Every recovery by anybody under the care of a homeopath was a cure achieved by the latter. If patients with diarrhoea or influenza recover after receiving pills made of some entirely inert substance they are said to have been cured by the homeopath. The natural courses of these diseases have had nothing to do with the matter.

Every substance administered by the homeopath had to be pure and not combined with any other substance. Many substances thought to be inert had therapeutic powers when prepared by the homeopathic method. There were several other principles, many even more ridiculous.

Holmes said that medical accuracy is not to be looked for "in the florid reports of benevolent associations, the assertions of illustrious patrons, the lax effusions of daily journals, or the effervescent gossip of the tea-table."[7]

He also attributed "a degree of ignorance as to the natural course of diseases" for the extravagant published claims of many homeopaths.[8] A young woman affected with jaundice is mentioned in the German "Annals of Clinical Homoeopathy" as having been cured in 29 days by "pulsatilla and nux vomica".[9] Another case of jaundice recovered in 34 days after homeopathic doses of pulsatilla, aconite, and cinchona. Holmes had a case in his own household, in whom the jaundice lasted about ten days and this was longer than he had repeatedly seen in hospital practice. A Dr. Munneche of Lichtenburg in Saxony was called to a patient with a sprained ankle who had been receiving palliative treatment for a fortnight. The patient recovered by the use of arnica in a little more than a month longer, and this extraordinary fact was published in the French "Archives of Homoeopathic Medicine."[10]

In the same journal a case was reported of a young patient who with nothing more than influenza went shopping on the sixth day! Lucky her. A case of croup was reported in the *Homoeopathic Gazette* of Leipsig, in which "leeches, blistering, inhalation of hot vapour and powerful internal medicine" had been employed, and yet the merit was all attributed to one drop of homeopathic fluid.[11]

In homeopathic journals and gossip one can never, or next to never, find anything but successful cases.[12]

The strong interactions between water molecules are what cause water to be a liquid, despite its low molecular weight. As a result liquid water does indeed have structures, and these structures will be altered by dissolved molecules, but these structures persist for a very short time only. Because of the rapid thermal motion of the water molecules, a structure that is formed at one moment will be completely gone a few picoseconds later. A picosecond is 0.000000000001 seconds. A millionth of a millionth of a second; that is the length of the "memory" of water. The memory of water an expression much loved by the homeopaths has a rather short shelf life but recent work[13] suggests that the "memory" may be even shorter than this, more like 50 femtoseconds.

As a member of the Australian Council Against Health Fraud once remarked: "Strangely, the water offered as treatment does not remember the bladders it has been stored in, or the chemicals that may have come into contact with its molecules, or the other contents of the sewers it may have been in, or the cosmic radiation which has blasted through it. I suppose you might say that the medicinal water of the homeopath has a selective memory."[14]

<u>Should homeopathy be available on Government Health Services?</u>

The medical correspondent of the Weekly Telegraph, Kate Devlin, reported in July 2010 that doctors at the British Medical Association (BMA) annual conference had voted for over-the-counter medicines to be clearly identified as having no provable clinical effect. Chemists should be forced to clearly mark "nonsense"[15] homeopathic remedies as placebos to stop customers being misled, the doctors had said. The remedies should only be sold in chemists and other shops if they were clearly marked "placebo".

The call to scrap homeopathy on the National Health Service drew an outraged response from supporters of the treatment, dozens of whom picketed the conference centre. Dr Tom Dolphin of the British Medical Association Junior Doctors Committee told the conference that he had previously described homeopathy as witchcraft but now wanted to apologise to witches. "Homeopathy is not witchcraft, it is nonsense on stilts" he said.

The delegates said the National Health Service should no longer pay for homeopathic remedies that did not work and could endanger patients' health. Millions of pounds of health service funds should not be wasted on the treatments, the conference in Brighton heard. They said that there was no scientific evidence that the treatments were any better than dummy pills and diverting patients from conventional medicine could cause their health to deteriorate. During the BBC2 TV program mentioned previously, Kathy Sykes, the presenter showed that she had visited the Centre for Frontier Medicine in Biofield Science at the University of Arizona in the USA. She determined there that the National Institutes of Health provided $1.8 million of United States taxpayers' money for this project which seemed not to do real research at all.[16] Sykes commented that this "research" was not so much trying to find the evidence for "healing energy", but was rather working on the basis that there was one. This is not proper research.

The Council for Healthcare Regulatory Excellence (CHRE) is a statutory overarching body, covering all of the United Kingdom and separate from Government.[17] The organisation gets over £2 million per year of taxpayer's money. Established in April 2003, it promotes best practice and consistency in the regulation of healthcare professionals by nine regulatory bodies including not only the General Medical Council and the General Dental Council, but also the two forms of alternative medicine that have so far succeeded in obtaining "regulated" status, the General Chiropractic Council and the General Osteopathic Council.[18]

What does the Royal London Homeopathic Hospital (RLHH) cost the taxpayer? With the help of the Freedom of Information Act 2000, David Colquhoun was able to make some good guesses. At least £18 million had been spent on refurbishing the RLHH. The recurrent costs were not so easy to discover. The direct cost of running the RLHH is £3.379 million per year of which £3.175 million per year was paid by the National Health Service.[19] Approximately 75 per cent of the direct costs are for salaries.[20]

These are the salary costs of staff working at the RLHH. The staff are medical, nursing, pharmacy, administrative and managerial, and ancillary. The balance of cost is for purchase of drugs, laboratory tests, use of patient beds in other Trust hospitals, building and office running costs. As well as this, the NHS pays also for indirect services, but nobody seems to know the cost of these (and still less, their value). Indirect services are those not charged directly to the RLHH and will include the following: Payroll, payment and income services, accountancy, recruitment, training, personnel, governance and clinical audit, Research and Development (R and D) management and governance,[21] medical and nursing education, training and professional support, communications, I.M. and T., estates maintenance management and planning, catering, cleaning, security, insurance, depreciation, payment of public dividend. These services are supplied by the Finance Directorate, Workforce Directorate, Chief Nurse Directorate, Capital Investment Directorate, IM and T Directorate, R and D Directorate, Governance Directorate, Directorate of Corporate Services and Communications Directorate.[22]

For the UCLH Trust as a whole, indirect costs amount to 39.2 percent of direct costs. If that proportion applies to RLHH, then the total annual cost of RLHH would be £4.7 million. David Colquhoun said: "That sounds to me like a lot of money for a placebo effect."[23] According to Colquhoun it seems that Lord Winston made an error of fact when he defended the RLHH in the House of Lords[24] by saying "My Lords, perhaps I may be allowed to break with tradition and come to the assistance of my noble friend. Is it not the case that the national homeopathic hospital conducts perfectly normative medicine and is it not justified in doing that, irrespective of the efficacy or otherwise of homeopathy, which I believe is only a small part of its practice?" 53.2 per cent of items dispensed at the hospital were homeopathic, a further 13.5 per cent were herbal or homeopathic creams or ointments and a still further 7.8 per cent were supplements/homeopathic (New Era Products). These figures obtained from an audit taken in August 2004 and provided under the Freedom of Information Act refer to the number of items dispensed. The value of the items was unable to be determined. This number of items dispensed totals 74.5 per cent and the remaining 25.5 per cent was made up of herbal tinctures and potencies, Iscador products, Aromatherapy, Marigold products, Tablets/nutritionals, Nutraceuticals, Anthroposophicals medicine, Allopathic products and Weleda Flower essence in various proportions. Judged by its prescription patterns homeopathy provides a huge part and hardly "only a small part of its practice." The RLHH is, in fact, 97.7 percent homeopathic.[25] Their web site lists eight consultants; all described as "homeopathic consultants" and a ninth has been added recently.

Mark Henderson and Fran Yeoman wrote that Members of Parliament had insisted that the NHS must audit spending on alternative therapy. They quoted that "The Department of Health admitted that it had no idea how much taxpayers' money was being spent on non-conventional therapies".[26]

Phil Willis, chairman of the Commons Science and Technology Select Committee, said the department had a duty to collect accurate information on the extent of NHS support.[27] Homeopathy in Britain has been in a state of steady decline over recent years. The number of NHS prescriptions for homeopathic remedies dropped by over 85 per cent between 2000 and 2010 (from 134,000 to 16,359), with homeopathy accounting for only 0.001 per cent of the total 2010 prescribing budget.[28]

The Tunbridge Wells Homeopathic Hospital, then one of four homeopathic hospitals operated by the NHS and which treated up to 1,000 patients a year, was closed in 2009 following a drop in referrals and a review by the West Kent Primary Care Trust of funding of homeopathy.[29]

This would save The South West Kent Primary Care Trust (PCT) £160,000 per year, which would be available for effective treatments. James Thallon, of the

PCT said "Homeopathy has been around since the 18th Century and has got a large body of very convinced adherents, but in the era of evidence-based medicine it's beginning to struggle a little bit, so I'm afraid that we're reflecting this in our decision."

In September 2010 another of the four, the Royal London Homoeopathic Hospital, was renamed as the Royal London Hospital for Integrated Medicine to more accurately reflect the nature of its work.[30] A fifth homeopathic hospital run by the NHS, the Hahnemann Hospital in Liverpool, had been closed in 1976.[31] The Liverpool Department of Homeopathic Medicine is now at the Old Swan Health Centre, Old Swan.[32] In 2011 the British Homeopathic Association said that 400 General Practitioners used homeopathy in their everyday practice.[33, 34] The British Homeopathic Dental Association (BHDA) claimed to have 69 dentists,[35] while the British Association of Homeopathic Veterinary Surgeons had 36 vets listed as members.[36] There were over 41,000 general practitioners[37] and around 24,000 registered veterinary surgeons[38] in the UK, and almost 23,000 dentists doing National Health Service work in England.[39]

Studies from the 1990s suggest that between 5.9 and 7.5 per cent of English NHS general practitioners have prescribed homoeopathy, while less than one per cent have prescribed herbal remedies. Current levels of prescribing are unknown but are thought to have increased. Sixty percent of Scottish general practices[40] now prescribe homoeopathic or herbal remedies and recognised drug–herb interactions are identified in four per cent of patients prescribed oral herbal remedies.

Around 2009, a few UK universities started closing or reviewing their courses on homeopathy and complementary medicine, after accusations that they were teaching pseudoscience.[41] These courses had been attracting bad publicity and criticism for the universities teaching them. In May 2010 it was announced that junior doctors' training would no longer include placements at the Glasgow Homeopathic Hospital.[42]

A freedom of Information Act request by David Colquhoun, elicited the following cost of CAM in Glasgow. The running costs for the Glasgow Homeopathic Hospital were: £1,658,000 and £1,881,000 in 2004/05 and 2005/06 respectively. There is no record of specific costs associated with General Practitioners or others employed by the National Health Service Board providing complementary and alternative medicine.[43] If homoeopathy, hypnosis, acupuncture or any other form of complementary medicine is provided it is not as a costed, discrete service.

Boots and other pharmacies

Boots the Chemists is a very big business in the UK. There are 1,450 Boots stores in the UK, employing over 68,000 people.[44] At one time they were sufficiently ethical not to deal in homeopathy but no longer according to David Colquhoun. He visited several Boots stores, sought out the most senior pharmacist that he could find, and asked them to recommend a natural remedy for a five year old son who has had diarrhoea for three days. In every case but one, the pharmacist reached for a copy of the Boots pamphlet on homeopathy, and thumbed through it, while desperately, but unsuccessfully, trying to retain an air of professional authority.[45]

Then one or another homeopathic treatment from the booklet was recommended. In only one case out of six did the pharmacist even mention rehydration and a consultation with a family medical practicioner. One pharmacist, who turned out to have qualified in Germany, was very insistent that homeopathic treatment was inappropriate and that rehydration and a visit to the doctor was essential. The other five, including one who had an impressive-looking badge saying "consultant pharmacist", did not even mention rehydration. Colquhoun concluded that the education of the pharmacists was clearly insufficient for them to give reliable advice. On the contrary, their advice was downright dangerous.

Boots also run an "educational" web site for children, the "Boots learning store" where one can find out about "vital forces".[46] This meaningless medieval gobbledygook, according to Colquhoun, is being peddled as "education" by the biggest retail pharmacy chain in the UK. The "Student Notes" include the following direct claim that homeopathy can cure diseases: "in many cases the properly chosen 'alternative' healing technique, plus properly chosen lifestyle changes, can heal both acute (sudden and severe disease of short duration) and chronic (slowly developing and long lasting illnesses. In other cases, 'conventional' medicine is only needed in emergencies or it may still form the major part of a Holistic Healing Plan".

One can also take the examination, the first question of which was; "What would we call Hahnemann's 'proving' today". The multiple choice answer gave the three possible answers as Placebo trials, Clinical trials or Experimental trials. The answer given was Clinical trials. If Hahnemann's "proving" could be described as a "clinical trial", Colquhoun considers that this might go a long way "to explain the quality of their learning store, and the quality of the advice given by their pharmacists."[47]

This example is particularly worrying where the latest government money-saving measures in the United Kingdom mean that nurses and pharmacists will be able to prescribe treatments for more serious conditions such as heart disease and diabetes, traditionally the domain of general practitioners.[48]

The Health Secretary Patricia Hewitt at the time said: "Nurse and pharmacist independent prescribing is a huge step forward in improving patient accessibility to medicines from highly skilled and well trained staff"[49,50] and Chief Pharmaceutical Officer, Dr Keith Ridge has added: "For pharmacists, this is the dawn of a new era. It will help transform the public's perception of pharmacy and the services they deliver to patients." It certainly will and maybe not for the better.

Boots have donated £160,000 to the Exeter University Development Campaign, to be used to fund a Research Fellowship in the Centre for Complementary Health Studies.[51] Professor Edzard Ernst, Director of the Centre, approached Boots, bearing in mind their recent strong commercial interest in homeopathy and herbal remedies.[52] The Research Fellow will concentrate particularly on these two subjects.

Homeopathic remedies are now available from many pharmacies. Yet instead of giving clear guidance to those members who are beginning to stock such products, the Royal Pharmaceutical Society (RPS) have quietly withdrawn their recommendation to inform consumers of the lack of evidence of efficacy for these products.[53] An RPS Council Statement issued in 1986 was quite clear about the Society's position on homeopathy. It advised members, "to inform any persons seeking advice on homeopathic products that there is no scientific evidence for their efficacy, beyond that to be expected from a placebo response."

The form in which the statement was subsequently incorporated into the RPS code on Medicines, Ethics and Practice was rather more liberal. Paragraph 1.6 states, "A pharmacist must not give an impression to a potential purchaser that any product associated with maintenance of health or a food supplement is efficacious when there is no evidence of efficacy." The only specific mention of homeopathy relates to homeopathic vaccines, advising against supply without medical prescription.

Does merely stocking a product constitute giving an impression that it is efficacious? HealthWatch believes that, in the case of pharmacies, it does. Because pharmacists are qualified health professionals who consumers are encouraged to consult for advice on everyday medical conditions, the very presence of a product on a chemist's shelves implies a form of tacit medical endorsement - considerably more so than in a supermarket or health food shop. "If homeopathic remedies didn't work," believe consumers, "Boots wouldn't stock them."

A spot check carried out by HealthWatch on five pharmacy outlets discovered that homeopathic remedies were stocked in both the Unichem and Boots outlets - the latter as part of a prominent display of alternative medicines. Of two independent chemists, one stocked Bach Flower Remedies with an explanatory placard telling one what they did along with the advice that, for serious conditions a homeopathic physician should be consulted.[54] The other planned to stock them "when he had room", and when pressed agreed that while there was no evidence of efficacy, it was not unethical to sell them as, "they did no harm." Only one pharmacist, running a small outlet attached to a supermarket, confided that she thought it was not appropriate to stock homeopathic remedies. On this basis HealthWatch believed that the RPS code of ethics, para 1.6, was being widely disregarded in the competition for trade between high street pharmacies and health food shops.[55] They called on the RPS to clarify their position with regard to homeopathic remedies, and to carry out their own spot checks to see whether the code was being applied.[56]

The internet and homeopathy

Katya Schmidt and Edzard Ernst determined that homeopaths were giving bad advice on the internet.[57] They found that homeopaths were advising against vaccination. So much for the argument that homeopathy at least does no harm. Schmidt and Ernst obtained addresses of United Kingdom homeopaths, chiropractors and general practitioners from online referral directories. They sent fictitious letters purporting to be from a patient asking for advice about the MMR vaccination. After sending a follow-up letter explaining the nature and aim of the project and offering the option of withdrawal, 26 per cent of all respondents withdrew their answers.[58] Homeopaths yielded a final response rate of 53 per cent compared to chiropractors 32 per cent. General Practitioners unanimously refused to give advice over the Internet. No homeopaths out of 77 and only one chiropractor out of 16 advised in favour of the MMR vaccination.[59]

Two homeopaths and three chiropractors indirectly advised in favour of MMR. They concluded that some CAM providers had a negative attitude towards immunisation and means of changing this should be considered. They considered that many CAM practitioners were supporters of the "anti-vaccination movement". The measles, mumps and rubella vaccination programme (MMR) has been of recent concern among professionals, parents and the general public alike mainly due to the infamous research conducted by Andrew Wakefield which has now been thoroughly discredited. His work, discussed in the chapter on Medical Quackery, together with that of Dr Spock and the Women's Health Initiative have all caused untold harm.

Chiropractors, homeopaths and naturopaths often advise their clients against immunisation.[60] In a survey investigating United States chiropractors' attitudes, one-third agreed that there is no scientific proof that immunisation prevents disease and that vaccinations cause more disease than they prevent.[61] In an Australian survey 83% of all Sydney homeopaths did not recommend immunisation [62] and a German survey found that active immunisations against the 'classic childhood diseases', including MMR are used with more restraint among homeopathic physicians .[63] In another study of 117 Austrian homeopaths only 33 rated immunisation as an important preventive procedure.[64] The chiropractic profession has also repeatedly expressed their negative view on vaccination.[65] Schmidt and Ernst concluded that their study confirmed previous investigations suggesting that some CAM providers have a negative attitude towards immunisation, specifically MMR, and that with the increasing popularity of CAM this could amount to a major threat to public health.

Is homeopathy harmful?

It is one thing to tolerate homeopathy as a harmless 19th century eccentricity for its placebo effect in minor self-limiting conditions like colds. It is quite another to have it recommended for seriously ill patients.

The Council for Healthcare Regulatory Excellence "promotes best practice and consistency in the regulation of healthcare professionals" including the General Chiropractic Council and the General Osteopathic Council. Inappropriate use of these two forms of alternative medicine must therefore fall under the general umbrella of the Council and indeed it did.

Dr. Marisa Viegas was suspended by the General Medical Council in the United Kingdom for advising a patient to stop heart medication which led to her death. The Amsterdam Medical Disciplinary Tribunal[66] struck off one doctor and suspended two others for their exclusive use of complementary treatments, including "vegatests," homeopathic medicine, and food supplements to treat Sylvia Millecam, the Dutch actress and comedian who died from breast cancer in

2001 at the age of 45.[67] The doctors were judged to have ignored existing standards for treating breast cancer, used unsatisfactory methods, and withheld information during their treatment of Ms Millecam.[68] She chose to forego regular treatment[69] and instead sought second opinions from several paranormal and alternative healers including the Dutch new age guru, Jomanda.[70] One doctor carried out a vegatest, which measures the electrical resistance of connective tissue under the skin, diagnosed a bacterial infection, which he treated with non-registered medicines,[71] thus leaving the cancer untreated for months. Millecam's condition steadily worsened and she was eventually moved to a regular hospital at a time when the tumor was so large as to be beyond medical treatment. She died in the hospital in Nijmegen two days later.[72] On 19 June 2007, three physicians who were involved in her treatment were prohibited to continue their work as physicians.

These are examples that show that homeopathy is not harmless. It can and does cost lives.

In 2004 two doctors working in private practice in the UK and treating their patients with complementary medicine were found guilty of serious professional misconduct by the General Medical Council.[73] Edzard Ernst commented[74] "The General Medical Council seems to be reminding us that the integration of complementary medicine has to be based on scientific evidence; otherwise it is in danger of amounting to professional misconduct". Unfortunately a great deal of such professional misconduct is still being funded by the National Health Service.[75]

In 2003, a Dr. Michelle Langdon risked the health of an 11-month-old girl and failed to get proper consent before using homeopathic medicine.[76] Dr Langdon, a partner at the Brunswick Medical Centre in Camden, North London, treated the baby's stomach infection by using a "dowsing" ritual to select a remedy. She was found guilty of serious professional misconduct and banned from practising medicine for three months.[77]

A bit of "serious professional misconduct" did not seem to have prevented Dr Langdon from being a committee member of the British Society for Integrated Medicine.[78] Their Founder President, Dr Julian Kenyon, wrote the following in their February 2006 newsletter. "Because we have to provide an evidence base for all the treatments we use, as demanded by the Health Care Commission (this is a statutory requirement), then technically the practice of homeopathy is currently illegal!"[79] Professor Ernst[80] said that "Evidence based complementary medicine must no longer remain a contradiction in terms. We need to be able to advise our patients responsibly about the risks and benefits of these treatments. Failing to take this challenge would be nothing less than disregarding the best interests of our patients."

Exeter's Department of Complementary Medicine, working with the Princess Elizabeth Orthopaedic Hospital and *BBC News West,* analysed questionnaires returned by 686 family practitioners and 121 members of the public and uncovered experiences of serious adverse effects ranging from paraplegia following neck manipulation, to the deaths of two children after homoeopaths advised changing or stopping essential medication. They concluded that "Serious adverse effects from CAM 'Natural' does not mean 'risk-free'."[81]

The public should be made aware that complementary and alternative therapies are not necessarily risk free, said the authors, and family practitioners need to be aware of risks when referring patients to CAM practitioners.

No fewer than 11 per cent of the family practitioners who returned questionnaires reported serious or potentially serious adverse effects. Of those which arose directly from the therapy, spinal manipulation was most often the cause; examples included severe whiplash injury with paralysis, and repeated manipulation of a thoracic tumour. Herbal treatments, various diets and acupuncture accounted for most of the remainder of direct effects reported. There were also reports of indirect effects, these usually involved interference with effective orthodox care for conditions such as asthma, diabetes and cancer.

The wife of a golfing friend of mine developed a particularly aggressive type of cancer which was diagnosed too late for any real prospect of a cure. Desperate, my friend took her to Columbia for some exotic unrecognised and very expensive homeopathic treatment. I could find no evidence at all that this particular form of treatment was effective in any way and it was not. She died shortly after her return. One cannot blame patients in any way whatsoever for seeking any form of treatment that might possibly help. When diagnosed with a terminal illness they have very little to lose but "quacks" who know that their treatment has no chance of success cannot be excused for raising false hopes and making huge financial gains out of other's misfortunes and lack of knowledge. Another friend spent much money on hyperbaric medicine for his intellectually challenged child. This did not help either.

Vaccinations

Many homeopaths believe that their remedies can help lessen the side effects of conventional vaccination. They offer "alternative vaccinations" which could leave patients vulnerable to potentially fatal diseases.[82] This was revealed by a BBC investigation.[83]

Three practitioners admitted giving patients a homeopathic medicine designed to replace the MMR vaccine.[84] An Inverness-based homeopath, Katie Jarvis, said she only offered "Homeopathic Prophylaxis"[85] to patients who expressed an interest but the discovery has prompted a shocked reaction from doctors.[86] When asked about the practice, Ms Jarvis said: "The alternative that I would offer would be a homeopathic remedy made from diseased tissue, that comes from someone with that disease, and then made into potentised form so that is given in a homeopathic remedy. It can be given instead of, or as well as, the vaccination. I'm not advocating that they do not take the vaccination, I am providing support for those who choose not to by giving them an alternative." she said.[87] When asked if the homeopathic remedy offered the same protection as the MMR vaccine, she replied: "I'd like to say that they were safer, but I can't prove that."[88]

The British Medical Association's director of science and ethics, Dr Vivienne Nathanson, said: [89] "Replacing proven vaccines, tested vaccines, vaccines that are used globally and we know are effective with homeopathic alternatives where there is no evidence of efficacy, no evidence of effectiveness, is extremely worrying because it could persuade families that their children are safe and protected when they're not." Some of those children will go on to get the illness, some may have permanent life-threatening sequelae or they may even die. When the family think they have protected their children that is a tragedy which should not be allowed to happen. Katie Jarvis said she had protected herself against flu with homeopathic treatment but that is different. She is an adult and entitled to choose. Ms Jarvis also claimed she could protect patients against other diseases, like polio, tetanus and diphtheria.[90]

The practice of replacing conventional vaccines with homeopathic alternatives has actually been condemned by the Faculty of Homeopathy.[91] They have stated that there was no evidence that homeopathic treatments protect against diseases and they have advised patients to use conventional medicines. What on earth are people like Katie Jarvis doing? Do they appreciate the harm they are causing? The politicians and others who support them for whatever reason are equally culpable.

The National Health Service, Highland, the health board covering Inverness, said it was considering withdrawing funding for homeopathic preparations.[92] Their chief operating officer Elaine Mead said:[93] "It is important that NHS Highland can demonstrate the quality and clinical effectiveness of all of the treatments currently provided at times of more scarce resource. It is right that we re-look at any investment in this area in the light of the current debate between clinical groups."

Immunisations work by enhancing the body's own immunity and it is mostly thanks to immunisation that diseases such as measles, polio, diphtheria, tetanus, and rubella are today rare in the developed world. They are an excellent example of preventative medicine. They are effective and should be accepted by everyone. Despite this there is resistance to vaccination. This resistance has been described by Edward R Friedlander from the University of Health Sciences College of Osteopathic Medicine in Kansas City.[94] Friedlander[95] examined several internet web sites which opposed childhood immunisations. He found rhetoric about "making informed choices," plus "a mass of half-truths and (at most sites) outright, obvious lies." The links were mostly to other "alternative" medicine sites. Those sites that contained citations to scientific papers misrepresented their contents. Several cite references were to 1990s-era publications in refereed medical journals but "none of the authors use their sources truthfully." One web site was typical.[96] The author's most obviously untrue claims; that immunisations had not made the diseases less common and that 29,972 Japanese died of smallpox despite having been immunised, were referenced only to the works of other anti-immunisation activists. The author also cited the Lancet[97] to claim that "Oman experienced a widespread polio outbreak six months after achieving complete vaccination." A check of the source showed this to be a cynical lie. Coverage was far from complete. Exposure was so massive where herd immunity was low that a few immunised children were not protected.

Outbreaks of disease can occur among communities who resist immunisation. This showcases the effectiveness of the vaccines and the consequences of non-vaccination. In 1985, measles raged through a Christian

Scientist school, with 125 cases and three deaths.[98] In 1991, there were at least 890 cases of rubella among the Amish in five states of the USA, and over a dozen babies with congenital rubella syndrome in Pennsylvania alone.[99] These cases would have been entirely preventable with immunisation. In a measles outbreak among the US Amish in 1987, there were 130 cases. The attack rate was 1.7 per cent among immunised individuals, and 73.8 per cent among unimmunised individuals. Two Amish died of measles in the following year.[100] In 1979, a polio outbreak paralysed 14 Amish people in the United States; the outbreak spread to unimmunised non-Amish neighbours.[101] In 1992, a Netherlands epidemic of polio began in a religious community affecting 68 people, paralysing 59, and killing two. None of the affected had been immunised.[102]

For some reason, diptheria-pertussis-tetanus (DPT) immunisation rates have been low for decades in Italy, with only about 50 per cent coverage. People bring the disease home to newborn babies who cannot yet be immunised and who are most vulnerable to severe disease.[103] One out of every 14 babies under one year of age is admitted to hospital for pertussis or whooping cough; of these, one in 850 dies.[104] Hundreds of thousands of children in the developing world die of pertussis each year.[105] Antibiotics are largely ineffective against it. The disease can last for months, and permanent brain damage occurs in up to four per cent of survivors from bleeding into the brain.[106] By the 1970s, because of vaccination, pertussis was rare in the developed nations. Because the immunity that the vaccine confers is incomplete, herd immunity is particularly important. In several countries, governments accepted the activist agenda. What followed is now history.[107] In 1974, a year in which there had been no pertussis deaths in Japan, the Japanese government stopped immunizing against pertussis due to the anti-immunisation "debate." In 1979 a pertussis epidemic resulted in over 13,000 cases and claimed 41 lives.

Measles is the most contagious of diseases. Unfortunately about ten per cent of people who receive the measles immunisation do not become immune. Only a high level of immunisation ensures neighborhood safety.[108] In the United States, 130 people died in the 1989-1991 outbreak alone. Among the urban poor, the cause is lack of immunisation due to social and economic problems.[109]

Elsewhere, the epidemics have begun among "exemptors" and spread to people who had not responded to the vaccine.[110] In the United States, 15 states now allow children to forgo immunisations because of their parents' "philosophical" objections.

Although many chiropractors oppose immunisation, many others strongly encourage their patients to accept immunisation.[111] The Faculty of Homeopathy in Great Britain has a formal statement acknowledging that homeopathic remedies do not affect antibodies, and hence it does not recommend that homeopathy be substituted for standard immunization. Unfortunately, according to Friedlander, many homeopaths ignore this statement.[112]

Recent US surveys of naturopaths and homeopaths,[113] and of chiropractors[114] revealed that some of each recommend immunisation, and others openly oppose immunisation. But in each category, the majority either declined to answer or said they left the decision to the family! This is hardly good enough.

Also in 1974, after the Wakefield debacle immunisation rates fell, and the annual incidence of pertussis increased from almost none to more than 100 per 100,000 per year.[115] Public confidence in the vaccine was reestablished in the mid-1980s and the disease has again become rare. Pertussis was extremely rare in Australia until an early 1990s antivaccine campaign. Immunisation rates dropped, and over 5000 people were sick in 1994 alone. Sweden stopped immunising in the late 1970s. During 1980-1983, the incidence of pertussis among children from birth to age four had increased to 3,370 per 100,000 per year, with rates of death and brain damage equal to those in the developing world.[116]There are many more examples that could be given. Friedlander mentions more of them in his review.

According to him in the early 1980s a television feature in the USA titled *Vaccine Roulette* and a book *A Shot in the Dark* informed audiences that the Pertussis vaccine caused permanent brain damage or death.[117] This was followed by lawsuits, manufacturers ceasing production, skyrocketing vaccine costs to cover liability, and the National Childhood Vaccine Injury Act of 1986. This compensation program has undoubtedly paid money to families whose children were not injured by vaccines, but this, Friedlander suggests, "seems to be wiser social policy than leaving juries to evaluate scientific questions."[118]

In 1994 the news media falsely reported that Miss America had become deaf as a result of the Pertussis vaccine. Her paediatrician later confirmed that the actual cause was hemophilus meningitis, which now has been mostly eliminated due to a vaccine.[119]

Susan C. Crump and Melanie Oxley the chair and vice-chair of the Society of Homeopaths felt that public confidence in homeopathy may have been dealt a blow by the reporting of Schmidt and Ernst. They argued that the survey seemed to have "used dubious and possibly unethical methods to extract potentially sensational information."[120] but they added that The Society of Homeopaths does not encourage its members to advise patients against vaccination. They acknowledged that there was much anecdotal and scientific evidence to support arguments both for and against vaccination. They believed that parents should be supported in making rational informed decisions about the short and long term implications of vaccination for their children. This was hardly a firm denial.

They did say that their members were fully insured, abided by a strict code of ethics and practice, and were expected to participate in regular activities for continuing professional development but, although they had stated that their Society did not encourage its members to advise patients against vaccination, they omitted to say whether their members adhered to this or not. Many obviously do not.

<u>Homeopathic malaria prophylaxis</u>

To argue that homeopathy does no harm is totally erroneous. It harms, if using homeopathy delays diagnosis of serious disease like cancer. It harms if homeopaths persuade one not to be vaccinated against smallpox, mumps or measles for example. It harms if one listens to the ill-informed advice that is given by many homeopaths about how to avoid malaria when you visit countries where it is common. This advice can be lethal. The malaria mortality rate being so high and living in a country with a relatively high incidence of malaria this subject is close to my heart.

The London School of Hygiene and Tropical Medicine was so concerned that it got together with the scientific pressure group "Sense about Science" to organise a survey of ten homeopathic practices mainly based in and around London.[121] They sent an undercover researcher in to say she was about to go in to a malaria infested country.[122] In each case, the researcher secretly recorded the conversations in order to document the consultation.[123]

The results were shocking. Seven out of the ten homeopaths failed to ask about the patient's medical background and also failed to offer any general advice about bite prevention. Worse still, ten out of ten homeopaths were willing to advise homeopathic protection against malaria instead of conventional treatment. This would have put the pretend traveler's life at risk. They all recommended doses of homeopathic remedies, 99.99 per cent water with an almost undetectable trace of effective remedies such as quinine.[124] None of them directed the researcher to a General Practitioner or Travel Clinic.

The homeopaths offered anecdotes to show that homeopathy was effective. One said: "Once somebody told me she went to Africa to work and she said the people who took malaria tablets got malaria, although it was probably a different subversive type not the full blown, but the people who took homeopathics didn't. They didn't get ill at all."[125] She also advised that homeopathy could protect against yellow fever, dysentery and typhoid.[126]

The television Newsnight team followed up this research with a program on *BBC2* TV (13th July 2006) after a marvelous bit of secret filming. A researcher with a hidden camera went to ten alternative health clinics.[127] She asked for advice on protecting herself from malaria on a holiday to Africa and each time was recommended homeopathic products instead of being directed to a general practitioner or conventional travel clinic. Homeopathic treatment was all that they recommended for malaria. Among the clinics and pharmacies visited[128] were the Vale Practice in East Dulwich, Helios in Covent Garden, and Nelsons Pharmacy which claims to be Britain's biggest manufacturer of homeopathic remedies off Oxford Street in London.[129] Even when the researcher said she planned to go to Malawi, a high risk area, Nelsons only suggested the addition of garlic, oil of citronella and vitamins rather than a trip to the doctors.[130] The Nelsons adviser told the researcher that the homeopathic compounds would protect her. "The remedies should lower your susceptibility; because what they do is they make it so your energy, your living energy, doesn't have a kind of malaria-shaped hole in it. The malarial mosquitoes won't come along and fill that in. The remedies sort it out."[131] This is absolutely ridiculous and potentially lethal. Do homeopaths really believe that they are not causing harm?

A spokesperson for Nelson's said staff were trained to provide responsible advice about malaria protection, and to advise that patients should consult a general practitioner before deciding on treatments.[132] "We are concerned to hear that this may not have happened in this case and have taken immediate steps to reiterate to the pharmacy team that this advice must be given."[133] A statement from Helios said: "We give advice on traditional homeopathic remedies which have been used by people for many decades in their attempt to avoid conventional treatment for malaria. There are many bibliographic references to the use of these remedies." They told *Newsnight*'s researcher she only needed their homeopathic compounds to protect her, saying "Yes you don't need to take anything else."[134]

What about evidence based medicine? Does it matter as long as the homeopathic product is being sold?

The Vale Practice said it was "a complementary therapy centre that does exactly that - complement the medical model.[135] This, however, can only be done after a thorough consultation. In this instance a consultation was refused and direct and leading questions were put to the homeopath which can be taken out of context. Unfortunately this example is unrepresentative of practice policies. The Vale Practice ... has a policy of referring to the GP whenever indicated."

The same Melanie Oxley mentioned above, the vice-chair of the Society of Homeopaths protested that members of her organisation did not advise against proper malaria prevention, or against vaccination. The filming revealed that they do. Apart from their inability to stop their members giving lethal advice, the regulators themselves are deluded. Even Peter Fisher from the Royal London Homeopathic Hospital said "I'm very angry about it because people are going to get malaria.[136] There is absolutely no reason to think that homeopathy works to prevent malaria and you won't find that in any textbook or journal of homeopathy so people will get malaria, people may even die of malaria if they follow this advice."[137] Fisher, the Queen's homeopathic physician has the sense to acknowledge that homeopathy does not work for serious conditions, yet persists in his delusion that it works for milder illnesses.

The homeopaths recommended Malaria nosodes 30C where the source material is so diluted that not a single molecule is left. The medicines therefore contain no medicine. They are nothing but sugar pills. The source material is, incidentally, not stated. One source says it is made from "African swamp water containing impurities, algae and plants as well as mosquito slough, larvae and eggs." It is lucky that there is none of it left in the pill one takes. To sell pills that contain nothing whatsoever and to pretend that they will protect you against malaria is nothing short of criminal. Malaria is a major risk to people travelling in the tropics and can kill within days of the first symptoms.[138]

In the European Union in 2000, 15,528 cases of malaria in returning travellers were reported to the World Health Organisation. Almost 2,000 people returned to Britain with malaria last year and 12 died.[139] According to the Department of Health, most cases resulted from people not taking the appropriate protective drugs. Dr Ron Behrens, director of the travel clinic at the Hospital for Tropical Diseases, said: "We have treated people ... who thought they were protected by homeopathic medicines and contracted malaria."

In 2005 the Health Protection Agency issued a warning because of people falling seriously ill when using homeopathic remedies. Its advisory committee on malaria said: "Herbal remedies have not been tested for their ability to prevent or treat malaria and are not licensed for these uses ... There is no scientific proof that homeopathic remedies are effective in either preventing or treating malaria."

The homeopaths also recommended China Off which is made from Cinchona bark which should contain some quinine China Sulph is made from quinine itself. Quinine is only recommended treatment in very exceptional cases of malaria and is not recommended as prophylaxis. These preparations, however, contain only minute amounts of quinine that could not possibly have any effect at all. To recommend this treatment as prophylaxis for malaria is no more than fraud. Natrum Muriaticum another recommendation of the homeopaths is nothing more than sodium chloride, common salt. This is being recommended and sold as prophylaxis for malaria.

Numerous cases of malaria have resulted from the false optimism and belief in these homeopathic forms of malaria prophylaxis [140,141,142] The newspapers rightly had a field day. "Malaria risk for tourists who trust alternative practitioners" wrote Mark Henderson, in *The Times* on July 14th. "Homoeopathy: voodoo on the NHS" wrote Jamie White in the same paper the next day."It is outrageous that the NHS should knowingly promote this. It is quackery. And it is knowingly; the NHS Direct website points out that homoeopathy is contrary to everything we know about chemistry and medicine, and that there is no experimental evidence to support its preposterous claims. Yet the NHS still promotes it, because "despite the lack of clinical evidence, homoeopathy remains one of the most popular complementary therapies in the UK" he wrote. "Homeopaths 'endangering lives' by offering malaria remedies" wrote *The Guardian*. "Do not rely on homeopathy to protect against malaria, doctors warn" was the advice in the *Daily Mail*. They quoted Dr Evan Harris (Lib Dem) of the all-party parliamentary malaria group, as saying "This sort of outrageous quackery is unacceptable. Vulnerable people are being duped into handing over cash for useless remedies and are having their health put at risk through grossly inadequate advice.[143] People need to consider homeopathy in the same way as they treat faith-healing and witchcraft - that is not to risk their life or health on it." But the gullible continue to be gullible.[144]

Alok Jha, the science correspondent of *The Guardian* said on Friday 14 July 2006 that doctors and scientists have warned holidaymakers not to use homeopathic remedies for malaria and other serious tropical diseases or their lives could be put at risk.[145] He quoted the BBC investigation which found ten homeopathic clinics and pharmacies allegedly reneging on government guidelines by recommending unproven remedies for malaria and other tropical diseases such as typhoid, dengue fever and yellow fever.[146] Scientists said the homeopaths' advice was reprehensible and likely to endanger lives. Professor Geoffrey Pasvol, a tropical medicine expert at Imperial College London, said: "Medical practitioners would be sued, taken to court and found guilty for far less. What this investigation has unearthed is appalling." Yet the gullible continue to be gullible.

An editorial in *The Lancet*[147] proclaimed "The end of homeopathy" as long ago as 2005. The editor claimed that this was the issue in which "a new evaluation was published". The authors of an article in the journal had pointed out the fact that it is unsurprising that homoeopathy fares poorly when compared with allopathy. Of greater interest was the fact that this debate continues, despite 150 years of unfavourable findings. The more dilute the evidence for homeopathy becomes, the greater seems its popularity. They argue that for too long: "a politically correct laissez-faire attitude has existed towards homoeopathy, …" The editorial continued: "Surely the time has passed for selective analyses, biased reports, or further investment in research to perpetuate the homeopathy versus allopathy debate.[148] Now doctors need to be bold and honest with their patients about homeopathy's lack of benefit, and with themselves about the failings of modern medicine to address patients' needs for personalised care."[149]

Regulation of homeopathy

The prevalence of homeopathy varies from country to country and so do the regulations concerning it.[150] In some countries such as Austria and Germany there are no specific legal regulations, while in others like France and Denmark licenses or degrees in conventional medicine from accredited universities are required.

In France, some parts of the United Kingdom, Denmark, and Luxembourg homeopathic treatment is covered by national insurance.[151] In Belgium and the Czech Republic homeopathy is not covered.[152] In Austria, public insurance requires scientific proof of effectiveness in order to reimburse medical treatments, but exceptions are made for homeopathy.[153] In 2004 Germany, which formerly offered homeopathy under its public health insurance scheme, withdrew this privilege with a few exceptions. In June 2005, the Swiss Government, after a 5-year trial, withdrew insurance coverage for homeopathy and four other complementary treatments, stating that they did not meet efficacy and cost-effectiveness criteria. However, following the result of a referendum in 2009 the five therapies were reinstated for a further 6-year trial period from 2012.[154]

To harmonize the market of homeopathic products in the European Union, the Council of the European Communities, directed the member states to implement certain changes in their national legislation by Directive 92/73/EEC.[155]

This was replaced by Directive 2001/83/EC on the Community code relating to medicinal products for human use.[156] Member states were required to ensure that homeopathic products (for oral or external use) could be registered without proof of therapeutic efficacy provided that there was a sufficient degree of dilution to guarantee the safety of the product.[157] Other homeopathic products could still be registered and products such as Arnica became legally available.[158] The labels of homeopathic products registered without proof of efficacy must include the words "homeopathic medicinal product without approved therapeutic indications" as well as "a warning advising the user to consult a doctor if the symptoms persist during the use of the medicinal product."

Homeopathic medicines in Britain are regulated by the Medicines and Healthcare products Regulatory Agency (MHRA).[159] This body and the British reaction to the Council of the European Communities directives have been fully discussed in the previous chapter.

In February 2010 the British House of Commons Science and Technology Committee concluded that: "the National Health Service (NHS) should cease funding homeopathy.[160] It also concludes that the Medicines and Healthcare products Regulatory Agency (MHRA) should not allow homeopathic product labels to make medical claims without evidence of efficacy. As they are not medicines, homeopathic products should no longer be licensed by the MHRA." Part of their conclusions stated that "When the NHS funds homeopathy, it endorses it.[161] Since the NHS Constitution explicitly gives people the right to expect that decisions on the funding of drugs and treatments are made 'following a proper consideration of the evidence', patients may reasonably form the [misleading] view [inferred from the fact of any NHS financial support] that homeopathy is an evidence-based treatment." Since no evidence of benefit has been found, other than the placebo effect, the report's recommendation was that "The Government should stop allowing the funding of homeopathy on the NHS."[162]

The government stated that this decision would be left open to the Primary Care Trusts, the smaller bodies in charge of regional NHS management, instead of being done by the government itself.[163]

In June 2010, the British Medical Association voted three to one in favour of a motion that homeopathy should be banned from the NHS, and kept from being sold as medicine in pharmacies.[164] In February 2011, out of 104 Primary Care Trusts who responded, 72 said they did not fund homeopathy, with ten of these having stopped funding homeopathy in the last four years.[165]

There have also been popular demonstrations against homeopathy as part of the 10:23 campaign, which began in January 2010.[166,167,168] This campaign started at 10:23am on January 30th 2010, when more than four hundred homeopathy sceptics nationwide took part in a mass homeopathic "overdose" in protest at Boots' continued endorsement and sale of homeopathic remedies, and to raise public awareness about the fact that homeopathic remedies have nothing in them. Sceptics and consumer rights activists each publicly swallowed an entire bottle of homeopathic "pillules" to demonstrate that these "remedies", prepared according to a long-discredited 18th century ritual, are nothing but sugar pills. The protest aimed to raise public awareness about the reality of homeopathy, and put further pressure on Boots to live up to its responsibilities as the "scientist on the high street" and stop selling treatments which did not work.[169, 170]

Although the legislation for homeopathic remedies in Germany is the same as that of the European Union, Germany is the only member state of the European Union in which homeopathic remedies based on minerals or plants, and produced only in very low quantities, do not need to be registered. In other member states only remedies individually prepared in a pharmacy are exempt.[171]

In the USA homeopathic drugs are generally considered to be biologically safe because they are so diluted to the point where there are no molecules from the original solution left in a dose of the final remedy.[172]

The FDA makes significant exemptions for homeopathic remedies as compared to other drugs.[173] Manufacturers of homeopathic remedies are not required to submit new drug applications to the FDA. They are "exempt from good manufacturing practice requirements related to expiration dating" and they are exempt from "finished product testing for identity and strength." Interestingly they may also "contain much higher amounts" of alcohol than other drugs, which may contain "no more than 10 percent ... and ... even less for children's medications."[174]

India has the largest homeopathic infrastructure in the world, with low estimates at about 64,000, but going as high as 300,000 practising homeopaths. In addition, there are 180 colleges teaching courses, and 7,500 government clinics and 307 hospitals which dispense homeopathic remedies.[175,176] In China and

Japan, homeopathy appears to be almost unknown.[177, 178,179] Any person wishing to practice homeopathy in any way whatsoever within the borders of South Africa must be registered with the Allied Health Professions Council of South Africa (AHPCSA).[180] Registration is a legal requirement and under South African Law it is a criminal offence to practice homeopathy without registration. Homeopathic registration in South Africa enjoys a standing, rights and privileges similar to that of conventional medical practitioners. This means that the legal scope of practice of a homeopathic practitioner is very similar to that of a conventional medical practitioner. All private Homeopathic colleges were closed during the late 1970s by the South African Department of Health and the only training recognised by the AHPCSA at the present time is a five year full-time Masters degree in Homeopathy offered at the University of Johannesburg[181] and Durban University of Technology.[182] The practice of homeopathy in South Africa requires medical training as a prerequisite for a degree in homeopathy. Medical practitioners may register as homeopathic practitioners only after successful completion of the post graduate diploma.[183]

Although the Dutch government funded CAM research between 1986 and 2003, it formally ended funding in 2006.[184] The French weighed in.[185] France's most august medical authority dismissed homoeopathic remedies in a damning report. The Académie de Médecine, an advisory body of distinguished physicians, has upset practitioners and the homoeopathic industry by saying that they subscribe to "mumbo jumbo." "In the latest episode of a 200-year-old quarrel over the treatment of illness with minute doses of natural medicines, the academy urged the state to stop subsidising homoeopathy through the National Health Service." The report said. "Homoeopathy is a method dreamed up two centuries ago, based on prejudices that were devoid of any foundation. It has survived as a doctrine completely outside the remarkable scientific movement which has been transforming medicine for two centuries."[186] Homeopathic treatments should not be viewed as medicines because they were not subject to clinical testing and no proof of their effectiveness was required, it said, adding that it was an aberration for the state to pay 35 per cent of patients' fees for consultations with homoeopaths.[187]

Even in England, Edzard Ernst,[188] came out very clearly against homeopathy in Trends in Pharmacological Sciences (2005). In it he said: "Homeopathy is a popular but implausible form of medicine. Contrary to many claims by homeopaths, there is no conclusive evidence that highly dilute homeopathic remedies are different from placebos. The benefits that many patients experience after homeopathic treatment are therefore most probably due to nonspecific treatment effects. Contrary to widespread belief, homeopathy is not entirely devoid of risk. Thus, the proven benefits of highly dilute homeopathic remedies, beyond the beneficial effects of placebos, do not outweigh the potential for harm that this approach can cause." This was also reported in *The Observer* of 18th Dec, 2005 under the title "Professor savages homeopathy."

The Department of Health view on homeopathy, referred to earlier, differs somewhat. A letter from Caroline Flint, Minister of State at the Department of Health who describes herself as "New Labour Member of Parliament for the Don Valley constituency in South Yorkshire," offered the opinion that homeopathy works and referred a writer to the Faculty of Homeopathy; "which has a network of advisors around the country who are pleased to offer advice to members of the public about homeopathic issues". Caroline Flint's qualification for offering this advice is her BA. Hons. degree in American Literature and History at the University of East Anglia. She is a former local government officer and senior researcher/political officer GMB 1991-7 yet feels confident to proffer the advice given.

David Colquhoun suggested that ill-informed views like these were certainly consistent with the view that the bizarre decision by the MHRA, to allow dishonest labelling of homeopathic products, was taken under instructions from the Department of Health.

In the letter, dated 2nd August, 2006, Caroline Flint stated "The Department of Health acknowledges that there are now numerous complementary therapies available in the UK. Some of these therapies have been known to alleviate the symptoms of certain illnesses in cases where orthodox medicine does not seem to have offered a complete solution. However, it is the responsibility of local NHS organisations to commission healthcare packages for NHS patients, be it complementary or orthodox. Complementary and alternative medicine treatments are clearly attractive to a number of people and so in principle could feature in a range of services offered by local NHS organisations. Primary Care trusts (PCTs) often have specific policies on the extent to which their patients can be given access to complementary medicines and within these policies, it is open to GPs to give access to specific therapies where they consider it is in the interests of the individual patient. The cost-effectiveness, availability and evidence in support of specific therapies are all issues that are taken into account when deciding what treatment to provide."

This type of advice on health matters is not confined only to the members of the Labour party. Even though homeopathy has been described as "witchcraft" spending on it in the National Health Service could rise despite the Health Service facing drastic cuts. Health Secretary Andrew Lansley rejected calls from MPs on the Commons science committee to ban funding of the unproven treatment.[189]

Homeopathy products will still be available on a tightening NHS budget. Speaking in July 2010, Lansley effectively gave the green light for spending on homeopathy to go up, because of his plans for patients to be able to "shop around" until they find a GP willing to prescribe complementary therapies.[190]

This means more patients will have access to such treatments. There will be no restrictions on the advertising of homeopathic treatments, he added. Taxpayers pay about £4 million a year for homeopathy on the NHS. Critics responded with fury at the prospect of an increase at a time when some local Trusts are cutting back on cataract operations, hip replacements and in vitro fertilisation treatment.

In answer to an e-mail from David Colquhoun sent in April 2007, Mike Penning M.P. wrote: "While I respect your concerns about the NHS expenditure on homeopathic hospitals, personally I think that as the NHS is in receipt of funding to the tune of over £100 billion it is not a case of not enough money to fund cancer treatments it is more a case of where and how it is spent. As you can see from the enclosed standard letter the Conservative Party's view is that there should be a small amount of money made available for homeopathic hospitals. I fully understand that you may not agree with this position but I thank you for sharing your concerns with me."[191] Another letter reflecting the government's position on homeopathy[192] stated: "I very much understand and sympathise with your concerns about the future of NHS homeopathic hospitals. Homeopathy and alternative treatments are a valuable resource for doctors to be able to draw upon when offering treatments.[193] Where a doctor and a patient believe that a homeopathic treatment may be of benefit to the patient, I believe doctors should be free to prescribe that medicine. It is worrying to me that Primary Care Trusts are seeking to cut funding which could threaten the future of homeopathic hospitals. The Government's management of NHS spending has produced a situation whereby the NHS budget has nearly doubled from £57 billion in 1998 to £96 billion this year, and yet last year up to 27,000 jobs were lost, hospitals up and down the country are closing or cutting back services[194] and the NHS as a whole is predicted to finish the year with a deficits totalling £1.3 billion. All the while Patricia Hewitt proclaims last year to be the 'best year ever' for the NHS. Weighed down with yet more targets from central government and seeing £1 billion 'top-sliced' from their budgets by the Department of Health to disguise the regional debts, trusts are being forced to cut back on services they have provided for years. Against this backdrop, it is not surprising that Trusts have decided to take the axe to homeopathic care, as a short term solution to their financial difficulties.[195] I am opposed to these short sighted cuts because, as you will well know, homeopathic care is enormously valued by thousands of people and in an NHS that the Government repeatedly tells us is 'patient-led' it ought to be available where it proves cost and clinically effective.[196] It is clear that the Government is giving no commitment to safeguard the future of homeopathic treatment on the NHS. I will also forward your letter to the Secretary of State for Health, Patricia Hewitt MP, so that she can be made aware of the value of homeopathic care to you as a patient. Let me assure you the Shadow Health Team will continue to hold the Government to account for its gross mishandling of the NHS."

In May, Dr Tom Dolphin told the British Medical Association's Junior Doctors Committee group's conference: "Homeopathy is witchcraft.[197] It is a disgrace that nestling between the National Hospital for Neurology and Great Ormond Street Hospital there is a homeopathic hospital paid for by the NHS."

The Commons science select committee called for funding for homeopathy by the NHS to cease and the Government's Chief Scientific Adviser, John Beddington, said he believed that the "evidence of efficacy and the scientific basis of homeopathy is highly questionable".[198] But the Department of Health nevertheless said that efficacy was not the only important factor when deciding whether scarce NHS resources should be spent on a treatment; patient choice was essential too.[199]

The British Medical Association head of science and ethics, Dr Vivienne Nathanson, added: "We believe that limited and scarce NHS resources should only be used to support medicines and treatment that have been shown to be effective. We are concerned that scarce funding will be spent on 'treatment' that has no evidence base and that may not work."[200]

There is still hope that the British government may see the light. The MHRA launched a formal public consultation on the consolidation of UK medicines legislation on the 25th October, 2011. Interested parties were encouraged to contribute to the development of the legislation which will greatly simplify and clarify the law regulating medicines in the UK.[201] The draft consolidated regulations will be presented to test that they are complete, accurate, user-friendly and do not introduce unintended changes. The consultation also proposes policy changes to ensure that medicines legislation remains fit for purpose and reflects modern practice.

MHRA Chief Executive, Sir Kent Woods, said: "Medicines legislation which has been amended many times over several decades can be greatly simplified by consolidation. The current need for this has received widespread support from both pharmacists and the pharmaceutical industry. It will amalgamate 40 years of outdated and fragmented legislation, reducing it by around two thirds, making it clearer and easier to understand as well as ensuring that medicines regulation is supported by a modern and straightforward legal framework."

The consolidation is the cornerstone of the MHRA's Regulatory Excellence program that will examine regulations to ensure that they remain fit for purpose and that the MHRA continues to deliver high-quality and proportionate regulation to safeguard public health.[202] The Association of British Pharmaceutical Industry (ABPI) Chief Executive, Stephen Whitehead, said: "The ABPI welcomes this opportunity to contribute to providing clearer legislation and encourages our members to actively participate in the consultation."

The Proprietary Association of Great Britain (PAGB) Director of Legal and Regulatory Affairs, Helen Darracott, also commented: "The work to consolidate the complex UK medicines legislation is very much welcomed by the over-the-counter medicines industry. We look forward to engaging in the consultation to deliver a more concise and simplified legal text that is clear, meaningful and user-friendly to work with." The consolidation will replace approximately 200 Statutory Instruments (SIs) relating to human medicines and much of the Medicines Act 1968 with uniform and simplified regulations named The Human Medicines Regulations. It was due to come into force in July 2012.

The MHRA have stated that no product is risk-free.[203] Underpinning all their work, lie robust and fact-based judgements to ensure that the benefits to patients and the public justify the risks. They keep watch over medicines and devices, and take any necessary action to protect the public promptly if there is a problem.[204] They encourage everyone – the public and healthcare professionals[205] as well as the industry – to tell them about any problems with a medicine or medical device, so that they can investigate and take any necessary action.[206]

Under the title Homeopathic "mumbo jumbo" the Physiological Society[207] have expressed the view that "alternative medicine" has, with very few exceptions, no scientific foundation, either empirical or theoretical. "As an extreme example, many homeopathic medicines contain no molecules of their ingredient, so they can have no effect (beyond that of a placebo). To claim otherwise it would be necessary to abandon the entire molecular basis of chemistry. The Society believes that any claim made for a medicine must be based on evidence, and that it is a duty of the regulatory authorities to ensure that this is done."

The World Health Organization (WHO) has warned that people with conditions such as HIV, TB and malaria should not rely on homeopathic treatments.[208] The organisation was responding to calls from young researchers who fear the promotion of homeopathy in the developing world could put people's lives at risk.[209]

Dr Robert Hagan,[210] a researcher in biomolecular science at the University of St Andrews and a member of Voice of Young Science Network, which is part of the charity Sense About Science campaigning for "evidence-based" care said: "We need governments around the world to recognise the dangers of promoting homeopathy for life-threatening illnesses."[211]

In a letter to the WHO in June,[212] the medics from the UK and Africa said: "We are calling on the WHO to condemn the promotion of homeopathy for treating TB, infant diarrhoea, influenza, malaria and HIV. Homeopathy does not protect people from, or treat, these diseases. Those of us working with the most rural and impoverished people of the world already struggle to deliver the medical help that is needed. When homeopathy stands in place of effective treatment, lives are lost. We hope that by raising awareness of the WHO's position on homeopathy we will be supporting those people who are taking a stand against these potentially disastrous practices."[213] The doctors also complained that homeopathy[214] was being promoted as a treatment for diarrhoea in children but a spokesman for the WHO department of child and adolescent health and development said: "We have found no evidence to date that homeopathy would bring any benefit.[215] Homeopathy does not focus on the treatment and prevention of dehydration, in total contradiction with the scientific basis and our recommendations for the management of diarrhoea."

Dr Mario Raviglione, director of the Stop TB department at the WHO, also said: "Our evidence-based WHO TB treatment/management guidelines, as well as the International Standards of Tuberculosis Care do not recommend use of homeopathy."[216]

Dr Nick Beeching, a specialist in infectious diseases at the Royal Liverpool University Hospital, said: "Infections such as malaria, HIV and tuberculosis all have a high mortality rate but can usually be controlled or cured by a variety of proven treatments, for which there is ample experience and scientific trial data.[217] There is no objective evidence that homeopathy has any effect on these infections, and I think it is irresponsible for a healthcare worker to promote the use of homeopathy in place of proven treatment for any life-threatening illness."

Do supporters of homeopathic practices realise how culpable they are? They obviously do not. Paula Ross,[218] the chief executive of the Society of Homeopaths, said it was right to raise concerns about promotion of homeopathy as a cure for TB, malaria or HIV and Aids but she added typically: "This is just another poorly wrapped attempt to discredit homeopathy by Sense About Science.[219] The irony is that in their efforts to promote evidence in medicine, they have failed to do their own homework. There is a strong and growing evidence base for homeopathy and most notably, this also includes childhood diarrhoea."
"Strong and growing" evidence and "also evidence homeopathy could help" are

not convincing enough words in my book. Certainly not convincing enough to replace "rehydration."

While there are many reports of controlled studies about alternative medicine, just two reviews are mentioned. From a meta-analysis of homeopathy it was concluded that "at the moment the evidence of clinical trials is positive but not sufficient to draw definite conclusions because most trials are of low methodological quality and because of the unknown role of publication bias." [220]

Dr Sara Eames, president of the faculty,[221] said people should not be deprived of effective conventional medicines for serious disease but she added: "Millions die each year as those affected have no access to these drugs. It therefore seems reasonable to consider what beneficial role homeopathy could play."[222] Then she stated that: "What is needed is further research and investment into homeopathy."

How much more research and investment is needed to show that ineffective treatment not only does not work but that it is also costing innocent people their lives. Who or which next ardent proponent of homeopathy will yet again be requesting further research and investment. When is enough, enough?

Edzard Ernst's concluding remarks[223] in his abovementioned article published in *Trends in Pharmacological Sciences* (2005) stated "Therapeutic decisions should be based foremost on an assessment of the potential risk versus proven benefit. For homeopathy, the benefit side of this equation is currently not clearly defined: the best available evidence does not convincingly show benefits over and above those of placebo. The risks of homeopathy are probably relatively small. But even small risks can weigh heavy if the benefit is uncertain, small or totally absent. If one adds to all this, the scientific implausibility of the basic concepts that underlie homeopathic thinking, the inescapable conclusion is not positive: 250 years after the birth of its 'inventor', homeopathy is not associated with a risk-benefit profile that is demonstrably positive." The honest words of a professor of alternative medicine.

References:

1. *David Colquhoun's Improbable Science page.* http://dcscience.net/. The quack page, http://www.ucl.ac.uk/pharmacology/dc-bits-old/quack4.html (accessed July 20, 2013). 2. *A Sceptic's Medical Dictionary* (BMJ publishing, 1997). Michael O'Donnell. Quoting Sir Peter Medawar. *Advice to a Young Scientist*. Published in 1979. 3. Ben Goldacre. "Bad Science". Fourth Estate. London. 2009. p 38. 4. Oliver Wendell Holmes. Homeopathy and Its Kindred Delusions. This essay was presented as two lectures to the Boston Society for the Diffusion of Useful Knowledge in 1842 and was reproduced in *Examining Holistic Medicine* (Prometheus Books, 1985). Posted on March 26, 1999. Homoeopathy And Its Kindred Delusions. Lecture II. Part 2, http://chestofbooks.com/health/general/Oliver-Wendell-Holmes-Medical-Essays/Homoeopathy-And-Its-Kindred-Delusions-Lecture-II-Part-2.html (accessed July 20, 2013). 5. Rouzé, M. (1993) *Oscillococcinum*, le joli grand canard. *Science et Pseudo-sciences, Cahiers bimestriels de l'Association Française pour l'Information Scientifique* 202. Accessed July 2006.
6. Barrett, S. (2003) *Homeopathy: The Ultimate Fake* Quackwatch.org. http://www.quackwatch.org/01QuackeryRelatedTopics/homeo.html. Accessed July

2006 7. Homeopathy and Its Kindred Delusions, http://www.quackwatch.com/01QuackeryRelatedTopics/holmes.html (accessed July 20, 2013).
8. Ibid.
9. Ibid.
10. Ibid.
11. Ibid.
12. Ibid.
13. Cowan et al. *Ultrafast memory loss and energy redistribution in the hydrogen bond network of liquid H_2O*. Nature 434. p 199-202. 10 March 2005.
14. The quack page, http://www.ucl.ac.uk/pharmacology/dc-bits-old/quack4.html (accessed July 20, 2013).
15. Kate Devlin. Alternative medicine "nonsense". The Weekly Telegraph July 7th-13th 2010. 16. The quack page, http://www.ucl.ac.uk/pharmacology/dc-bits-old/quack4.html (accessed July 20, 2013).
17. DC's Improbable Science page, http://dcscience.net/improbable.html (accessed July 20, 2013).
18. DC's Improbable Science page, http://dcscience.net/improbable.html (accessed July 20, 2013).
19. The quack page, http://www.ucl.ac.uk/pharmacology/dc-bits-old/quack4.html (accessed July 20, 2013).
20. Ibid.
21. Ibid.
22. Ibid.
23. Ibid.
24. Ibid.
25. Ibid.
26. Ibid.
27. Mark Henderson and Fran Yeoman. The Times 24th May, 2006. Home. A Close Look at "Alternative' Medicine." NHS told to abandon CAM. NHS must audit spending on alternative therapy, MPs say.
28. Beckford, M. (2011-08-30). "NHS spending on homeopathy prescriptions falls to £122,000". London: Daily telegraph. http://www.telegraph.co.uk/health/healthnews/8729588 /NHS-spending-on-homeopathy-prescriptions-falls-to-122000.html. Regulation and prevalence of homeopathy - Wikipedia, the free .., http://en.wikipedia.org/wiki/International_prevalance_and_regulation_of_homeopathy (accessed July 20, 2013).
29. Evidence Check 2: Homeopathy, Fourth Report of Session 2009–10, House of Commons Science and Technology Committee, 20 October 2009, parliament.uk. Regulation and prevalence of homeopathy.
30. "History of The Royal London Hospital for Integrated Medicine". University College London Hospitals NHS Foundation Trust. Regulation and prevalence of homeopathy - Wikipedia, the free .., http://en.wikipedia.org/wiki/International_prevalance_and_regulation_of_homeopathy (accessed July 20, 2013).
31. "The Liverpool Hahnemann Hospital and Homeopathic Dispensaries including Liverpool branch of the British Homeopathic Society". National Archives. http://www.nationalarchives.gov.uk/a2a/records.aspx?cat=138-614hah&cid=0#0.

32. http://www.liverpoolcommunityhealth.nhs.uk/health-services/Specialist Services/ Homeopathy.aspx . National Archives. http://www.nationalarchives.gov.uk/a2a/records.aspx?cat=138-614hah&cid=0#0. 33. ^ http://www.britishhomeopathic.org/getting_treatment/homeopathy_in_the_nhs/ . Regulation and prevalence of homeopathy - Wikipedia, the free .., http://en.wikipedia.org/wiki/International_prevalance_and_regulation_of_homeopathy (accessed July 20, 2013).

34. ^ http://www.facultyofhomeopathy.org/media/facts_about_hom/nhs_referrals.html http://www.rcvs.org.uk/about-us/about-the-veterinary-profession/. Retrieved 2011-12-11. Regulation and prevalence of homeopathy - Wikipedia, the free .., http://en.wikipedia.org/wiki/International_prevalance_and_regulation_of_homeopathy (accessed July 20, 2013).

35. ^ http://www.bhda.co.uk/list.php

36. ^ http://www.bahvs.com/findavet.htm

37. ^ "Briefing Paper - General Practitioners". British Medical Association. http://www.bma.org.uk/press_centre/pressgps.jsp. Retrieved 2011-12-19. Regulation and prevalence of homeopathy - Wikipedia, the free .., http://en.wikipedia.org/wiki/International_prevalance_and_regulation_of_homeopathy (accessed July 20, 2013).

38. ^ "About the veterinary profession". Royal College of Veterinary Surgeons. 39. ^ "NHS Dental statistics for England: 2010/11". NHS Information Centre. http://www.ic.nhs.uk/webfiles/publications/007_Primary_Care/Dentistry/Dental_Stats_Eng_2010_11/NHS_Dental_Statistics_for_England_2010_11_Report_v2.pdf. Retrieved 2011-12-11.

40. Ross, S., Simpson, C. R. and McLay, J. S. (2006). Homoeopathic and herbal prescribing in general practice in Scotland. British Journal of Clinical Pharmacology, 62: 647–652. doi: 10.1111/j.1365-2125.2006.02702.

41. ^ a b Alexandra Frean (2009-01-03). "Universities drop degree courses in alternative medicine". Times Online (London). http://www.timesonline.co.uk/tol/life_and_style/education/article5614896.ece. Regulation and prevalence of homeopathy - Wikipedia, the free .., http://en.wikipedia.org/wiki/International_prevalance_and_regulation_of_homeopathy (accessed July 20, 2013).

42. ^ Helen Puttick (2009-04-24). "NHS scraps doctors' training at Scots homeopathic hospital". heraldscotland. http://www.heraldscotland.com/news/health/nhs-scraps-doctors-training-at-scots-homeopathic-hospital-1.1029985.

43. The quack page, http://www.ucl.ac.uk/pharmacology/dc-bits-old/quack4.html (accessed July 20, 2013).

44. Ibid.

45. Boots Unconcerned About Nelsons Production Problems. | The .., http://www.quackometer.net/blog/2012/08/boots-unconcerned-about-nelsons-production-problems.html (accessed July 20, 2013).

46. The quack page, http://www.ucl.ac.uk/pharmacology/dc-bits-old/quack4.html (accessed July 20, 2013).

47. Ibid.

48. Ibid.

49. Ibid.

50. BBC NEWS | Health | Nurse drug prescribing extended, http://news.bbc.co.uk/2/hi/health/4955428.stm (accessed July 20, 2013). 51. Boots to fund research. HealthWatch Newsletter no 21: April 1996. http://www.healthwatch-uk.org/newsletters/nlett21.html (accessed July 20, 2013). 52. HealthWatch Newsletter no 21, http://www.healthwatch-uk.org/newsletters/nlett21.html (accessed July 20, 2013).
53. HealthWatch. *"RPS tones down homeopathy advice."* Newsletter no 21: April 1996 http://www.healthwatch-uk.org/newsletters/nlett21.html (accessed July 20, 2013). 54. HealthWatch Newsletter no 21, http://www.healthwatch-uk.org/newsletters/nlett21.html (accessed July 20, 2013).
55. Ibid.
56. Ibid.
57. Schmidt K. and Ernst E. *Complementary Medicine.* Peninsula Medical School, Universities of Exeter and Plymouth. (2003, *Vaccine* 21. 1044–1047). The quack page, http://www.ucl.ac.uk/pharmacology/dc-bits-old/quack4.html (accessed July 20, 2013).
58. The quack page, http://www.ucl.ac.uk/pharmacology/dc-bits-old/quack4.html (accessed July 20, 2013).
59. Ibid.
60. Ernst E. *Rise in popularity of complementary and alternative medicine: reasons and consequences for vaccination.* Vaccine 2002;20:S90–3.
61. Colley F, Haas M. *Attitudes on immunization: a survey of American chiropractors.* J Manipul Physiol Ther 1995;18:420–1.
62. Sulfaro F, Fasher B, Burgess MA. *Homeopathic vaccination. What does it mean?* Med J Austr 1994;161:305–7.
63. Lehrke P, Nuebling M, Hofmann F, Stoessel U. *Attitudes of homeopathic physicians towards vaccination.* Vaccine 2001;19:4859–64.
64. Rasky E, Friedl W, Haidvogl M, Stronegger JW. *Arbeits- und Lebensweise von homöopatisch tätigen Ärztinnen und Ärzten in Österreich.* Wien Med Wochenschr 1994;17:419–24.
65. Koren T. *The vaccine dilemma: another viewpoint on the issue.* Chiro J 1993;Sept:1–28. 66. *Dutch doctors suspended for use of complementary medicine.* British Medical Journal. 22 April, 2006. 332. (7547): 929. doi: 10.1136/bmj.332.7547.929-a The quack page, http://www.ucl.ac.uk/pharmacology/dc-bits-old/quack4.html (accessed July 20, 2013). 67. The quack page, http://www.ucl.ac.uk/pharmacology/dc-bits-old/quack4.html (accessed July 20, 2013).
68. Ibid.
69. Sylvia Millecam - Wikipedia, the free encyclopedia, http://en.wikipedia.org/wiki/Sylvia_Millecam (accessed July 20, 2013).
70. The quack page, http://www.ucl.ac.uk/pharmacology/dc-bits-old/quack4.html (accessed July 20, 2013).
71. Ibid.
72. Sylvia Millecam - Wikipedia, the free encyclopedia, http://en.wikipedia.org/wiki/Sylvia_Millecam (accessed July 20, 2013).
73. The quack page, http://www.ucl.ac.uk/pharmacology/dc-bits-old/quack4.html (accessed July 20, 2013).
74. Ibid.
75. Ibid.
76. Ibid.

77. Ibid.
78. Ibid.
79. NEWSLETTER, http://www.bsim.org.uk/Newsletter%20-%20February%202006.pdf (accessed July 20, 2013).
80. Annals of the Rheumatic Diseases 1999; 58: 69-70. Can complementary medicine ever be evidence based?, http://www.brightsurf.com/news/headlines/18937/Can_complementary_medicine_ever_be_evidence_based.html (accessed July 20, 2013).
81. Abbot NC, Hill M, Barnes J et al. International Journal of Risk & Safety in Medicine 1998; 11: 99–106.
82. DON'T BELIEVE THE LIES: Homeopathy--a genuine and traditional .., http://nationalsocialistbritain.blogspot.com/2010/09/homeopathy-genuine-and-traditional.html (accessed July 20, 2013).
83. Samantha Poling. Investigations correspondent. BMA homeopathy "vaccines" warning. BBC Scotland. Doctors warn over homeopathic "vaccines."13 September 2010.
84. Doctors warn over homeopathic 'vaccines' | SeekerBlog, http://seekerblog.com/2013/02/28/doctors-warn-over-homeopathic-vaccines/ (accessed July 20, 2013).
85. Ibid.
86. Herbal Remedies and Complementary Therapies in the News .., http://www.complementarytherapynews.co.uk/2010_09_01_archive.html (accessed July 20, 2013).
87. Doctors warn over homeopathic 'vaccines' | SeekerBlog, http://seekerblog.com/2013/02/28/doctors-warn-over-homeopathic-vaccines/ (accessed July 20, 2013).
88. Ibid.
89. Ibid.
90. Ibid.
91. Ibid.
92. Ibid.
93. Ibid.
94. Edward R. Friedlander. Opposition to Immunization: A Pattern of Deception. Scientific Review of Alt Med 5(1):18-23, 2001© 2001 Prometheus Books, Inc.
95. Edward R. Friedlander. Opposition to Immunization: A Pattern of Deception. Scientific Review of Alt Med 5(1):18-23, 2001© 2001 Prometheus Books, Inc. http://webspace.webring.com/people/il/lmorgan/fearmongers/opposition_to_immunization.htm (accessed July 20, 2013).
96. "Dispelling Vaccine Myths." www.unc.edu/~aphillip/www/vaccine/dvm1.htm. Doctors warn over homeopathic 'vaccines' | SeekerBlog, http://seekerblog.com/2013/02/28/doctors-warn-over-homeopathic-vaccines/ (accessed July 20, 2013).
97. Sutter RW, Patriarca PA, Brogan S. Outbreak of paralytic poliomyelitis in Oman: Evidence for transmission among fully vaccinated children. Lancet. 1991;338:715-720. Opposition To Immunization, http://webspace.webring.com/people/il/lmorgan/fearmongers/opposition_to_immunization.htm (accessed July 20, 2013).
98. Novotny T, Jennings CE, Doran M, et al. Measles outbreaks in religious groups exempt from immunization laws. Public Health Rep. 1988;103(1):49-54. Opposition To Immunization,

http://webspace.webring.com/people/il/lmorgan/fearmongers/opposition_to_immunization.htm (accessed July 20, 2013).
99. Mellinger AK, Cragan JD, Atkinson WL, et al. High incidence of congenital rubella syndrome after a rubella outbreak. Pediatr Infect Dis J. 1995;14(7):573-578. Opposition To Immunization, http://webspace.webring.com/people/il/lmorgan/fearmongers/opposition_to_immunization.htm (accessed July 20, 2013).
100. Sutter RW, Markowitz LE, Bennetch JM, Morris W, Zell ER, Preblud SR. Measles among the Amish. J Infect Dis. 1991;163(1):12-16. Opposition To Immunization, http://webspace.webring.com/people/il/lmorgan/fearmongers/opposition_to_immunization.htm (accessed July 20, 2013).
101. Follow-up on poliomyelitis. MMWR. 1979;28(29): 345-346. Opposition To Immunization, http://webspace.webring.com/people/il/lmorgan/fearmongers/opposition_to_immunization.htm (accessed July 20, 2013).
102. Oostvogel PM, van Wijngaarden JK, van der Avoort HG, et al. Poliomyelitis outbreak in an unvaccinated community in the Netherlands, 1992-1993. Lancet. 334:665-670.
103. Opposition To Immunization, http://webspace.webring.com/people/il/lmorgan/fearmongers/opposition_to_immunization.htm (accessed July 20, 2013).
104. Binkin NJ, Salmaso S, Tozzi AE, Scuderi G, Greco D, Greco D. Epidemiology of pertussis in a developed country with low vaccination coverage: Italian experience. Pediatr Infect Dis J. 1992;11:653-661. Opposition To Immunization, http://webspace.webring.com/people/il/lmorgan/fearmongers/opposition_to_immunization.htm (accessed July 20, 2013).
105. Opposition To Immunization, http://webspace.webring.com/people/il/lmorgan/fearmongers/opposition_to_immunization.htm (accessed July 20, 2013).
106. Galazka A. Control of pertussis in the world. World Health Stat Q. 1992;45:238-247. Opposition To Immunization, http://webspace.webring.com/people/il/lmorgan/fearmongers/opposition_to_immunization.htm (accessed July 20, 2013).
107. Gangarosa EJ, Galazka AM, Wolfe CK, et al. Impact of anti-vaccine movements on pertussis control: the untold story. Lancet. 1998;351:356-361.
108. Opposition To Immunization, http://webspace.webring.com/people/il/lmorgan/fearmongers/opposition_to_immunization.htm (accessed July 20, 2013).
109. Ibid.
110. Measles outbreak: Southwestern Utah. MMWR. 1997;46:766-769.
111. Anderson R. Chiropractors for and against vaccines. Med Anthropol. 1990;12:169-186. Opposition To Immunization, http://webspace.webring.com/people/il/lmorgan/fearmongers/opposition_to_immunization.htm (accessed July 20, 2013).
112. Opposition To Immunization, http://webspace.webring.com/people/il/lmorgan/fearmongers/opposition_to_immunization.htm (accessed July 20, 2013).
113. Lee ACC, Kemper KJ. Homeopathy and naturopathy: practice characteristics and pediatric care. Arch Pediatr Adolesc Med. 2000;154:75-80.

114. Lee ACC, Li DH, Kemper JH. Chiropractic care for children. Arch Pediatr Adolesc Med. 2000;154:401-407. Opposition To Immunization, http://webspace.webring.com/people/il/lmorgan/fearmongers/opposition_to_immunization.htm (accessed July 20, 2013).

115. Opposition To Immunization, http://webspace.webring.com/people/il/lmorgan/fearmongers/opposition_to_immunization.htm (accessed July 20, 2013).

116. Romanus V, Jonsell R, Bergquist SO. Pertussis in Sweden after the cessation of general immunization in 1979. Pediatr Infect Dis J. 1987;6(6):364. Opposition To Immunization, http://webspace.webring.com/people/il/lmorgan/fearmongers/opposition_to_immunization.htm (accessed July 20, 2013).

117. Opposition To Immunization, http://webspace.webring.com/people/il/lmorgan/fearmongers/opposition_to_immunization.htm (accessed July 20, 2013).

118. Evans G. Vaccine liability and safety: a progress report. Pediatr Infect Dis J. 1996;14(6):477-478. Opposition To Immunization, http://webspace.webring.com/people/il/lmorgan/fearmongers/opposition_to_immunization.htm (accessed July 20, 2013).

119. Freed GL, Katz SL, Clark SL. Safety of vaccinations. JAMA. 1996;276(23):1869. Opposition To Immunization, http://webspace.webring.com/people/il/lmorgan/fearmongers/opposition_to_immunization.htm (accessed July 20, 2013).

120. Susan C Crump and Melanie Oxley. Society of Homeopaths does not advise against vaccination. BMJ 2003;326:164 *doi: 10.1136/bmj.326.7381.164 (Published 18 January 2003.)*

121. BBC NEWS | Programmes | Newsnight Home | Malaria advice .., http://news.bbc.co.uk/2/hi/programmes/newsnight/5178122.stm (accessed July 20, 2013). 122. Ibid.

123. Homeopathy: What's the harm? - Ground Up Strength, http://www.gustrength.com/health:homeopathy-what-s-the-harm (accessed July 20, 2013).

124. BBC NEWS | Programmes | Newsnight Home | Malaria advice .., http://news.bbc.co.uk/2/hi/programmes/newsnight/5178122.stm (accessed July 20, 2013).

125. Homeopathy: What's the harm? - Ground Up Strength, http://www.gustrength.com/health:homeopathy-what-s-the-harm (accessed July 20, 2013).

126. Ibid.

127. Ban Homeopathy, http://banhomeopathy.blogspot.in/ (accessed July 20, 2013).

128. Ibid.

129. BBC NEWS | Programmes | Newsnight Home | Malaria advice .., http://news.bbc.co.uk/2/hi/programmes/newsnight/5178122.stm (accessed July 20, 2013).

130. Ibid.

131. Homeopathy: What's the harm? - Ground Up Strength, http://www.gustrength.com/health:homeopathy-what-s-the-harm (accessed July 20, 2013).

132. Ban Homeopathy, http://banhomeopathy.blogspot.in/ (accessed July 20, 2013).

133. Ibid.

134. BBC NEWS | Programmes | Newsnight Home | Malaria advice .., http://news.bbc.co.uk/2/hi/programmes/newsnight/5178122.stm (accessed July 20, 2013).
135. Ban Homeopathy, http://banhomeopathy.blogspot.in/ (accessed July 20, 2013).
136. BBC NEWS | Programmes | Newsnight Home | Malaria advice .., http://news.bbc.co.uk/2/hi/programmes/newsnight/5178122.stm (accessed July 20, 2013).
137. Ibid.
138. Ban Homeopathy, http://banhomeopathy.blogspot.in/ (accessed July 20, 2013).
139. Ibid.
140. Carlsson, T., Bergqvist, L., Hellgren, U. *False safety with homeopathic agents. Swedes became ill with malaria in spite of prophylaxis.* Lakartidningen. 1995;92:4467–4468. Carlsson et al. *J Travel Med.* 1996 Mar 1;3(1):62. (PMID: 9815426)
141. BMJ. 2000 November 18; 321(7271): 1288.
142. Jelinek. T. *Importation of falciparum malaria from Thailand: should current recommendations for chemoprophylaxis be adapted?* Eurosurveillance, Volume 11, Issue 22, 01 June 2006.
143. Don't rely on homeopathy to beat malaria, doctors warn | Mail .., http://www.dailymail.co.uk/news/article-395568/Dont-rely-homeopathy-beat-malaria-doctors-warn.html (accessed July 20, 2013).
144. Ibid.
145. Ban Homeopathy, http://banhomeopathy.blogspot.in/ (accessed July 20, 2013).
146. Ibid.
147. Editorial. Aijing Shang et al. The Lancet. 2005. 336. p 690. The quack page, http://www.ucl.ac.uk/pharmacology/dc-bits-old/quack4.html (accessed July 20, 2013). 148. The quack page, http://www.ucl.ac.uk/pharmacology/dc-bits-old/quack4.html (accessed July 20, 2013).
149. Ibid.
150. Wikipedia, the free encyclopedia. Accesed December 28, 2011. This page was last modified on 19 December 2011. Regulation and prevalence of homeopathy - Wikipedia, the free .., http://en.wikipedia.org/wiki/International_prevalance_and_regulation_of_homeopathy (accessed July 20, 2013).
151. Regulation and prevalence of homeopathy - Wikipedia, the free .., http://en.wikipedia.org/wiki/International_prevalance_and_regulation_of_homeopathy (accessed July 20, 2013).
152. Ibid.
153. "Legal Status of Traditional Medicine and Complementary/Alternative Medicine: A Worldwide Review" (PDF). *World Health Organization.* 2001. Note that the document specifically states that it is not an official document of the WHO. 154. Dacey J (14 January 2011). "Alternative therapies are put to the test". swissinfo.ch. http://www.swissinfo.ch/eng/swiss_news/Alternative_therapies_are_put_to_the_test.html?cid=29242484. Retrieved 2011-11-24
155. ^ Council Directive 92/73/EEC of 22 September 1992 widening the scope of Directives 65/65/EEC and 75/319/EEC on the approximation of provisions laid down by Law, Regulation or Administrative Action relating to medicinal products and laying down additional provisions on homeopathic medicinal products. Regulation and prevalence of homeopathy - Wikipedia, the free ..,

http://en.wikipedia.org/wiki/International_prevalance_and_regulation_of_homeopathy (accessed July 20, 2013).

156. ^ a b Directive 2001/83/EC of the European Parliament and of the Council of 6 November 2001 on the Community code relating to medicinal products for human use. Regulation and prevalence of homeopathy - Wikipedia, the free .., http://en.wikipedia.org/wiki/International_prevalance_and_regulation_of_homeopathy (accessed July 20, 2013).

157. Regulation and prevalence of homeopathy - Wikipedia, the free .., http://en.wikipedia.org/wiki/International_prevalance_and_regulation_of_homeopathy (accessed July 20, 2013).

158. Ibid.
159. Ibid.
160. Ibid.
161. Ibid.

162.^ UK Parliamentary Committee Science and Technology Committee – "Evidence Check 2: Homeopathy". Regulation and prevalence of homeopathy - Wikipedia, the free .., http://en.wikipedia.org/wiki/International_prevalance_and_regulation_of_homeopathy (accessed July 20, 2013).

163. http://www.official-documents.gov.uk/document/cm79/7914/7914.pdf

164. Boseley, Sarah (2010-06-29). "Ban homeopathy from NHS, say doctors". *The Guardian* (London). http://www.guardian.co.uk/society/2010/jun/29/ban-homeopathy-from-nhs-doctors. Regulation and prevalence of homeopathy - Wikipedia, the free .., http://en.wikipedia.org/wiki/International_prevalance_and_regulation_of_homeopathy (accessed July 20, 2013).

165. ^ "Third of NHS trusts fund homeopathy". *BBC News*. 2011-02-18. http://www.bbc.co.uk/news/health-12492742.

166. "Liverpool anti-homeopathy campaigners stage protest". BBC News. 2010-01-30. http://news.bbc.co.uk/2/hi/uk_news/england/merseyside/8488946.stm. The Big Swallow: 30 January 2010 | manicstreetpreacher, http://edthemanicstreetpreacher.wordpress.com/2010/01/20/10-23-big-swallow/ (accessed July 20, 2013).

167. "Overdose' protest against homeopathy". BBC News. 2010-01-30. http://news.bbc.co.uk/2/hi/uk_news/scotland/glasgow_and_west/8488286.stm.

168. "Mass 'overdose' in Leicester city centre". Leicester Mercury. 2010-01-30. http://www.thisisleicestershire.co.uk/news/Mass-overdose-Leicester-city-centre/article-1782650-detail/article.html.

169. The 10:23 Event - 1023.org.uk - RichardDawkins.net, http://www.richarddawkins.net/articles/4934 (accessed July 20, 2013).

170. The Big Swallow: 30 January 2010 | manicstreetpreacher, http://edthemanicstreetpreacher.wordpress.com/2010/01/20/10-23-big-swallow/ (accessed July 20, 2013).

171. Report of a 2007 European Medicines Agency workshop on homeopathic medicinal products, including a presentation by the European Committee for Homeopathy. Regulation and prevalence of homeopathy - Wikipedia, the free .., http://en.wikipedia.org/wiki/International_prevalance_and_regulation_of_homeopathy (accessed July 20, 2013).

172. Milgrom LR (2007). "Conspicuous by its absence: the memory of water, macro-entanglement, and the possibility of homeopathy". *Homeopathy* 96 (3): 209–19.

doi:10.1016/j.homp.2007.05.002. PMID 17678819. Regulation and prevalence of homeopathy - Wikipedia, the free .., http://en.wikipedia.org/wiki/International_prevalance_and_regulation_of_homeopathy (accessed July 20, 2013).

173. Isadora Stehlin, Food and Drug Administration Public Affairs Officer, "Homeopathy: Real Medicine or Empty Promises?", *FDA Consumer*, December 1996. Regulation and prevalence of homeopathy - Wikipedia, the free .., http://en.wikipedia.org/wiki/International_prevalance_and_regulation_of_homeopathy (accessed July 20, 2013).

174. Regulation and prevalence of homeopathy - Wikipedia, the free .., http://en.wikipedia.org/wiki/International_prevalance_and_regulation_of_homeopathy (accessed July 20, 2013).

175. Dr. Raj Kumar Manchanda & Dr. Mukul Kulashreshtha, *Cost Effectiveness and Efficacy of Homeopathy in Primary Health Care Units of Government of Delhi- A study* Regulation and prevalence of homeopathy - Wikipedia, the free .., http://en.wikipedia.org/wiki/International_prevalance_and_regulation_of_homeopathy (accessed July 20, 2013).

176. Arokiasamy, P; M. Guruswamy, T.K. Roy, H. Lhungdim, *et al.*. "World Health Survey, 2003" (PDF). *International Institute for Population Sciences*. http://www.who.int/healthinfo/survey/whs_hspa_book.pdf. Retrieved 2007-09-07.

177. Alternative Systems of Medicine: Homeopathy, Traditional Chinese Medicine, and Ayurveda, retrieved March 21, 2008

178. [ab]WHO: Legal Status of Traditional Medicine and Complementary/Alternative Medicine: A Worldwide Review, 2001, retrieved March 21, 2008

179. ^Interview to Dr. Luc after a three weeks visit to china, 2005, retrieved March 21, 2008.

180. Regulation and prevalence of homeopathy - Wikipedia, the free .., http://en.wikipedia.org/wiki/International_prevalance_and_regulation_of_homeopathy (accessed July 20, 2013).

181. http://www.uj.ac.za/Default.aspx?alias=www.uj.ac.za/homoeopathy . Regulation and prevalence of homeopathy - Wikipedia, the free .., http://en.wikipedia.org/wiki/International_prevalance_and_regulation_of_homeopathy (accessed July 20, 2013).

182. http://www.dut.ac.za/site/awdep.asp?depnum=22609

183. Regulation and prevalence of homeopathy - Wikipedia, the free .., http://en.wikipedia.org/wiki/International_prevalance_and_regulation_of_homeopathy (accessed July 20, 2013).

184. Renckens, C. N. (December 2009). *"A Dutch view of the science of CAM 1986—2003". Eval Health Prof* 32 (4): 431–50. doi:10.1177/0163278709346815. PMID 19926606.

185. Charles Bremner. *Académie de Médecine condemns homeopathy. The Times.* September 08, 2004. The quack page, http://www.ucl.ac.uk/pharmacology/dc-bits-old/quack4.html (accessed July 20, 2013).

186. The quack page, http://www.ucl.ac.uk/pharmacology/dc-bits-old/quack4.html (accessed July 20, 2013).

187. Ibid.

188. Ernst, Edzard. Trends in Pharmacological Sciences. Vol 26. No. 11. November 2005. www.sciencedirect@2005 Elsevier. Ltd. Doi:10.1016/j.tips.2005.09.003. The quack page, http://www.ucl.ac.uk/pharmacology/dc-bits-old/quack4.html (accessed July 20, 2013).

189. More homeopathy on NHS as health cash is squeezed | Mail Online, http://www.dailymail.co.uk/health/article-1297910/More-homeopathy-NHS-health-cash-squeezed.html (accessed July 20, 2013).
190. Ibid.
191. The quack page, http://www.ucl.ac.uk/pharmacology/dc-bits-old/quack4.html (accessed July 20, 2013).
192. State Sponsored Quackery | The Quackometer Blog, http://www.quackometer.net/blog/2007/08/state-sponsored-quackery.html (accessed July 20, 2013).
193. MP David Tredinnick is Wrong about the Homeopathy Report .., http://www.quackometer.net/blog/2010/03/mp-david-tredinnick-is-wrong-about-the-homeopathy-report.html (accessed July 20, 2013).
194. State Sponsored Quackery | The Quackometer Blog, http://www.quackometer.net/blog/2007/08/state-sponsored-quackery.html (accessed July 20, 2013).
195. Ibid.
196. Homoeopathy: Help explain it to our credulous .., http://forums.randi.org/archive/index.php/t-88184.html (accessed July 20, 2013). 197. Is homeopathy the modern equivalent of witchcraft? - Yahoo .., http://uk.answers.yahoo.com/question/index?qid=20100518045246AAZI0gK (accessed July 20, 2013).
198. More homeopathy on NHS as health cash is squeezed | Mail Online, http://www.dailymail.co.uk/health/article-1297910/More-homeopathy-NHS-health-cash-squeezed.html (accessed July 20, 2013).
199. More homeopathy on NHS as health cash is squeezed | Mail Online, http://www.dailymail.co.uk/health/article-1297910/More-homeopathy-NHS-health-cash-squeezed.html (accessed July 20, 2013).
200. Ibid.
201. Press releases: MHRA - Medicines and Healthcare products .., http://www.mhra.gov.uk/NewsCentre/Pressreleases/CON132052 (accessed July 20, 2013).
202. Ibid.
203. Pharmacy Links, http://www.lexonuk.com/site/lexon_links.php (accessed July 20, 2013).
204. Press releases: MHRA - Medicines and Healthcare products .., http://www.mhra.gov.uk/NewsCentre/Pressreleases/CON132052 (accessed July 20, 2013).
205. Ibid.
206. Pharmacy Links, http://www.lexonuk.com/site/lexon_links.php (accessed July 20, 2013).
207. Austin Elliott. Editor. Physiology News. Summer 2005. No. 59. Senator Tom Harkin: NCCAM and inviting the Four Horsemen of .., http://scienceblogs.com/insolence/2009/03/03/senator-tom-harkin/ (accessed July 20, 2013).
208. BBC NEWS | Health | Homeopathy not a cure, says WHO, http://www.bbc.co.uk/2/hi/health/8211925.stm (accessed July 20, 2013).
209. WHO warns against homeopathy use — OneWorld South Asia, http://southasia.oneworld.net/news/who-warns-against-homeopathy-use (accessed July 20, 2013).
210. Ibid.

211. Ibid.
212. Ibid.
213. Ibid.
214. Ibid.
215. BBC NEWS | Health | Homeopathy not a cure, says WHO, http://www.bbc.co.uk/2/hi/health/8211925.stm (accessed July 20, 2013).
216. WHO warns against homeopathy use — OneWorld South Asia, http://southasia.oneworld.net/news/who-warns-against-homeopathy-use (accessed July 20, 2013).
217. Ibid.
218. Ibid.
219. BBC News Online | Homeopathy not a cure, says WHO, http://news.bbc.co.uk/2/mobile/health/8211925.stm (accessed July 20, 2013).
220. Kleijnen J, Knipschild P, ter Riet G. Clinical trials of homeopathy. *BMJ*. 1991;302:316–323.
221. WHO warns against homeopathy use — OneWorld South Asia, http://southasia.oneworld.net/news/who-warns-against-homeopathy-use (accessed July 20, 2013).
222. Ibid.
223. Ernst, Edzard. Trends in Pharmacological Sciences. Vol 26. No. 11. November 2005. www.sciencedirect@2005 Elsevier. Ltd. Doi:10.1016/j.tips.2005.09.003. ebm-first - Research papers, http://www.ebm-first.com/homeopathy/research-papers.html (accessed July 20, 2013).

CHAPTER FIVE - QUACKERY - TRADITIONAL CHINESE MEDICINE

History

"Chinese medicine," or "traditional Chinese medicine "(TCM), encompasses a vast array of folk medical practices based on mysticism. The belief is that the body's vital energy (chi or qi) circulates through channels, called meridians that have branches connected to bodily organs and functions. Supporters of acupuncture like to use the word "energy" in association with the term chi, but "the core concept of chi bears no resemblance to the western concept of energy."[1]

Illness is attributed to imbalance or interruption of chi. Ancient practices such as acupuncture, based on ancient Chinese philosophy, [2] Qigong, and the use of various herbs are claimed to restore balance. Qigong is also claimed to influence the flow of "vital energy."

In translation from the original Chinese manuscripts the translators, being insufficiently acquainted with English usage, consistently and most amusingly, maybe even appropriately, translated the word "patient" as "victim." Acupuncture's origins are uncertain. It was believed that some soldiers with chronic afflictions who received wounds in battle were believed to have been cured by the arrow wounds [3] but there are variations on this idea.[4] According to Wikipedia, sharpened stones known as Bian shi were originally used as well as sharpened bones. The practice may date to the Neolithic[5] or possibly even earlier in the Stone Age.[6]

Hieroglyphs and pictographs have been found dating from the Shang Dynasty (1600–1100 BCE) which suggest that acupuncture was practiced along with moxibustion.[7] Moxibustion was the burning of cone-shaped preparations of *Artemisia vulgaris* (mugwort) on or near the skin, often but not always near or on an acupuncture point. Traditionally acupuncture was used to treat acute conditions while moxibustion was used for chronic diseases. It has also been suggested that acupuncture has its origins in bloodletting[8] or demonology.[9] The bloodletting was because, in early times, the Chinese thought disease was closely related to the vascular system. Despite improvements in metallurgy over centuries, it was not until the second century BCE during the Han Dynasty that stone and bone needles were replaced with metal.[10] The earliest Chinese medical text to describe acupuncture is the *Huangdi Neijing*, the legendary Yellow Emperor's *Classic of Internal Medicine (History of Acupuncture)* which was compiled around 305–204 BCE.[11] The *Huangdi Neijing* does not distinguish between acupuncture and moxibustion and gives the same indication for both treatments.

Other sources state that the first description of acupuncture as a therapeutic technique was in the Shi-chi text in the year 90 B.C.E. although it is accepted that earlier texts do describe the use of objects such as sharp stones to drain blood or infection.[12]

In Chinese medicine, there are six pulses, which allegedly measure not heartbeats but energy flow. These are taken at two levels of pressure on both wrists. The tongue may also provide diagnostic clues in its color and texture! Traditional acupuncture now involves the insertion of stainless steel needles into various body areas.[13]

In relation to Chinese medicine, most people have heard of the terms "yin" and "yang." Originally the terms meant the shady (yin) and sunny (yang) sides of a hill and if one was ill one was considered to be out of balance with nature and these two opposing forces.[14] It was the rise and fall of these opposite, but complementary forces that was believed to produce most of the natural cyclical events but, not unlike homeopathy, there was also an element of belief that like corresponds to like. Not unlike voodoo, it was also believed that hurting a picture of a person would result in real harm to the person.[15] It was even believed that eating food that looked like a particular body organ would be beneficial to that organ.[16]

There were many other different philosophies involved in the history of Chinese medicine many of them contradicting each other.[17] Bloodletting was eliminated from the procedure of acupuncture through the adoption of more modern physiology but surgery was prohibited for a long time in China since it was regarded as unacceptable to open the body in this way.[18]

In 1822, an edict from the Chinese Emperor banned the practice and teaching of acupuncture within the Imperial Academy of Medicine outright, as it was considered unfit to be practiced by gentlemen-scholars.[19] At this point, acupuncture was still cited in Europe "with both scepticism and praise, with little study and only a small amount of experimentation."[20] It should be remembered that acupuncture arose at a time when there was no understanding of modern physiology, biochemistry, or healing mechanisms.[21] If a person, treated with acupuncture, improved, it was assumed that the treatment had caused the improvement.[22]

There was no formal study of diseases and their natural history, and no attempt was made to determine whether the person would have improved without the treatment. The improvement of symptoms was readily assumed to be caused by the treatment received even though it may not have been causally related. In this way, many specific treatments, including acupuncture, have been passed on untested to this day.[23]

By the early twentieth century the Chinese looked more and more to "Western" or conventional medicine. The early Chinese Communist Party, in particular, expressed considerable antipathy toward traditional Chinese medicine, ridiculing it as superstitious, irrational, and backward.[24] It was said of Chinese doctors that "Our men of learning do not understand science; thus they make use of yin-yang signs and beliefs in the five elements to confuse the world ... Our doctors do not understand science: they not only know nothing of human anatomy, but also know nothing of the analysis of medicines; as for bacterial poisoning and infections they have not even heard of them ... We will never comprehend the chi even if we were to search everywhere in the universe. All of these fanciful notions and irrational beliefs can be corrected at their roots by science."[25] Acupuncture and other traditional techniques became marginalized and were mostly restricted to the rural areas.[26,27,28]

Medical journals made little mention of traditional Chinese medicine at this time and during the period 1927-36 there was not a single paper on acupuncture published in the *Chinese Journal of Physiology*.[29]

Ear acupuncture which is based on the assumption of reflexological representation of the entire body in the outer ear was later developed in France.[30]

Mao Tse-tung saved traditional Chinese medicine, including acupuncture, by politicizing it[31, 32, 33, 34] even though, it is claimed, he personally rejected it allegedly saying, on one occasion when he himself was sick, "even though I believe we should promote Chinese medicine, I personally do not believe in it. I don't take Chinese medicine."[35] Acupuncture and other traditional therapies were powerful political tools and were used to judge support for the Cultural Revolution.[36, 37] Doctors and patients came under considerable political pressure to use traditional techniques, and critics were harshly treated.[38] This pressure also impacted upon the medical literature, with the *Chinese Medical Journal* (CMJ) being replaced in October 1966 by a frankly political journal *China's Medicine* whose banner included the words "official organ of the Chinese Medical Association."[39]

The editorial of the first edition proclaimed: "We will hold still higher the great red banner of Mao Tse-tung's thought, creatively study and apply Chairman Mao's works and continuously advance the revolutionization of our ideology and work so that we may better serve the Chinese people and the revolutionary people of the world."[40]

In 1987, a paper reviewing the history of the *Chinese Medical Journal* (CMJ) stated "It is sad to recollect the gloomy days of the 'Cultural Revolution,' which lasted 10 years, starting in 1966. *China's Medicine* which appeared from 1966 to 1968, filled with political documents, but very few medical papers ... Although our Journal resumed publication in 1975, many authors still started their scientific articles with superfluous political sloganeering... Low quality papers were also accepted. Fortunately, normalcy was gradually restored in the Journal after 1979."[41]

The quality of research into TCM in China has been extremely poor.[42] A recent analysis of 2,938 reports of clinical trials reported in Chinese medical journals stated that no conclusions could be drawn from the vast majority of them.[43] The researchers stated: "In most of the trials, disease was defined and diagnosed according to conventional medicine; trial outcomes were assessed with objective or subjective (or both) methods of conventional medicine, often complemented by traditional Chinese methods. Over 90 per cent of the trials in non-specialist journals evaluated herbal treatments that were mostly proprietary Chinese medicines". The methodological quality of these trials is described in detail by Tang and others.[44]

Acupuncture "gained attention in the United States" when President Richard Nixon visited China in 1972.[45] During one part of the visit, the delegation was shown a patient undergoing major surgery while fully awake, ostensibly receiving acupuncture rather than anesthesia. Later it was found that the patients selected for the surgery had both a high pain tolerance and had received heavy indoctrination before the operation; these demonstration cases were also frequently receiving morphine surreptitiously through an intravenous drip that observers were told contained only fluids and nutrients.[46]

Technique of acupuncture

The technique of acupuncture involves the puncturing of the skin with needles.[47] The needles are used to stimulate various points located over the body and by this means the body's balance can be restored.

The needles are usually inserted and twirled and may be left in for short periods. The points chosen for stimulation depend upon the patient's symptoms, the season, the weather, and the result of taking the pulse at the wrist. Some modern practitioners use low-level laser light instead of needles. If effective, this would be a useful noninvasive alternative to puncturing the skin but unfortunately for users (and recipients) of this technique, the evidence supporting its use is "pretty much nonexistent." [48,49,50]

Acupuncture and surgery

In addition to President Nixon's visit the early 1970s were a period during which medical visits to China were popular, and these usually involved demonstrations of the almost miraculous effectiveness of acupuncture. These visits were then written up in Western medical journals more as journalistic pieces than as critical scientific reviews.[51,52,53]

The rapid increase in popularity of acupuncture in the West followed on from the reports of these visits, and it had captured the public's imagination long before scientific studies began to question the validity of the anecdotes. An excellent example of this phenomenon, and a reminder of the importance of objective testing, is a published review of the use of acupuncture in sensorineural hearing loss.[54] This paper described how easily an unproven remedy may be unquestioningly promoted and how scientific assessment usually occurs as an afterthought. It described the following process: A visit to China by a well-known, and respected, ear-nose-and-throat specialist. Demonstrations for this person of apparent cures effected by acupuncture. No inquiry made as to whether the patients "cured" had had pre and post-treatment audiometric testing. Return to the U.S.A whereupon reports of cures began to reach the public via the media, particularly popular newspapers and magazines.[55] Public demand for the treatment to be made available as a result of the media reports of these "cures" and the apparently high success rates being achieved by trained local practitioners. The lack of objective scientific evidence for the reported cures is noted with concern, and research is conducted. Formal studies show that acupuncture has no effect upon hearing levels of individuals with sensorineural hearing loss.[56]

The specialist who originally traveled to China, and wrote of the remarkable demonstrations he saw there, wrote the following just three years later: "It is a tragic mistake to take a child or an adult for that matter for acupuncture treatment for neurosensory deafness to any of the so-called acupuncture centers. There has not been one case of improvement demonstrated audiometrically, when a child or any deaf patient was tested before undergoing treatment and then afterwards by any reputable otologist. There have only been unreliable and perhaps planted testimonials."[57]

The use of acupuncture as anesthesia for surgery has also apparently fallen out of favor with scientifically trained surgeons in China. A delegation of the Committee for Skeptical Inquiry reported in 1995: "We were not shown acupuncture anesthesia for surgery, this apparently having fallen out of favor with scientifically trained surgeons.[58] Dr. Han, for instance, had been emphatic that he and his colleagues see acupuncture only as an analgesic (pain reducer), not an anesthetic (an agent that blocks all conscious sensations)."[59]

Posner and Sampson[60] described an article on acupuncture written by Dr. Isadore Rosenfeld,[61] the health editor of the magazine, *Parade*. Dr Rosenfeld, a well-known cardiologist, professor of clinical medicine and author, published an article in the magazine supplement of the paper in 1998. The magazine supplement was provided to Sunday newspapers across the United States and claimed a weekly adult readership of 82 million. In the article Rosenfeld described an operation that he witnessed more than 20 years previously during a visit to China. In addition to the *Parade* article, one of his books also contained a description of the same incident.[62] The operation was that of "open-heart surgery" and the only "anesthetic" was an acupuncture needle in the female patient's right earlobe "connected to an electrical source." Very few acupuncture enthusiasts even now would profess its efficacy for this type of operation and Posner and Sampson were "unable to reconcile Rosenfeld's anecdote with scientific experience or common sense. They could not understand how a patient could have survived an open-chest, open-heart operation performed as described. There was no ventilatory support, no heart-bypass machine and an absence of intravenous access sites.[63] They questioned whether the patient had received only acupuncture anesthesia or, had Dr. Rosenfeld and his party been treated to something more akin to "psychic surgery," a technique commonly employed by conjuring practitioners in the Philippine Islands?[64]

According to Posner and Sampson, thousands of people from all over the world fly to the Philippines each year to have their bodies "opened" without a scalpel.[65] They have cancer or other tissue removed and their state of health returned to "normal." This is done within minutes and without discomfort, all by various sleight-of-hand techniques. In other words, it is a sham operation. Peter Sellers, the movie comedian of the 1960s and 1970s, reportedly opted for such a procedure over traditional cardiac bypass with predictably disastrous consequences.[66] Most, if not all, of these patients go home to die of their diseases.[67]

In his book, Dr. Rosenfeld dismisses the possibility that he could have been "duped by Chairman Mao" but would trained physicians' eyes be expected to have spotted such a fraud? Arthur Taub, a member of an acupuncture evaluation committee, has said that major surgical procedures thought to be performed under acupuncture alone entailed administration of meperidine and barbiturates.[68] Victor Herbert, professor of medicine at the Mt. Sinai School of Medicine, found that patients supposedly having acupuncture anesthesia for simpler operations were actually receiving morphine at the time.[69] Chinese surgeons have admitted that only suggestible people were selected for "acupuncture anesthesia," and that abdominal and chest operations were not done under acupuncture because the musculature must be sufficiently relaxed in order to expose an operative field large enough in which to work.[70]

This relaxation is standard practice in the Western world and is usually achieved by the use of muscle relaxant drugs. This necessitates artificial ventilation through an endotracheal tube and is why patients, after major surgery, often complain of a sore throat. Physicians might not make the best observers to detect elaborate hoaxes. Such hoaxes generally are unveiled not by practitioners in the field of medicine, but by experts in conjuring. For instance, the magician and scientific sceptic, James Randi [71,72,73] has done more to expose the Philippine "psychic surgeons" than has that nation's medical community. In his thirties, Randi worked in Philippine night clubs and all across Japan.[74] He witnessed many tricks that were presented as being supernatural. One of his earliest reported experiences is that of seeing an evangelist using a version of the "one-ahead"[75] routine to convince churchgoers of his divine powers.

Randi, who identified himself as an atheist, has stated that many accounts in religious texts, including the virgin birth, the miracles of Jesus Christ, and the parting of the Red Sea by Moses, are not believable.[76] For example, Randi referred to the Virgin Mary as being "impregnated by a ghost of some sort, and as a result produced a son who could walk on water, raise the dead, turn water into wine, and multiply loaves of bread and fishes" and he questioned how Adam and Eve "could have two sons, one of whom killed the other, and yet managed to populate the earth without committing incest." He wrote that, compared to the Bible, "*The Wizard of Oz* is more believable. And more fun."[77] To this, I would add that Adam has been depicted as having a navel. If true, how can that be explained?

According to Posner and Sampson, only one physician took the trouble to expose this sham, the late William Nolen, MD.[78]

In India, the so-called God Men, who claim miraculous powers, were exposed by the doyen of the Indian rationalist movement, B. Premanand. Before his death at the age of 79 Premanand had offered one Lakh Rupees to anyone who could demonstrate psychic abilities under fraud-proof conditions. There were few takers. In the United States, it was again Randi who, after physicists had tested his demonstrations and vouched for Uri Geller's apparent paranormal abilities, explained his mystique rationally.[79] Geller sued Randi for $15 million in 1991 and lost.[80]

In the book The Faith Healers Randi explained his anger and criticism of faith healers as arising out of compassion for the helpless victims of fraud.

Referring to psychic surgery as practiced by João de Deus (John of God), a self-proclaimed psychic surgeon who had received international attention, Randi said "To any experienced conjurer, the methods by which these seeming miracles are produced are very obvious."[81]

In 1988 while in China as part of a scientific delegation, Randi discovered how "Chi" or "Qigong" masters, who claimed to cure ills from a distance with a mere wave of their hands, used magic tricks to fool their audiences. Sampson was in the follow-up delegation in 1995 and heard about such deceptive practices from Chinese scientists.[82]

The ability of humans to withstand severely painful procedures without anaesthesia has been well documented. Skrabanek and McKormick have recorded operations done in Europe including amputations, thyroidectomies, and mastectomies without anaesthetic or acupuncture needles. Many reports have demonstrated that it is possible for people to bear the pain of surgery. In 1843, an American surgeon, Peter Parker, performed a mastectomy on a Chinese patient, who, when the operation was over, "raised herself from the table without assistance, jumped upon the floor, and made a bow to the gentlemen present ... as though nothing had occurred."[83]

Another surgeon wrote in 1863 that a large proportion of those (in China) on whom operations were performed had no chloroform ... Some did not even clench their hands or teeth, but lay upon the table perfectly motionless, while their muscles were being cut by the knife and their bones divided by the saw."[84]

In Dr. Rosenfeld's book he says "I took a color photograph of that memorable scene: the open chest, the smiling patient, and the surgeon's hands holding her heart. I show it to anyone who scoffs at acupuncture" but Posner and Sampson were denied permission to reproduce the actual photograph in their article.[85] Dr. Rosenfeld did acknowledge that not being a surgeon, he "did not pay any particular attention at the time to the surgical technique used."[86] He said that his motivation in publicising his story was simply "to draw attention to the possible use of acupuncture to alleviate chronic pain and suffering ... I thought acupuncture was worth looking into. I still do, as does a panel convened recently by the NIH ... I continue to keep an open mind on the subject."[87]

Posner and Sampson, while appreciating Dr Rosenfeld's position conveyed their concern that many of *Parade*'s 80-plus-million readers, as well as some practitioners who might be inclined towards dabbling with acupuncture for major surgical anesthesia, could easily have drawn a conclusion that Dr. Rosenfeld says he did not intend; that acupuncture appears to possess mysterious and unexplained analgesic properties.[88]

An even more famous "acupuncture" anecdote concerns the late *New York Times* writer James "Scotty" Reston. While in China in 1971, Reston required an emergency appendectomy.[89] Reports circulated that the surgery had been performed with acupuncture anaesthesia. In reality, his surgical anaesthesia had been quite conventional, though he did receive acupuncture for post-operative discomfort.[90]

"Tooth fairy" science

The American Medical Association takes no position specifically on acupuncture; the AMA groups it with other alternative treatments, saying "there is little evidence to confirm the safety or efficacy of most alternative therapies."[91]

Harriet Hall[92] a retired family practitioner who is interested in quackery, has summed up the significance of acupuncture research in an interesting way: "Acupuncture studies have shown that it makes no difference where you put the needles. Or whether you use needles or just pretend to use needles (as long as the subject believes you used them). Many acupuncture researchers are doing what I call Tooth Fairy science: measuring how much money is left under the pillow without bothering to ask if the Tooth Fairy is real." Hall coined the expression "Tooth Fairy science" which seeks explanations for things before establishing that those things actually exist.

Classic examples of Tooth Fairy science abound in CAM. Hall said that "A grocer claims to have cured a janitor's deafness by manipulating his spine and chiropractic is born, but was the man really deaf to begin with? Was he really deaf but remained deaf?[93] Data is collected and many studies are done to show how spinal manipulation, by affecting vital energy, cures not only deafness but many other things as well. A healer claims to have cured someone's cancer by chanting and consulting a great crow in the Himalayas, but did the patient really have cancer to begin with? Studies are done and statistically significant results are achieved that show chanting and crow consultation work better than chance. When the studies show that prayer doesn't heal or that applied kinesiology or dowsing doesn't work under controlled conditions do their advocates reject a belief in spirits or energies? No. They know their fairies exist. That's their story and they're sticking to it no matter what the evidence. They have tons of anecdotal evidence that outweighs any scientific studies that don't confirm their beliefs. Tooth Fairy science is a magnet for those who believe that the plural of anecdotes is scientific data."

The King's Fund in the UK has called for "New research methods needed to build evidence base on effectiveness of popular complementary therapies." This is surely the cart before the horse. It is scientific cheating which they call a "new research method."[94] Hall says that the "whole idea of double-blind, randomised, placebo-controlled studies is to avoid deluding ourselves.[95] CAM folks apparently want us to delude ourselves so we can continue to believe in fairies" what she calls a very unhealthy, unscientific approach to research. Her article concludes that it is possible that Santa Claus really does fly around the world in a reindeer-powered sleigh and deliver presents to millions of households in a single night, but there might be a simpler explanation for all those gifts appearing on Christmas morning. Zeus might have delivered them, of course, with help from the fairies.[96]

Popularity of acupuncture

In the early 1970s a real increase in the use of acupuncture occurred in the United States and around the world. A study published by the National Centre for Complementary and Alternative Medicine (NCCAM), found that 3.1 million adults and 150,000 children used acupuncture in 2007, seeking relief from ailments including headache or back pain, insomnia and attention-deficit disorders.[97] That was about one million more adults than in 2002, when the last NCCAM survey was done. In 2007, NCCAM spent about $9.1 million on acupuncture research.

A poll of American doctors in 2005 showed that 59 per cent believed acupuncture was at least somewhat effective for treatment of pain.[98] More than half of the physicians believed that acupuncture could be effective "to some extent." As of 2004, nearly 50 per cent of Americans who were enrolled in employer health insurance plans were covered for acupuncture treatments.[99,100]

Both medical and nonmedical "acupuncturists" started to put needles into everybody. Even in Zimbabwe, where there is no control on acupuncturists as there is for normal medical practice, doctors and other people went on courses to learn the technique. In the United States, today, some states restrict the practice of acupuncture to physicians or others operating under their direct supervision.[101] In about 20 states only, can people who lack medical training perform acupuncture without medical supervision.[102]

This is not true in Zimbabwe where acupuncture may be performed by qualified doctors, lay people or anyone who so desires. All that is necessary is to have attended a two week course and then to put up a certificate in one's consulting rooms.

In the USA those who specialise in acupuncture and oriental medicine are usually referred to as "licensed acupuncturists", or L.Ac.'s.[103] The abbreviation "Dipl. Ac." stands for "Diplomate of Acupuncture" and signifies that the holder is board-certified by the NCCAOM.[104] Twenty-three states require certification, according to that body.[105]

In 1996, the United States Food and Drug Administration changed the status of acupuncture needles from Class III to Class II medical devices, meaning that the needles are regarded as safe and effective when used appropriately by licensed practitioners.[106,107,108] They are required to be labelled for single use and used only by practitioners who are legally authorised to use them.

Is acupuncture effective?

A BBC article claimed on December 1st 1999 that "Scientists prove acupuncture works." The BBC noted that researchers had found that acupuncture produced statistically significant pain relief in two separate studies.[109] In addition, a meta-analysis of seven acupuncture studies conducted by the National Cancer Institute showed significant benefits from the treatment. The summary of the meta-analysis stated that "Four randomized controlled trials, a nonrandomized clinical study and two case series found that acupuncture enhanced or regulated immune function."[110]

Proponents of acupuncture believe that it promotes general health, relieves pain, treats infertility and treats and prevents certain diseases,[111] among other benefits such as cessation of smoking, but scientific research has not found it to be effective for anything but the relief of some types of pain and nausea.[112,113, 114,115,116,117]

Nausea and vomiting

For the prevention of postoperative nausea and vomiting systemic reviews have found conflicting results.[118,119] A 2004 Cochrane Review initially concluded that acupuncture appeared to be more effective than antiemetic drugs in treating postoperative nausea and vomiting,[120] but the authors subsequently retracted this conclusion which they said was due to a publication bias in Asian countries that had skewed their results.[121] A later review in 2008 examined randomised controlled trials on the effects of the P6 point, as well as points thought to rely on the same meridian, at preventing postoperative nausea and vomiting within the first 24 hours of surgery.[122] Three of the ten studies found statistically significant evidence that acupuncture could prevent this postoperative nausea and vomiting[123] though comparison of the studies is difficult due to the use of varied methodologies (different patient groups, different ways of stimulating the P6 point such as a needle versus finger pressure versus a special bracelet, timing and length of application of pressure, the use of one versus both arms, whether a general anaesthetic was used, and the mixture of men and women in the studies).[124]

The reviewer ultimately concluded that "due to the lack of robust studies, [this review] found that neither acupressure nor acupuncture was effective in preventing or managing postoperative nausea and vomiting in adults" and suggested further research to clarify issues such as the length and type of stimulation applied, training of those applying stimulation and gathering data, risk factors for postoperative nausea and vomiting, inclusion of proper placebos, and the analysis of specific populations.[125] The author also suggested disagreement with previous systemic reviews were due to their inclusion of older studies with poorer methodologies, while the more recent, better quality studies included in the review offered more negative results.[126]

An updated Cochrane Review published in 2009 concluded that both penetrative and non-penetrative stimulation of the P6 acupuncture point was approximately equal to, but not better than, preventive antiemetic drugs for postoperative nausea and vomiting though only ten per cent of the studies had adequate information on patient blinding regarding receiving standard or nonstandard acupuncture.[127] A 2011 Cochrane Review on the treatment of vomiting after the start of chemotherapy concluded that acupuncture point stimulation with needles and electro acupuncture reduced the number of times subjects vomited on the day of treatment, but were no help regarding immediate or delayed nausea.[128]

Acupressure was found to reduce the short-term severity of nausea, but was no help over the long term and did not influence vomiting. All of the experiments reviewed also used medication to control vomiting, though trials involving electro acupuncture did not use the newest drugs available.[129]

Relief of pain

Acupuncture may have a small effect in the short-term management of some types of pain [130,131,132] though a very recent 2011 review concluded that acupuncture was of doubtful efficacy in treating pain other than neck pain.[133] Together with many other similar papers published in the 1970's Lee and others[134] described how after 979 applications of acupuncture, a substantial number of their patients stated that they had relief immediately following a series of four acupuncture treatments each. It did not matter whether the needles were placed in the traditional meridian locations or in arbitrary fixed control points.[135] Four weeks following treatment, 65 per cent of their 261 patients with chronic pain reported little or no reduction in the intensity of their pain, 17 per cent reported a 50 per cent reduction, and 18 per cent at least a 75 per cent reduction. Much later, in 2009, a review of the highest quality clinical trials of acupuncture in the treatment of pain, published in the *British Medical Journal*, reported a "small analgesic effect of acupuncture was found, which seems to lack clinical relevance and cannot be clearly distinguished from bias.[137]

Whether needling at acupuncture points, or at any site, reduces pain independently of the psychological impact of the treatment ritual is unclear."[138] A 2011 review of fifty-seven systematic reviews of the topic, published in the Journal of the International Association for the Study of Pain found there is "little truly convincing evidence that acupuncture is effective in reducing pain."[139] A review of Cochrane Collaboration articles on pain concluded that "Their results suggest that acupuncture is effective for some but not all types of pain" and singled out migraines, neck disorders, tension headaches, and peripheral joint osteoarthritis as having evidence supporting acupuncture's use, while results were inconclusive for shoulder pain, lateral elbow pain, and low back pain and negative for rheumatoid arthritis."[140]

For chronic low back pain, acupuncture is more effective than other CAM treatments, but no more effective than conventional and alternative treatments for short-term pain relief and improving function.[141] However, when combined with other conventional therapies, the combination is slightly better than conventional therapy alone.[142,143] A review for the American Pain Society/American College of Physicians found fair evidence that acupuncture is effective for chronic low back pain.[144]

In November 1997, the National Institute of Drug Abuse, (NIDA) held a Consensus Conference on Acupuncture.[145] The conference was set up by Alan Trachtenberg, MD, a former acting director of the Office of Alternative Medicine (OAM) and an advocate of acupuncture. The conference was cosponsored by the Office of Medical Applications of Research (OMAR) with the OAM in a supporting role. According to Sampson,[146] the editor of the Scientific Review of Alternative Medicine, the organising committee was made up largely of National Institute of Health staff and extramural members known to be interested in "alternative" methods of medicine. Predictably there was an absence of speakers known to have obtained negative results from acupuncture research. Authors who had not found positive results from their research on acupuncture had not been invited. Sampson listed the panel that was asked to evaluate the presentations and suggested that they seemed to be "weighted toward social advocacy, rather than evaluative science."[147] The chairman for example was David Ramsey, President of the University of Maryland, Baltimore, which received ongoing grants exceeding $1 million for its pain and acupuncture program from the Laing Foundation of the U.K. and from the OAM itself.[148] Howard Fields, MD, PhD, a pain physiologist from the University of California, San Francisco, and probably the one best-qualified expert on the panel did not attend the Congress because of illness.[149] Sampson spoke to him later and, according to Sampson, Fields stated that he did not support the recommendations arrived at by the Conference and that the best understanding of acupuncture's perceived effects was as a placebo!

The panel's report was composed before the conference and changed somewhat after the presentations.[150] The report recommended acupuncture for musculoskeletal pain, some headaches, and nausea. It did concede that placebo effects may be operative in acupuncture but accepted the proposition that acupuncture has more specific, non-placebo physiologic effects as well. It concluded that despite research on acupuncture being difficult to conduct, there was sufficient evidence to encourage further study and expand its use.[151] The report virtually acknowledged that acupuncture was difficult to evaluate by double-blind controlled studies because sham acupuncture produces similar changes.[152]

From this most authorities and even people in the street would conclude that if "sham" acupuncture points can be almost anywhere on the body, and if "real" acupuncture and "sham" acupuncture show no consistent, significant differences, then why use "real" acupuncture at all?[153] Sampson asks "Why not just prick oneself periodically with a small-gauge disposable needle and leave it in place for 20 minutes?[154] Why go to a licensed individual who spent one year learning where to place needles in the "right" places, especially when that individual knows little about disease, cannot tell the difference between a serious illness and somatization, does not know the natural history of disease and its alterations by therapies, and has little or no understanding of what scientific biomedicine is about?"

Sampson was concerned about what constituted fairness in evaluation of what he called "aberrant medicine." The Consensus Conference had underplayed the most obvious and probable reasons for perceived effects.[155] Those were, according to Sampson; natural history of disease, regression to the mean, suggestion, counter-irritation, distraction, expectation, consensus, identifying with and aiding in the desires of a dominant figure (the Stockholm effect), fatigue, habituation, ritual, reinforcement, and other well-known psychological mechanisms.[156] With such an array of obvious alternative explanations and such fertile areas for productive research, Sampson concluded that "one must have a set of strong biases to have agreed to the conference conclusions."[157] He considered that acupuncture research and the conference's conclusions showed not only bias but signs of pseudoscientific thinking.

Subsequent to the Conference a number of studies had been done for conditions such as asthma and nausea. Two analyses of the research into acupuncture in 1988 and 1990 showed that the best quality papers were almost uniformly negative, and the weakest or most poorly performed studies were mostly positive.[158,159]

In 2006 the National Institute of Health's National Centre for Complementary and Alternative Medicine stated that it continued to abide by the recommendations of the 1997 NIH consensus statement, "even if research is still unable to explain its mechanism."[160]

A World Health Organisation (WHO) 2005 report was also criticised in a 2008 book *Trick or Treatment*[161] for, in addition to being produced by a panel that included no critics of acupuncture at all, also containing two major errors;[162] including too many results from low-quality clinical trials, and including a large number of trials originating in China where, probably due to publication bias, no negative trials have ever been produced! In contrast, studies originating in the West include a mixture of positive, negative and neutral results. Ernst and Singh, the authors of the book, described the report as "highly misleading", a "shoddy piece of work that was never rigorously scrutinized" and stated that the results of high-quality clinical trials do not support the use of acupuncture to treat anything but pain and nausea.[163]

Ernst also described the statement in a 2006 peer reviewed article as "Perhaps the most obviously over-optimistic overview [of acupuncture]", noting that of the 35 conditions that the WHO stated acupuncture was effective for, 27 of the systematic reviews that the WHO report was based on found that acupuncture was not effective for treating the specified condition.[164]

The National Health Service of the United Kingdom[165] has stated that there is "reasonably good evidence that acupuncture is an effective treatment" for nausea, vomiting, osteoarthritis of the knee and several types of pain but "because of disagreements over the way acupuncture trials should be carried out and over what their results mean, this evidence does not allow us to draw definite conclusions". The NHS stated that there was evidence against acupuncture being useful for rheumatoid arthritis, smoking cessation and weight loss, and inadequate evidence for most other conditions that acupuncture is used for.[166]

Many carefully designed and conducted scientific studies have so far failed to demonstrate that the use of traditional Chinese acupuncture is associated with more effective pain relief than either placebo or counterirritant stimulation such as transcutaneous electrical stimulation (TENS). [167,168,169,170,171,172,173,174,175,176,177,178,179,180,181,182,183,184,185,186,187,188,189,190]

Many of these numerous trials have compared "real" acupuncture needles inserted according to one of the traditional theories and "sham" acupuncture needles inserted at other sites.[191] In some cases these "other" sites were those which, according to traditional theory, were least likely to reduce pain. No difference in effectiveness between the two methods was found.[192,193,194,195,196,197] Many of the studies were conducted with the cooperation and participation of professionals trained in traditional acupuncture.[198]

They cannot all be part of some imaginary anti-acupuncture conspiracy as proponents of the procedure would like to believe.

Counterirritant techniques may be useful for the relief of pain.[199,200,201] The view that acupuncture has an action or effect that is different to that seen with these placebo or counterirritant techniques is not supported by evidence. In view of this some modern practitioners of acupuncture have abandoned the older theories, including even the presence of precise acupuncture points.[202] The British practitioner Felix Mann has been noted to observe wryly that if the modern texts are to be believed there is "no skin left which is not an acupuncture point."[203]

Other medical conditions

The Danish Knowledge and Research Centre for Alternative Medicines have listed all the Cochrane Collaboration reviews regarding acupuncture[204] and the overall conclusion is that in the "majority of the Cochrane reviews about acupuncture, acupressure, electroacupuncture and moxibustion [concluded] there exists no solid evidence to determine the effectiveness of the treatments. The reviews point out that many of the studies suffer from methodological defects and shortcomings. Furthermore, the number of trial subjects has been limited. Thus most of the overall conclusions are uncertain."[205]

The Cochrane Collaboration or other review articles have concluded there was insufficient evidence to determine whether acupuncture is beneficial, often because of the paucity and poor quality of the research,[206] and that further research is needed in: chronic asthma,[207] Bell's palsy,[208] cocaine dependence,[209] depression,[210] drug detoxification[211,212,213] epilepsy[214] fibromyalgia[215] glaucoma,[216,217] insomnia[218] irritable bowel syndrome[219] induction of childbirth[220] rheumatoid arthritis[221] shoulder pain[222] schizophrenia[223] acute stroke[224] and stroke rehabilitation,[225] tennis elbow[226] and vascular dementia.[227]

The effectiveness of acupuncture in managing the pain of primary dysmenorrhea was investigated in a randomised and controlled prospective clinical study by Helms as long ago as 1987.[228] In his study there was a 41 per cent reduction of extra analgesic medication used by the women who had received acupuncture and no change or increased use of medication seen in the other groups not receiving true acupuncture but The Danish Knowledge and Research Centre for Alternative Medicines[229] mentioned above was of the opinion that acupuncture was not of proven benefit in the treatment of dysmenorrhoea.[230]

Some acupuncturist proponents believe that acupuncture can assist with fertility, pregnancy and childbirth, attributing various conditions of health and difficulty with the flow of qi through various meridians.[231]

There is no evidence to support the view that acupuncture is of use in various systemic disorders such as asthma[232, 233] and psoriasis.[234] Its use in such situations is highly questionable and of benefit only to the acupuncturist and then only financially.

Smoking

A Cochrane review looked into acupuncture and related interventions for smoking cessation.[235] The review looked at trials comparing active acupuncture with sham acupuncture (using needles at other places in the body not thought to be useful) or control conditions. The review did not find consistent evidence that active acupuncture or related techniques increased the number of people who could successfully stop smoking. They did find, however, that acupuncture might be better than doing nothing, at least in the short term; and that there was not enough evidence to dismiss the possibility that acupuncture might have an effect greater than placebo.[236] There was no consistent, bias-free evidence that acupuncture, acupressure, laser therapy or electro stimulation were effective for smoking cessation, but lack of evidence and methodological problems meant that no firm conclusions could be drawn. Further, the authors considered that well-designed research into acupuncture, acupressure and laser stimulation was justified since these were popular interventions and safe when correctly applied, though these interventions alone were likely to be less effective than evidence-based interventions.[237]

Pain of labour

The use of acupuncture to manage pain in labour started, like so many of its other uses, in the 1970s but the evidence of its benefits remains unconvincing.[238]

However, its use and that of other forms of complementary and alternative medicine (CAM) continue to be popular in pregnancy. Amy Norton reporting for Reuters Health Information from New York in February 2011 described a paper in the British Journal of Obstetrics and Gynaecology[239] as casting doubt on the efficacy of acupuncture for the pain of labour.

While many women may want a drug-free way to ease the pain of childbirth, she said, a study had suggested that acupuncture was not the answer. The researchers found that among 105 women having their first babies and undergoing induction of labour at term, those given acupuncture before their contractions started showed no benefit when it came to relief of pain. Two-thirds of the women ended up requesting epidural analgesia during their labours. That compared with 56 per cent of women who received a sham version of acupuncture and 77 per cent of those given no acupuncture at all. The differences among the three groups were not statistically significant. They concluded that there was no analgesic benefit with acupuncture for pain relief during induced labour in nulliparae.

The findings followed another study by researchers in South Korea and the United Kingdom.[240] They performed a systematic review and meta-analysis of trials of acupuncture use published in 19 electronic databases from around the world. Ten randomised controlled trials (five from Europe, three from China and two from Iran) were identified as meeting the inclusion criteria and the results were analysed.[241] The researchers noted that the heterogeneity of the studies (large variation in the results from one study to another) made interpretation difficult but the results showed that there was little convincing evidence that women who had acupuncture experienced less labour pain than those who received no pain relief, a conventional analgesia, a placebo or sham acupuncture.[242] Dr Hyangsook Lee, the principal author, said "In our previous systematic review of three randomised controlled trials (RCTs) in 2004, acupuncture appeared to be a promising analgesic option for women in labour. In this current review, acupuncture did not seem to have any impact on other maternal or fetal outcomes, nor was it associated with harm. However, there was no convincing evidence that women receiving acupuncture experience less labour pain than those in the control groups. To summarise, the current evidence does not appear to recommend the use of acupuncture for labour pain."[243]

Co-author Professor Edzard Ernst said "Our analyses show that the effects of acupuncture perceived by women are largely due to placebo. Acupuncture has many qualities that maximise placebo effects: it involves touch and is invasive and, psychologically, is attached to the mysticism of the East. Our findings are in keeping with much of the recent research on acupuncture which demonstrates that the more one controls for such confounders, the smaller the effect of acupuncture gets."

It was interesting to note that the primary endpoint in this trial was the rate of epidural analgesia requested by the patients during their labours. Based on this study and past ones, the researchers concluded that acupuncture could not be recommended for wider use. They felt that the evidence from randomised controlled trials does not support the use of acupuncture for controlling labour pain. They said that the primary studies were diverse and often flawed and, yes, yet again they said that "Further research seems warranted."

On the other hand a single Swedish trial[244] of acupuncture treatment during labour "significantly reduced the need of epidural analgesia;" a relative risk of 12 per cent vs 22 per cent. The authors of this study concluded that their results "suggested" that acupuncture could be a good alternative or complement to those parturients who seek an alternative to pharmacological analgesia in childbirth. Yet again they requested "further trials."

In another Swedish study[245] acupuncture was administered by midwives who had undertaken a four-day course on the use of acupuncture during labour. This study found that "women who received acupuncture were half as likely to request an epidural during labor, and less likely to ask for other types of pain relief, such as nerve stimulation therapy or a warm rice bag." However, the treatment appeared to have no significant effect on how much pain the women said they were feeling.[246]

<u>Migraine and tension-type headaches</u>

A study of 302 patients with migraine headaches concluded "Acupuncture was no more effective than sham acupuncture in reducing migraine headaches although both interventions were more effective than a waiting list control." [247]

A trial by Melchart and colleagues on 270 patients showed conclusively that acupuncture could indeed produce amelioration of tension-type headache when compared with no treatment.[248] The trial was initiated at the request of the German health authorities. They had requested a randomised trial including a sham control condition with an observation period of at least six months to decide whether acupuncture should be included in routine reimbursement. The acupuncture was well tolerated, and improvements lasted several months after completion of treatment but the relief was produced whether or not needles were inserted at "acupuncture points". Very similar results were found with "superficial needling at non-acupuncture points."[249] Yet again it is shown that the mumbo-jumbo of meridians and magic points is nonsense. Yet again, that is a good reason why universities cannot be expected to train acupuncturists. The function of medicine is to minimise mumbo-jumbo, not to propagate it.

In a similar trial[250] thirty patients with tension-type headache were randomly chosen to undergo a trial of traditional Chinese acupuncture and sham acupuncture. The frequency of headache episodes, analgesic consumption and the headache index (but not the duration or intensity of headache episodes) significantly decreased over time; however, no difference between acupuncture and placebo treatment was found.[251]

Osteoarthritis

Like Glucosamine and chondroitin sulphate which will be discussed in a later chapter, there is conflicting evidence that acupuncture may be useful for osteoarthritis of the knee, with both positive[252, 253] and negative[254, 255, 256] results. The Osteoarthritis Research Society International released a set of consensus recommendations in 2008 that concluded acupuncture may be useful for treating the symptoms of osteoarthritis of the knee.[257] Results for osteoarthritis in other joints suggest insignificant effects in short-term pain relief, which may be due to placebo or expectation effects.[258]

In 2004, researchers at the Centre for Integrative Medicine at the University of Maryland[259] tested the effects of acupuncture on 570 people over 50 with osteoarthritis in the knee. The patients were split into three groups: The group that received education about their condition recorded a 22 percent improvement in function; those who received sham acupuncture improved 31 percent and those who were treated with true acupuncture recorded improvement of 40 percent. The benefits of the actual acupuncture showed up over time, with most of those who obtained relief feeling it after 14 weeks of treatment.

However, other studies have found no difference between sham acupuncture and the real thing. An analysis of 13 studies of pain treatment with acupuncture, published online by the British Medical Journal, concluded there was little difference in the effect of real, sham and no acupuncture.[260]

Rheumatoid arthritis

David and others,[261] after conducting a trial of acupuncture and rheumatoid arthritis, concluded that acupuncture could not be considered as a useful adjunct to therapy in patients with rheumatoid arthritis. Ernst[262], in a systemic review of acupuncture as a symptomatic treatment of osteoarthrosis, found that both acupuncture and sham needling were effective at alleviating pain in axial and peripheral joint osteoarthrosis.

Risks of acupuncture

There is general agreement that acupuncture is safe when administered by well-trained practitioners using sterile needles.[263,264,265,266] Acupuncture is a painful and unpleasant treatment[267] and some patients have found the insertion of needles in acupuncture too painful to endure.[268] It is an invasive procedure, and therefore not without risk.

Injuries are rare among patients treated by trained practitioners.[269,270] Sometimes, needles are required by law to be sterile, disposable and used only once; in some places, needles may be reused if they are re-sterilised. When needles are contaminated, risk of bacterial or other blood-borne infection increases, as with re-use of any type of needle.[271]

Estimates of adverse effects due to acupuncture range from 671 to 1,137 per 10,000 treatments.[272] The majority of adverse effects reported are minor, mainly slight haemorrhage (2.9 per cent), haematoma (2.2 per cent), and dizziness (1 per cent) [273] but acupuncture can cause severe adverse effects including death.[274] Fainting and convulsions may occur as well as local infections, contact dermatitis, nerve damage and even bacterial endocarditis.

A 2010 systematic review found that acupuncture has been associated with a possible total of up to 86 deaths over the years surveyed, most commonly due to pneumothorax.[275]

A 2011 review that included many case reports of injuries stated that "ninety-five cases of severe adverse effects including five fatalities" were evident in the literature reviewed. "Pneumothorax and infections were the most frequently reported adverse effects."[276] Some 50 cases of bacterial infections and more than 80 cases of hepatitis B have been reported since 1970.[277,278]

Other risks of serious injury include: nerve injury, brain damage or stroke, which is possible with very deep needling at the base of the skull,[279] kidney damage from deep needling in the low back; Haemopericardium, or puncture of the protective membrane surrounding the heart, which may occur with needling over a sternal foramen.[280]

Providing alternative or complementary medicine in place of standard modern medical care may always result in inadequate diagnosis or treatment of conditions for which modern medicine has a better treatment record.[281]

As with other alternative medicines, unethical or naïve practitioners may also induce patients to exhaust financial resources by pursuing ineffective treatment[282,283] but this may equally be true of practitioners of standard medical care.

Risks of acupuncture are not common and usually not serious but they are present [284,285,286,287,288,289,290] and, if this is so the question must be asked as to why, if equally effective counter-irritant techniques are available that do not involve puncturing the skin, acupuncture continues to be used. "Acupuncture is an elaborate but unnecessarily complicated means of achieving analgesia when a clinically safer and easier method is available."[291,292]

It should also be borne in mind that traditional Chinese medicine, if not acupuncture, is a threat to certain animal species.[293] For example, black bears, valued for their gall bladders, have been hunted nearly to extinction in Asia, and poaching of black bears is a serious problem in North America.

Conclusion

Acupuncture has been the subject of active scientific research both in regard to its basis and therapeutic effectiveness since the late 20th century, but it remains controversial among medical researchers and clinicians.[294] Research on acupuncture points and meridians has not demonstrated their existence or properties.[295] Clinical assessment of acupuncture treatments, due to its invasive and easily detected nature, makes it difficult to use proper scientific controls for placebo effects.[296,297,298,299,300]

There is no general agreement on the efficacy of acupuncture as a medical procedure.[301,302,303,304.] Positive results from some studies on the efficacy of acupuncture may be as a result of poorly designed studies, the placebo effect or publication bias.[305,306,307,308] This strong publication bias occurs mainly from certain countries; a review of studies on acupuncture found that trials originating in China, Japan, Hong Kong and Taiwan were uniformly favourable to acupuncture, as were ten out of 11 studies conducted in Russia.[309]

Edzard Ernst and Simon Singh state that (as the quality of experimental tests of acupuncture have increased over the course of several decades through better blinding, the use of sham needling as a form of placebo control, etc.) the "more that researchers eliminate bias from their trials, the greater the tendency for results to indicate that acupuncture is little more than a placebo."[310] Far too many research studies involving acupuncture conclude that "further research is needed", but opinion is divided as to whether this is a good investment on which to spend limited research funds.[311,312,313,314,315,316]

Accompanied by the numerous calls for more research, the call that repeatedly seems to go through the whole of CAM, the use of acupuncture for certain conditions has been tentatively endorsed by the United States National Institutes of Health[317] and National Centre for Complementary and Alternative Medicine,[318] the National Health Service of the United Kingdom,[319] and the World Health Organization,[320] though most of these endorsements have been criticized [321, 322, 323] and it has been questioned whether research on acupuncture is a good use of limited research funding.[324, 325, 326, 327, 328, 329]

The National Council Against Health Fraud stated in 1990 that acupuncture's "theory and practice are based on primitive and fanciful concepts of health and disease that bear no relationship to present scientific knowledge."[330]

In 1993 neurologist Arthur Taub called acupuncture "nonsense with needles."[331] The website *Quackwatch* criticises TCM as having unproven efficacy and an unsound scientific basis.[332]

Physicist John P. Jackson,[333] Steven Salzberg, director of the Centre for Bioinformatics and Computational Biology and professor at the University of Maryland,[334] Yale University professor of neurology, and founder and executive editor of the blog *Science Based Medicine*, Steven Novella,[335] and Wallace Sampson,[336] clinical professor emeritus of medicine at Stanford University and editor-in-chief at the *Scientific Review of Alternative Medicine,* have all characterized acupuncture as pseudoscience[337] or pseudomedical.[338]

Acupuncturist Felix Mann,[339] who was the author of the first comprehensive English language acupuncture textbook *Acupuncture: The Ancient Chinese Art of Healing,* has stated that "The traditional acupuncture points are no more real than the black spots a drunkard sees in front of his eyes" and compared the meridians to the meridians of longitude used in geography , an imaginary human construct.

A systematic review of acupuncture for pain concluded that "A small analgesic effect of acupuncture was found, which seems to lack clinical relevance and cannot be clearly distinguished from bias.[340] Whether needling at acupuncture points, or at any site, reduces pain independently of the psychological impact of the treatment ritual is unclear."[341]

One of the major challenges in acupuncture research is in the design of an appropriate placebo control group.[342] Because of the problem of invasiveness retracting needles were used as the form of placebo.[343] With the use of these devices the results of acupuncture have now been shown in a much larger number of studies to be due to the placebo effect.

Acupuncture itself is also a very strong placebo, and can provoke extremely high expectations from patients and test subjects; this is particularly problematic for health problems like chronic low back pain, where conventional treatment is often relatively ineffective and may have been unsuccessfully used in the past. In situations like these, it may be inappropriate to consider "conventional care" a proper control intervention for acupuncture since patient expectations for conventional care are quite low.[344]

In 1997, the American Medical Association Council on Scientific Affairs[345] stated: Critics contend that acupuncturists, including many traditionally trained physicians, merely stick needles in patients as a way to offer another form of treatment for which they can be reimbursed, since many insurance companies will do so. Critical reviews of acupuncture summarized by Hafner and others conclude that no evidence exists that acupuncture affects the course of any disease ... Much of the information currently known about these therapies makes it clear that many have not been shown to be efficacious. Well-designed, stringently controlled research should be done to evaluate the efficacy of alternative therapies.[346] According to Stephen Barrett,[347] The National Council Against Health Fraud has concluded that acupuncture is an unproven modality of treatment, its theory and practice are based on primitive and fanciful concepts of health and disease that bear no relationship to present scientific knowledge, research during the past 20 years has not demonstrated that acupuncture is effective against any disease and perceived effects of acupuncture are probably due to a combination of expectation, suggestion, counter-irritation, conditioning, and other psychological mechanisms.[348]

The public should have access to accurate information about acupuncture's current scientific status.[349] There is a marked difference between the claims of some practitioners of acupuncture and the findings of the clinical research. In short, scientific research has failed to confirm traditional Chinese acupuncture as a separate entity, and it appears to be just one of many "counterirritant" techniques demonstrated to have a mild analgesic effect.[350]

As it is an invasive technique, and safer means are available to achieve the same effect, how is its ongoing use to be justified? [351]

References.

1. Unschuld, P. U. Medicine in China: A History of Ideas. Berkeley, CA: University of California Press; Los Angeles and London, 1985, 8vo, pp. x, 423. Acupuncture: A History - Allegheny College: Webpub, http://webpub.allegheny.edu/employee/l/lcoates/CoatesPage/FS101/Articles_PDF/Acupuncture/acupuncture_history.pdf (accessed July 21, 2013).
2. Unschuld, P. U. Nan-Ching: The Classic of Difficult Issues, with Commentaries by Chinese and Japanese Authors from the Third Through the Twentieth Century. (Comparative Studies of Health Systems and Medical Care). Berkeley:University of California Press (September 10, 1986). p.5. ISBN-10: 0520053729. ISBN-13: 978-0520053724
3. Tiran, D; Mack S (2000). Complementary therapies for pregnancy and childbirth. Elsevier Health Sciences. pp. 79. ISBN 0702023280.
4. White, A; Ernst E (1999). Acupuncture: a scientific appraisal. Elsevier Health Sciences. pp. 1. ISBN 0750641630.
5. ^ a b Chiu, M (1993). Chinese acupuncture and moxibustion. Elsevier Health Sciences. p. 2. ISBN 0443042233.
http://books.google.ca/books?id=V5PAB4d5qmgC&pg=PA2.
6. ^ Ma, K.-W. (1992). "The roots and development of Chinese acupuncture: from prehistory to early 20th century". Acupuncture in Medicine 10: 92–9. doi:10.1136/aim.10.Suppl.92.
7. ^ Robson, T (2004). An Introduction to Co mplementary Medicine. Allen & Unwin. pp. 90. ISBN 1741140544.
8. ^ Epler Jr, D. C. (1980). "Bloodletting in early Chinese medicine and its relation to the origin of acupuncture". Bulletin of the history of medicine 54 (3): 337–367. PMID 6998524. edit
9. ^ a b c d e Prioreschi, P (2004). A history of Medicine, Volume 2. Horatius Press. pp. 147–8. ISBN 1888456019.
10. ^ a b Chiu, M (1993). Chinese acupuncture and moxibustion. Elsevier Health Sciences. p. 2. ISBN 0443042233.
http://books.google.ca/books?id=V5PAB4d5qmgC&pg=PA2
11. ^ a b c d e Prioreschi, P (2004). A history of Medicine, Volume 2. Horatius Press. pp. 147–8. ISBN 1888456019.
12. Unschuld P. U. Medicine in China: A History of Ideas. Berkeley, CA: University of California Press; Los Angeles and London, 1985.
13. Stephen Basser, M.D. The Skeptical Guide to Acupuncture History, Theories, and Practices. The Scientific Review of Alternative Medicine. Spring/Summer 1999 issue. Originally posted on February 22, 2005.
14. Unschuld P. U. Medicine in China: A History of Ideas. Berkeley, CA: University of California Press; Los Angeles and London, 1985.
15. Acupuncture: A History - Allegheny College: Webpub, http://webpub.allegheny.edu/employee/l/lcoates/CoatesPage/FS101/Articles_PDF/Acupuncture/acupuncture_history.pdf (accessed July 21, 2013).
16. Ibid.

17. Keiji Yamada. The formation of the Huang-ti Nei-ching. Acta Asiatica. 1979. Wellcome Library for the History and Understanding of Medicine; History of Science, Technology, and Medicine Database
18. Epler, Bloodletting in early Chinese medicine. J Hist Med Allied Sci (1995) 50 (1): 11-46. doi: 10.1093/jhmas/50.1.11
19. History Of Acupuncture, http://healthaaa.com/AT/History_Of_Acupuncture.html (accessed July 21, 2013).
20. Linda L. Barnes. American Acupuncture and Efficacy: Meanings and Their Points of Insertion. Medical Anthropology Quarterly. September 2005, Volume 19, Issue 3pp. 308–9. doi: 10.1525/maq.2005.19.3.239. Article first published online: 8 Jan 2008
History Of Acupuncture, http://healthaaa.com/AT/History_Of_Acupuncture.html (accessed July 21, 2013).
21. Acupuncture: A History - Allegheny College: Webpub, http://webpub.allegheny.edu/employee/l/lcoates/CoatesPage/FS101/Articles_PDF/Acupuncture/acupuncture_history.pdf (accessed July 21, 2013).
22. Ibid.
23. Stephen Basser, M.D. The Skeptical Guide to Acupuncture History, Theories, and Practices. The Scientific Review of Alternative Medicine. Spring/Summer 1999 issue. Originally posted on February 22, 2005. Acupuncture: A History - Allegheny College: Webpub, http://webpub.allegheny.edu/employee/l/lcoates/CoatesPage/FS101/Articles_PDF/Acupuncture/acupuncture_history.pdf (accessed July 21, 2013).
24. Rosenthal MM. Health Care in the People's Republic of China: Moving Toward Modernisation. Colorado: Westview Press; 1987.
25. Kwok DW. Scientism in Chinese Thought. New Haven; Yale University Press, 1965:135. Acupuncture: A History - Allegheny College: Webpub, http://webpub.allegheny.edu/employee/l/lcoates/CoatesPage/FS101/Articles_PDF/Acupuncture/acupuncture_history.pdf (accessed July 21, 2013).
26. Crozier, Traditional Medicine in Modern China. Acupuncture - Wikipedia, the free encyclopedia, http://en.wikipedia.org/wiki/Jhenjiou (accessed July 21, 2013).
27. Rosenthal, Health Care in the People's Republic of China.
28. Lampton D. The Politics of Medicine in China. Colorado: Westview Press; 1977. Acupuncture: A History - Allegheny College: Webpub, http://webpub.allegheny.edu/employee/l/lcoates/CoatesPage/FS101/Articles_PDF/Acupuncture/acupuncture_history.pdf (accessed July 21, 2013).
29. Acupuncture: A History - Allegheny College: Webpub, http://webpub.allegheny.edu/employee/l/lcoates/CoatesPage/FS101/Articles_PDF/Acupuncture/acupuncture_history.pdf (accessed July 21, 2013).
30. Crozier, Traditional Medicine in Modern China. Acupuncture - Wikipedia, the free encyclopedia, http://en.wikipedia.org/wiki/Jhenjiou (accessed July 21, 2013). 31. Ibid.
32. Lampton, The Politics of Medicine in China. Colorado: Westview Press; 1977. Thank you! Share Grammarly on Facebook!
33. Huard P, Wong M. Chinese Medicine. London: Weidenfeld and Nicolson; 1968.
34. Sidel VW. Health services in the People's Republic of China. In: Bowers JZ, Purcell EF, eds. Medicine and Society in China. New York, NY: Josia Macey Jr. Foundation; 1974. 35. Li Z. The Private Life of Chairman Mao: The Inside Story of the Man Who Made Modern China. London: Chatto & Windus; 1994:84.
Acupuncture: A History - Allegheny College: Webpub,

http://webpub.allegheny.edu/employee/l/lcoates/CoatesPage/FS101/Articles_PDF/Acupuncture/acupuncture_history.pdf (accessed July 21, 2013).Thank you! Share Grammarly on Facebook!

36. Unschuld P. U. Medicine in China: A History of Ideas. Berkeley, CA: University of California Press; Los Angeles and London, 1985.

37. Lampton, The Politics of Medicine in China. Acupuncture: A History - Allegheny College: Webpub, http://webpub.allegheny.edu/employee/l/lcoates/CoatesPage/FS101/Articles_PDF/Acupuncture/acupuncture_history.pdf (accessed July 21, 2013).

38. Acupuncture: Past and Present, http://www.acuwatch.org/hx/basser.shtml (accessed July 21, 2013).

39. Sidel, Health services in the People's Republic of China. Acupuncture: A History - Allegheny College: Webpub, http://webpub.allegheny.edu/employee/l/lcoates/CoatesPage/FS101/Articles_PDF/Acupuncture/acupuncture_history.pdf (accessed July 21, 2013).

40. Ibid.

41. Bao-xing C. A centennial review of the history of the Chinese Medical Journal. Chinese Medical Journal. 1987;100(6):438-439. Acupuncture: A History - Allegheny College: Webpub, http://webpub.allegheny.edu/employee/l/lcoates/CoatesPage/FS101/Articles_PDF/Acupuncture/acupuncture_history.pdf (accessed July 21, 2013).

42. Health Information, http://quackwatchinfo.blogspot.com/ (accessed July 21, 2013).

43. Acupuncture - Through the Maze, Christian Apologetics Ministry, http://www.mazeministry.com/resources/books/doombook/graphpix/quackwatch.htm (accessed July 21, 2013).

44. Unschuld, P. U. Nan-Ching: The Classic of Difficult Issues, with Commentaries by Chinese and Japanese Authors from the Third Through the Twentieth Century. (Comparative Studies of Health Systems and Medical Care). Berkeley:University of California Press (September 10, 1986). p.5. ISBN-10: 0520053729. ISBN-13: 978-0520053724. Health Information, http://quackwatchinfo.blogspot.com/ (accessed July 21, 2013).

45. History Of Acupuncture, http://healthaaa.com/AT/History_Of_Acupuncture.html (accessed July 21, 2013).

46. ^ a b Beyerstein, BL; Sampson W (1996). "Traditional Medicine and Pseudoscience in China: A Report of the Second CSICOP Delegation (Part 1)". Skeptical Inquirer (Committee for Skeptical Inquiry) 20 (4). http://www.csicop.org/si/show/china_conference_1/. History Of Acupuncture, http://healthaaa.com/AT/History_Of_Acupuncture.html (accessed July 21, 2013). 47. Stephen Basser, M.D. The Skeptical Guide to Acupuncture History, Theories, and Practices. The Scientific Review of Alternative Medicine. Spring/Summer 1999 issue. Originally posted on February 22, 2005.

48. Strauss S. Is laser therapy a sham? Medical Observer. April 30, 1993.

49. Haker E, Lundeberg T. Laser treatment applied to acupuncture points in lateral humeral epicondylagia: a double-blind study. Pain. 1990;43:243-247.

50. Gam AN, Thorsen H, Lonnberg F. The effect of low-level laser therapy on musculoskeletal pain: a meta-analysis. Pain. 1993;52:63-66.

51. Modell JH. Observations of "acupuncture anaesthesia" in the People's Republic of China. Archives of Surgery. 1974; 109:731-733.

52. Dimond EG. Acupuncture anaesthesia: Western medicine and Chinese traditional medicine. JAMA. 1971;218:1558-1563.
53. Bonica JJ. Therapeutic acupuncture in the People's Republic of China: implications for American medicine. JAMA. 1974;228(12):1544-1551.
54. Taub HA. Acupuncture and sensorineural hearing loss: a review. Journal of Speech and Hearing Disorders. 1975;40:427-433.
55. Acupuncture: A History - Allegheny College: Webpub, http://webpub.allegheny.edu/employee/l/lcoates/CoatesPage/FS101/Articles_PDF/Acupuncture/acupuncture_history.pdf (accessed July 21, 2013).
56. Acupuncture: Past and Present, http://www.acuwatch.org/hx/basser.shtml (accessed July 21, 2013).
57. Taub HA. Acupuncture and sensorineural hearing loss: a review. Journal of Speech and Hearing Disorders. 1975;40: p.433.
58. Acupuncture - Wikipedia, the free encyclopedia, http://en.wikipedia.org/wiki/Jhenjiou (accessed July 21, 2013).
59. ^ a b Beyerstein, BL; Sampson W (1996). "Traditional Medicine and Pseudoscience in China: A Report of the Second CSICOP Delegation (Part 1)". Skeptical Inquirer (Committee for Skeptical Inquiry) 20 (4). http://www.csicop.org/si/show/china_conference_1/.
60. Gary P. Posner, M.D. and Wallace Sampson, M.D. Chinese Acupuncture For Heart Surgery Anesthesia. The Scientific Review of Alternative Medicine. Fall/Winter 1999
61. Rosenfeld I. Acupuncture goes mainstream (almost). Parade. August 16, 1998: 10-11.
62. Rosenfeld I. Dr. Rosenfeld's Guide to Alternative Medicine. New York, NY: Fawcett Columbine; 1996: 30-32.
63. Rosenfeld's Acupuncture Claim - Gary Posner's Home Page, http://www.gpposner.com/Rosenfeld_sram.html (accessed July 21, 2013).
64. Ibid.
65. Ibid.
66. Ibid.
67. Nolen W. Healing: A Doctor in Search of a Miracle. New York, NY: Random House; 1974.
68. Taub A. Acupuncture. In: The Health Robbers. Barrett S, Jarvis W, eds. Amherst, NY: Prometheus Books; 1993.
69. Herbert V. Personal communication with Wallace Sampson. Rosenfeld's Acupuncture Claim - Gary Posner's Home Page, http://www.gpposner.com/Rosenfeld_sram.html (accessed July 21, 2013).
70. Rosenfeld's Acupuncture Claim - Gary Posner's Home Page, http://www.gpposner.com/Rosenfeld_sram.html (accessed July 21, 2013).
71.^ H.W. Wilson Company (1987). Current Biography Yearbook. Silverplatter International. p. 455.
72.^ "Sullivan", Walter (July 27, 1988). "Water That Has a Memory? Skeptics Win Second Round". The New York Times. http://www.nytimes.com/1988/07/27/us/water-that-has-a-memory-skeptics-win-second-round.html.
73.^ Cohen, Patricia (February 17, 2001). "Poof! You're a Skeptic: The Amazing Randi's Vanishing Humbug". The New York Times. http://www.nytimes.com/2001/02/17/arts/17RAND.html. Retrieved May 5, 2010. [dead link]

74. ^ "Filipino Justice". Randi.org. May 19, 2006. http://www.randi.org/jr/2006-05/051906sylvia.html#i13. Retrieved June 15, 2009. James Randi - Wikipedia, the free encyclopedia, http://en.wikipedia.org/wiki/Randi,_James (accessed July 21, 2013).

75.^ Jaroff, Leon (June 24, 2001). "Fighting Against Flimflam". Time. http://www.time.com/time/magazine/article/0,9171,149448,00.html?iid=chix-sphere. Retrieved June 18, 2007.

76. James Randi - Wikipedia, the free encyclopedia, http://en.wikipedia.org/wiki/Randi,_James (accessed July 21, 2013).

77.^ a b Philip B., Jr., Taft (July 5, 1981). "A Charlatan in Pursuit of Truth". New York Times. James Randi - Wikipedia, the free encyclopedia, http://en.wikipedia.org/wiki/Randi,_James (accessed July 21, 2013).

78. Nolen W. Healing: A Doctor in Search of a Miracle. New York, NY: Random House; 1974. Rosenfeld's Acupuncture Claim - Gary Posner's Home Page, http://www.gpposner.com/Rosenfeld_sram.html (accessed July 21, 2013).

79. Randi J. Flim-Flam. Amherst, NY: Prometheus Books; 1982.

80. ^ Petit, Charles (May 23, 1991). "Bay Magicians Back Uri Geller's Critic". San Francisco Chronicle: p. A27.

81. ^ Randi, James (2006). "An Encyclopedia of Claims, Frauds, and Hoaxes of the Occult and Supernatural: Psychic surgery". St. Martin's Press. James Randi - Wikipedia, the free encyclopedia, http://en.wikipedia.org/wiki/Randi,_James (accessed July 21, 2013).

82. Beyerstein B, Sampson W. Traditional medicine and pseudoscience in China: a report of the second CSICOP delegation. Part 1. Skeptical Inquirer. 1996;20(4):18-26. Rosenfeld's Acupuncture Claim - Gary Posner's Home Page, http://www.gpposner.com/Rosenfeld_sram.html (accessed July 21, 2013).

83. Rosenfeld's Acupuncture Claim - Gary Posner's Home Page, http://www.gpposner.com/Rosenfeld_sram.html (accessed July 21, 2013).

84. Skrabanek P, McCormick J. Fads and Fallacies in Medicine. Amherst, NY: Prometheus Books; 1990.

85. Gary P. Posner, M.D. and Wallace Sampson, M.D. Chinese Acupuncture For Heart Surgery Anesthesia. The Scientific Review of Alternative Medicine. Fall/Winter 1999. Rosenfeld's Acupuncture Claim - Gary Posner's Home Page, http://www.gpposner.com/Rosenfeld_sram.html (accessed July 21, 2013).

86. Rosenfeld's Acupuncture Claim - Gary Posner's Home Page, http://www.gpposner.com/Rosenfeld_sram.html (accessed July 21, 2013).

87. Ibid.

88. Ibid.

89. Ibid.

90. Gary P. Posner, M.D. and Wallace Sampson, M.D. Chinese Acupuncture For Heart Surgery Anesthesia. The Scientific Review of Alternative Medicine. Fall/Winter 1999.

91. Acupuncture popularity soars despite thin evidence - The .., http://www.sfnewmexican.com/HealthandScience/Acupuncture--popularity-soars-despite-thin-evidence (accessed July 21, 2013).

92. Harriet Hall in "Be Wary of Acupuncture, Qigong, and Chinese Medicine." Stephen Barrett, M.D. Quackwatch. Be Wary of Acupuncture, Qigong, and "Chinese Medicine", http://www.quackwatch.org/01QuackeryRelatedTopics/acu.html (accessed July 21, 2013). 93. Tooth Fairy science - The Skeptic's Dictionary - Skepdic.com, http://skepdic.com/toothfairyscience.html (accessed July 21, 2013).

94. Ibid.
95. Ibid.
96. Ibid.
97. Acupuncture popularity soars despite thin evidence - The .., http://www.sfnewmexican.com/HealthandScience/Acupuncture--popularity-soars-despite-thin-evidence (accessed July 21, 2013).
98. ^ "Physicians Divided on Impact of CAM on U.S. Health Care; Aromatherapy Fares Poorly; Acupuncture Touted". HCD Research. 9 September 2005. Archived from the original on 2006-01-10. http://web.archive.org/web/20060110033955/http://publish.hcdhealth.com/P1007/CumulativeReport.htm.
99. ^ Report: Insurance Coverage for Acupuncture on the Rise. Michael Devitt, Acupuncture Today, January, 2005, Vol. 06, Issue 01
100. ^ Claxton, Gary; Isadora Gil, Ben Finder, Erin Holve, Jon Gabel, Jeremy Pickreighn, Heidi Whitmore, Samantha Hawkins, and Cheryl Fahlman (2004). The Kaiser Family Foundation and Health Research and Educational Trust Employer Health Benefits 2004 Annual Survey. Kaiser Family Foundation. pp. 106–7. ISBN 0-87258-812-2. http://www.kff.org/insurance/7148/upload/2004-Employer-Health-Benefits-Survey-Full-Report.pdf. Acupuncture - Basic Medical Terms - Diseases Symptoms, http://www.diseases-diagnosis.com/virtual/acupuncture (accessed July 21, 2013).
101. Be Wary of Acupuncture, Qigong, and "Chinese Medicine", http://www.quackwatch.org/01QuackeryRelatedTopics/acu.html (accessed July 21, 2013).
102. Ibid.
103. Acupuncture - Basic Medical Terms - Diseases Symptoms, http://www.diseases-diagnosis.com/virtual/acupuncture (accessed July 21, 2013).
104. ^ nccaom.org.
105. ^ State Licensure Table.
106. ^ Updates-June 1996 FDA Consumer.
107. ^ US FDA/CDRH: Premarket Approvals.
108. Acupuncture needle status changed. FDA Talk Paper T96-21, April 1, 1996. Updates-June 1996 FDA Consumer and ^ US FDA/CDRH: Premarket Approvals. Acupuncture - Basic Medical Terms - Diseases Symptoms, http://www.diseases-diagnosis.com/virtual/acupuncture (accessed July 21, 2013).
109.^ http://news.bbc.co.uk/2/hi/health/545019.stm
110.http://www.cancer.gov/cancertopics/pdq/cam/acupuncture/healthprofessional/Page5^ a b c d e f g "Acupuncture". US National Center for Complementary and Alternative Medicine. 2006. http://nccam.nih.gov/health/acupuncture/. Retrieved 2006-03-02.
111. ^ Novak, Patricia D.; Dorland, Norman W.; Dorland, William Alexander Newman (1995). Dorland's Pocket Medical Dictionary (25th ed.). Philadelphia: W.B. Saunders. ISBN 0-7216-5738-9. OCLC 33123537.
112. ^ a b c d e f g Ernst, E.; Pittler, MH; Wider, B; Boddy, K (2007). "Acupuncture: its evidence-base is changing.". The American Journal of Chinese Medicine 35 (1): 21–5. doi:10.1142/S0192415X07004588. PMID 17265547.
113. ^ Cherkin, D. C.; Sherman, K. J.; Avins, A. L.; Erro, J. H.; Ichikawa, L.; Barlow, W. E.; Delaney, K.; Hawkes, R. et al. (2009). "A Randomized Trial Comparing Acupuncture, Simulated Acupuncture, and Usual Care for Chronic Low Back Pain".

Archives of Internal Medicine 169 (9): 858–866. doi:10.1001/archinternmed.2009.65. PMC 2832641. PMID 19433697. edit

114. ^ a b c d e f g h Ernst, E. (2006). "Acupuncture - a critical analysis". Journal of Internal Medicine 259 (2): 125–137. doi:10.1111/j.1365-2796.2005.01584.x. PMID 16420542. edit

115. ^ Shapiro R (2008). Suckers: How alternative medicine makes fools of us all. Vintage Books. OCLC 267166615.

116. ^ a b c d e f g h i Goddard B (2008). "2. The Truth about Acupuncture". In Singh S, Ernst E. Trick or Treatment: The Undeniable Facts about Alternative Medicine. pp. 39–90.

117. ^ a b c d e f Ernst, E.; Lee, M. S.; Choi, T. Y. (2011). "Acupuncture: Does it alleviate pain and are there serious risks? A review of reviews" (pdf). PAIN 152 (4): 755–764. doi:10.1016/j.pain.2010.11.004. PMID 21440191. http://www.dieutridau.com/thongtin/detai/acupuncture-does-it.pdf. edit

118. ^ a b Abraham, J. (2008). "Acupressure and acupuncture in preventing and managing postoperative nausea and vomiting in adults". Journal of perioperative practice 18 (12): 543–551. PMID 19192550. edit

119. ^ a b c d Lee A, Fan, LTY (2009). Lee, Anna. ed. "Stimulation of the wrist acupuncture point P6 for preventing postoperative nausea and vomiting". Cochrane Database of Systematic Reviews (Online) (2): CD003281. doi:10.1002/14651858.CD003281.pub3. PMID 15266478. http://www.cochrane.org/reviews/en/ab003281.html.

120. ^ Lee A, Done ML (2004). Lee, Anna. ed. "Stimulation of the wrist acupuncture point P6 for preventing postoperative nausea and vomiting". Cochrane Database of Systematic Reviews (Online) (3): CD003281. doi:10.1002/14651858.CD003281.pub2. PMID 15266478. http://www.cochrane.org/reviews/en/ab003281.html.

121. ^ a b c Lee A, Copas JB, Henmi M, Gin T, Chung RC (2006). "Publication bias affected the estimate of postoperative nausea in an acupoint stimulation systematic review". J Clin Epidemiol. 59 (9): 980–3. doi:10.1016/j.jclinepi.2006.02.003. PMID 16895822. Online Wellness Network Information Resource: Acupuncture .., http://www.onlinewellnessnetwork.com/resource_descriptions.asp?mdid=136 (accessed July 21, 2013).

122. Acupuncture test & product | parasitology center inc, http://www.parasitetesting.com/Acupuncture.cfm (accessed July 21, 2013).

123. Ibid.

124. Texas State Acupuncture & Herbal Clinic | Houston, TXTexas .., http://houston-acupuncture.com/specific-conditions/ (accessed July 21, 2013).

125. Online Wellness Network Information Resource: Acupuncture .., http://www.onlinewellnessnetwork.com/resource_descriptions.asp?mdid=136 (accessed July 21, 2013).

126. ^ a b Abraham, J. (2008). "Acupressure and acupuncture in preventing and managing postoperative nausea and vomiting in adults". Journal of perioperative practice 18 (12): 543–551. PMID 19192550. edit. Online Wellness Network Information Resource: Acupuncture .., http://www.onlinewellnessnetwork.com/resource_descriptions.asp?mdid=136 (accessed July 21, 2013).

127. ^ a b c d Lee A, Fan, LTY (2009). Lee, Anna. ed. "Stimulation of the wrist acupuncture point P6 for preventing postoperative nausea and vomiting". Cochrane Database of Systematic Reviews (Online) (2): CD003281.

doi:10.1002/14651858.CD003281.pub3. PMID 15266478.
http://www.cochrane.org/reviews/en/ab003281.html. Acupuncture test & product | parasitology center inc, http://www.parasitetesting.com/Acupuncture.cfm (accessed July 21, 2013).
128. Online Wellness Network Information Resource: Acupuncture .., http://www.onlinewellnessnetwork.com/resource_descriptions.asp?mdid=136 (accessed July 21, 2013).
129. ^ Ezzo, JM; Richardson, MA; Vickers, A; Allen, C; Dibble, SL; Issell, BF; Lao, L; Pearl, M et al. (2006). Ezzo, Jeanette. ed. "Acupuncture-point stimulation for chemotherapy-induced nausea or vomiting". Cochrane Database of Systematic Reviews (Online) (2): CD002285. doi:10.1002/14651858.CD002285.pub2. PMID 16625560. http://www.cochrane.org/reviews/en/ab002285.html.
130. ^ a b c d e f g h Ernst, E. (2006). "Acupuncture - a critical analysis". Journal of Internal Medicine 259 (2): 125–137. doi:10.1111/j.1365-2796.2005.01584.x. PMID 16420542. edit 131. ^ a b c d e Furlan, Andrea D; Van Tulder, Maurits W; Cherkin, Dan; Tsukayama, Hiroshi; Lao, Lixing; Koes, Bart W; Berman, Brian M (2005). Furlan, Andrea D. ed. "Acupuncture and dry-needling for low back pain" (pdf). Cochrane Database Syst Rev (1): CD001351. doi:10.1002/14651858.CD001351.pub2. PMID 15674876. http://www.thecochranelibrary.com/userfiles/ccoch/file/Acupuncture_ancient_traditions/CD001351.pdf.
132. ^ a b c d e f Madsen, M. V.; Gotzsche, P. C; Hrobjartsson, A. (2009). "Acupuncture treatment for pain: systematic review of randomised clinical trials with acupuncture, placebo acupuncture, and no acupuncture groups". BMJ 338: a3115. doi:10.1136/bmj.a3115. PMC 2769056. PMID 19174438.
133. ^ a b c d e f Ernst, E.; Lee, M. S.; Choi, T. Y. (2011). "Acupuncture: Does it alleviate pain and are there serious risks? A review of reviews" (pdf). PAIN 152 (4): 755–764. doi:10.1016/j.pain.2010.11.004. PMID 21440191. http://www.dieutridau.com/thongtin/detai/acupuncture-does-it.pdf. edit
134. Peter Ky Lee, MD, Thorkild W. Andersen, MD, Jerome H. Modell, MD and Segundina A. Saga, MD. Treatment of Chronic Pain With Acupuncture. (JAMA 232:1133-1135, 1975) doi: 10.1001/jama.1975.03250110015013. JAMA Network | JAMA | Treatment of Chronic Pain With Acupuncture, http://jama.jamanetwork.com/article.aspx?articleid=336776 (accessed July 21, 2013).
135. Ibid.
136. JAMA Network | JAMA | Treatment of Chronic Pain With Acupuncture, http://jama.jamanetwork.com/article.aspx?articleid=336776 (accessed July 21, 2013).
137. Texas State Acupuncture & Herbal Clinic | Houston, TXTexas .., http://houston-acupuncture.com/specific-conditions/ (accessed July 21, 2013).
138. ^ a b c d e f Madsen, M. V.; Gotzsche, P. C; Hrobjartsson, A. (2009). "Acupuncture treatment for pain: systematic review of randomised clinical trials with acupuncture, placebo acupuncture, and no acupuncture groups". BMJ 338: a3115. doi:10.1136/bmj.a3115. PMC 2769056. PMID 19174438.
139. ^ a b c d e f Ernst, E.; Lee, M. S.; Choi, T. Y. (2011). "Acupuncture: Does it alleviate pain and are there serious risks? A review of reviews" (pdf). PAIN 152 (4): 755–764. doi:10.1016/j.pain.2010.11.004. PMID 21440191. http://www.dieutridau.com/thongtin/detai/acupuncture-does-it.pdf. edit
140. ^ Lee, M. S.; Ernst, E. (2011). "Acupuncture for pain: An overview of Cochrane reviews". Chinese Journal of Integrative Medicine 17 (3): 187–189. doi:10.1007/s11655-011-0665-7. PMID 21359919. edit

141. Acupuncture - Sources Media Relations Experts News Releases .., http://www.sources.com/SSR/Docs/SSRW-Acupuncture.htm (accessed July 21, 2013).
142. ^ a b c d e Furlan, Andrea D; Van Tulder, Maurits W; Cherkin, Dan; Tsukayama, Hiroshi; Lao, Lixing; Koes, Bart W; Berman, Brian M (2005). Furlan, Andrea D. ed. "Acupuncture and dry-needling for low back pain" (pdf). Cochrane Database Syst Rev (1): CD001351. doi:10.1002/14651858.CD001351.pub2. PMID 15674876. http://www.thecochranelibrary.com/userfiles/ccoch/file/Acupuncture_ancient_traditions/CD001351.pdf.
143. ^ Manheimer E, White A, Berman B, Forys K, Ernst E (2005). "Meta-analysis: acupuncture for low back pain" (PDF). Ann Intern Med 142 (8): 651–63. PMID 15838072. http://www.annals.org/cgi/reprint/142/8/651.pdf.
144. ^ Chou, R.; Huffman, L. H.; American Pain, S.; American College Of, P. (2007). "Nonpharmacologic therapies for acute and chronic low back pain: A review of the evidence for an American Pain Society/American College of Physicians clinical practice guideline". Annals of internal medicine 147 (7): 492–504. PMID 17909210. edit
145. Veterinarywatch: On the NIDA Consensus Conference on Acupuncture, http://www.veterinarywatch.com/NIDA.htm (accessed July 21, 2013).
146. Wallace Sampson, Editor. On the National Institute of Drug Abuse Consensus Conference on Acupuncture. Scientific Review of Alternative Medicine, v2,n1, 1998
147. Veterinarywatch: On the NIDA Consensus Conference on Acupuncture, http://www.veterinarywatch.com/NIDA.htm (accessed July 21, 2013).
148. Ibid.
149. Ibid.
150. Wallace Sampson, Editor. On the National Institute of Drug Abuse Consensus Conference on Acupuncture. Scientific Review of Alternative Medicine, v2,n1, 1998.
151.^ a b c d e f g h i j k l m n o p q r s NIH Consensus Development Program (November 3–5, 1997). "Acupuncture --Consensus Development Conference Statement". National Institutes of Health. http://consensus.nih.gov/1997/1997Acupuncture107html.htm. Retrieved 2007-07-17. Veterinarywatch: On the NIDA Consensus Conference on Acupuncture, http://www.veterinarywatch.com/NIDA.htm (accessed July 21, 2013). Thank you! Share Grammarly on Facebook!
University of San Clemente - Courses, Programs, Degrees .., http://corporatefitnessorangecounty.com/ (accessed July 21, 2013).
152. Veterinarywatch: On the NIDA Consensus Conference on Acupuncture, http://www.veterinarywatch.com/NIDA.htm (accessed July 21, 2013).
153. Ibid.
154. Ibid.
155. Ibid.
156. Ibid.
157. Ibid.
158. Ter Reit G, Kleijnen J, Knipschild P. Acupuncture and chronic pain: a criteria-based meta-analysis. J Clin Epidem. 1990:43 1191-1199.
159. National Council Against Health Fraud (Sampson W, ed.) Acupuncture: riw position paper of the National Council Against Health Fraud. Clin J of Pain. 1991;7(2) 162-166.
160. ^ a b c d e f g "Acupuncture". US National Center for Complementary and Alternative Medicine. 2006. http://nccam.nih.gov/health/acupuncture/. Retrieved

2006-03-02. Acupuncture - Sources Media Relations Experts News Releases ..,
http://www.sources.com/SSR/Docs/SSRW-Acupuncture.htm (accessed July 21,
2013).
161. Online Wellness Network Information Resource: Acupuncture ..,
http://www.onlinewellnessnetwork.com/resource_descriptions.asp?mdid=136
(accessed July 21, 2013).
162. University of San Clemente - Courses, Programs, Degrees ..,
http://corporatefitnessorangecounty.com/ (accessed July 21, 2013).
163. Singh & Ernst. Trick or Treatment 2008, p. 277-8.
164. ^ a b c d e f g h Ernst, E. (2006). "Acupuncture - a critical analysis". Journal of Internal Medicine 259 (2): 125–137. doi:10.1111/j.1365-2796.2005.01584.x. PMID 16420542. edit
165. Acupuncture - Basic Medical Terms - Diseases Symptoms, http://www.diseases-diagnosis.com/virtual/acupuncture (accessed July 21, 2013).
166. ^ a b "Acupuncture: Evidence for its effectiveness". National Health Service. 2010-03-18. http://www.nhs.uk/Conditions/Acupuncture/Pages/Evidence.aspx. Retrieved 2010-08-10. Acupuncture - Basic Medical Terms - Diseases Symptoms, http://www.diseases-diagnosis.com/virtual/acupuncture (accessed July 21, 2013).
167. Thomas M, Eriksson SV, Lundeberg T. A comparative study of diazepam and acupuncture in patients with osteoarthritis pain: a placebo controlled study. American Journal of Chinese Medicine. 1991;19(2):95-100.
168. Godfrey CM, Morgan P. A controlled trial of the theory of acupuncture in musculoskeletal pain. Journal of Rheumatology. 1978;5(2):121-124.
169. Fox EJ, Melzack R. Transcutaneous electrical stimulation and acupuncture: comparison of treatment for low back pain. Pain. 1976;2(2):141-148.
170. Helms JM. Acupuncture for the management of primary dysmenorrhea. Obstetrics and Gynaecology. 1987;69:51-56.
171. Ghia J N, et al. Acupuncture and chronic pain mechanisms. Pain. 1976;2(3):285-299.
172. Gaw AC, Chang LW, Shaw LC. Efficacy of acupuncture on osteoarthritic pain. NEJM. 1975;293:375-378.
173. Edelist G, Gross AE, Langer F. Treatment of low back pain with acupuncture. Canadian Anaesthetic Society Journal. May 1976; 23(3):303-306.
174. Lee PK, et al. Treatment of chronic pain with acupuncture.JAMA. 1975;232:1133-1135.
175. Lewith GT, Field J, Machin D. Acupuncture compared with placebo in post-herpetic pain. Pain. 1983;17:361-368.
176. Tavola T, et al. Traditional Chinese acupuncture in tension type headache: a controlled study. Pain. 1992;48(3):325-329.
177. Moore ME, Berk SN. Acupuncture for chronic shoulder pain: an experimental study with attention to the role of placebo and hypnotic suggestibility. Annals of Internal Medicine. 1976;84(4):381-384.
178. Laitinen J. Treatment of cervical syndrome by acupuncture. Scandinavian Journal of Rehabilitation Medicine. 1975;7(3): 114-117.
179. Mendelson G, et al. Acupuncture treatment of chronic back pain: a double-blind placebo-controlled trial. American Journal of Medicine. 1983; 4(1):49-55.
180. Cheng RSS, Pomeranz B. Electrotherapy of chronic musculoskeletal pain: comparison of electroacupuncture and acupuncture-like trans cutaneous electrical nerve stimulation. Clinical Journal of Pain. 1987;2:143-149.

181. Tandon MK, Soh PFT, Wood AT. Acupuncture for bronchial asthma? A double-blind crossover study. Medical Journal of Australia. 1991;154: 409-412.
182. Day RL, et al. Evaluation of acupuncture anaesthesia: a psychophysical study. Anaesthesiology. 1975;43:507-517.
183. Ekblom A, et al. Increased postoperative pain and consumption of analgesics following acupuncture. Pain. 1991;44: 241-247.
184. Haker E, Lundeberg T. Acupuncture treatment in epicondylagia: a comparative study of two acupuncture techniques. Clinical Journal of Pain. 1990;6(3):221-226.
185. Gemmell HA, Jacobsen BH. Time-series study of auriculotherapy in the treatment of shoulder pain. Journal of the Australian Chiropractors' Association. 1990;20(3):82-84. 186. Richardson PH, Vincent CA. Acupuncture for the treatment of pain: a review of evaluative research. Pain. 1986;24(1): 15-40.
187. Bhatt-Sanders D. Acupuncture and rheumatoid arthritis: an analysis of the literature. Seminars in Arthritis and Rheumatism. 1985;14(4):225-231.
188. Ter Riet G, Kleijnen J, Knipschild P. Acupuncture and chronic pain: A criteria based meta-analysis. Journal of Clinical Epidemiology. 1990;43(11):1191-1996.
189. Patel M, et al. A meta-analysis of acupuncture for chronic pain. International Journal of Epidemiology. 1989;18(4):900-906
190. Aldridge D, Pietroni PC. Clinical assessment of acupuncture in asthma therapy: discussion paper. Journal of the Royal Society of Medicine. 1987;80(4):222-224.
191. Acupuncture: Past and Present, http://www.acuwatch.org/hx/basser.shtml (accessed July 21, 2013).
192. Godfrey CM, Morgan P. A controlled trial of the theory of acupuncture in musculoskeletal pain. Journal of Rheumatology. 1978;5(2):121-124.
193. Ghia J N, et al. Acupuncture and chronic pain mechanisms. Pain. 1976;2(3):285-299.
194. Gaw AC, Chang LW, Shaw LC. Efficacy of acupuncture on osteoarthritic pain. NEJM. 1975;293:375-378.
195. Edelist G, Gross AE, Langer F. Treatment of low back pain with acupuncture. Canadian Anaesthetic Society Journal. May 1976; 23(3):303-306.
196. Lee PK, et al. Treatment of chronic pain with acupuncture. JAMA. 1975;232:1133-1135.
197. Tavola T, et al. Traditional Chinese acupuncture in tension type headache: a controlled study. Pain. 1992;48(3):325-329.
198. Acupuncture: Past and Present, http://www.acuwatch.org/hx/basser.shtml (accessed July 21, 2013).
199. Deyo RA, et al. A controlled trial of trans cutaneous electrical nerve stimulation (TENS) and exercise for chronic low back pain .NEJM. 1990;322(23):1627-1634.
200. Langley GB, et al. The analgesic effects of trans cutaneous electrical nerve stimulation and placebo in chronic pain patients. Rheumatol. Int. 1984;2:1-5.
201. Thornsteinsson G, et al. The placebo effect of transcutaneous electrical stimulation. Pain. 1978;5:31-41.
202. Acupuncture: Past and Present, http://www.acuwatch.org/hx/basser.shtml (accessed July 21, 2013).
203. Botek ST. One doctor's acupuncture odyssey. Medical Tribune. May 2, 1984,
204. ^ "Cochrane and Alternative Medicine - Acupuncture". Danish Knowledge and Research Center for Alternative Medicines. 2011-09-28. http://www.vifab.dk/uk/cochrane+and+alternative+medicine/acupuncture?. Retrieved 2011-10-19. Online Wellness Network Information Resource: Acupuncture ..,

http://www.onlinewellnessnetwork.com/resource_descriptions.asp?mdid=136 (accessed July 21, 2013).
205. Ibid.
206. Ibid.
207. ^ McCarney, RW; Brinkhaus, B; Lasserson, TJ; Linde, K; McCarney, Robert W (2003). McCarney, Robert W. ed. "Acupuncture for chronic asthma". Cochrane Database of Systematic Reviews 2003 (3): CD000008. doi:10.1002/14651858.CD000008.pub2. PMID 14973944. http://www.cochrane.org/reviews/en/ab000008.html. Retrieved 2008-05-02.
208. ^ He, L; Zhou, MK; Zhou, D; Wu, B; Li, N; Kong, SY; Zhang, DP; Li, QF et al. (2004). He, Li. ed. "Acupuncture for Bell's palsy". Cochrane Database of Systematic Reviews 2007 (4): CD002914. doi:10.1002/14651858.CD002914.pub3. PMID 17943775. http://www.cochrane.org/reviews/en/ab002914.html. Retrieved 2008-05-02.
209. ^ Gates, S; Smith, LA; Foxcroft, DR; Gates, Simon (2006). Gates, Simon. ed. "Auricular acupuncture for cocaine dependence". Cochrane Database of Systematic Reviews 2006 (1): CD005192. doi:10.1002/14651858.CD005192.pub2. PMID 16437523. http://www.cochrane.org/reviews/en/ab005192.html. Retrieved 2008-05-02.
210. ^ Smith, CA; Hay, PP; Smith, Caroline A (2004-03-17). Smith, Caroline A. ed. "Acupuncture for depression". Cochrane Database of Systematic Reviews 2004 (3): CD004046. doi:10.1002/14651858.CD004046.pub2. PMID 15846693. http://www.cochrane.org/reviews/en/ab004046.html. Retrieved 2008-05-02.
211. ^ Jordan, J (2006). "Acupuncture treatment for opiate addiction: A systematic review". Journal of Substance Abuse Treatment 30 (4): 309–14. doi:10.1016/j.jsat.2006.02.005. PMID 16716845.
212. ^ Gates, Simon; Smith, Lesley A; Foxcroft, David (2006). Gates, Simon. ed. "Auricular acupuncture for cocaine dependence". Cochrane Database Syst Rev (1): CD005192. doi:10.1002/14651858.CD005192.pub2. PMID 16437523.
213. ^ Bearn, Jennifer; Swami, Anshul; Stewart, Duncan; Atnas, Catherine; Giotto, Lisa; Gossop, Michael (2009). "Auricular acupuncture as an adjunct to opiate detoxification treatment: Effects on withdrawal symptoms". Journal of Substance Abuse Treatment 36 (3): 345–9. doi:10.1016/j.jsat.2008.08.002. PMID 19004596
214. ^ Cheuk, DK; Wong, V; Cheuk, Daniel (2006). Cheuk, Daniel. ed. "Acupuncture for epilepsy". Cochrane Database of Systematic Reviews 2006 (2): CD005062. doi:10.1002/14651858.CD005062.pub2. PMID 16625622. http://www.cochrane.org/reviews/en/ab005062.html. Retrieved 2008-05-02.
215. ^ Mayhew E; Ernst E (2007). "Acupuncture for fibromyalgia—a systematic review of randomized clinical trials". Rheumatology (Oxford, England) 46 (5): 801–4. doi:10.1093/rheumatology/kel406. PMID 17189243.
216. ^ Law, SK; Li, T; Law, Simon K (2007). Law, Simon K. ed. "Acupuncture for glaucoma". Cochrane Database of Systematic Reviews 2007 (4): CD006030. doi:10.1002/14651858.CD006030.pub2. PMID 17943876. http://www.cochrane.org/reviews/en/ab006030.html. Retrieved 2008-05-02.
217. Acupuncture - Sources Media Relations Experts News Releases .., http://www.sources.com/SSR/Docs/SSRW-Acupuncture.htm (accessed July 21, 2013).
218. ^ Cheuk, DK; Yeung, WF; Chung, KF; Wong, V; Cheuk, Daniel KL (2007). Cheuk, Daniel KL. ed. "Acupuncture for insomnia". Cochrane Database of Systematic Reviews 2007 (3): CD005472. doi:10.1002/14651858.CD005472.pub2.

PMID 17636800. http://www.cochrane.org/reviews/en/ab005472.html. Retrieved 2008-05-02.
219. ^ Lim, B; Manheimer, E; Lao, L; Ziea, E; Wisniewski, J; Liu, J; Berman, B; Manheimer, Eric (2006). Manheimer, Eric. ed. "Acupuncture for treatment of irritable bowel syndrome". Cochrane Database of Systematic Reviews 2006 (4): CD005111. doi:10.1002/14651858.CD005111.pub2. PMID 17054239. http://www.cochrane.org/reviews/en/ab005111.html. Retrieved 2008-05-06.
220. ^ Smith, CA; Crowther, CA; Smith, Caroline A (2004). Smith, Caroline A. ed. "Acupuncture for induction of labour". Cochrane Database of Systematic Reviews 2004 (1): CD002962. doi:10.1002/14651858.CD002962.pub2. PMID 14973999. http://www.cochrane.org/reviews/en/ab002962.html. Retrieved 2008-05-06.
221. ^ Casimiro, L; Barnsley, L; Brosseau, L; Milne, S; Robinson, VA; Tugwell, P; Wells, G; Casimiro, Lynn (2005). Casimiro, Lynn. ed. "Acupuncture and electroacupuncture for the treatment of rheumatoid arthritis". Cochrane Database of Systematic Reviews 2005 (4): CD003788. doi:10.1002/14651858.CD003788.pub2. PMID 16235342. http://www.cochrane.org/reviews/en/ab003788.html. Retrieved 2008-05-06.
222. ^ Green, S; Buchbinder, R; Hetrick, S; Green, Sally (2005). Green, Sally. ed. "Acupuncture for shoulder pain". Cochrane Database of Systematic Reviews 2005 (2): CD005319. doi:10.1002/14651858.CD005319. PMID 15846753. http://www.cochrane.org/reviews/en/ab005319.html. Retrieved 2008-05-06.
223. ^ Rathbone, J; Xia, J; Rathbone, John (2005). Rathbone, John. ed. "Acupuncture for schizophrenia". Cochrane Database of Systematic Reviews 2005 (4): CD005475. doi:10.1002/14651858.CD005475. PMID 16235404. http://www.cochrane.org/reviews/en/ab005475.html. Retrieved 2008-05-06.
224. ^ Zhang, SH; Liu, M; Asplund, K; Li, L; Liu, Ming (2005). Liu, Ming. ed. "Acupuncture for acute stroke". Cochrane Database of Systematic Reviews 2005 (2): CD003317. doi:10.1002/14651858.CD003317.pub2. PMID 15846657. http://www.cochrane.org/reviews/en/ab003317.html. Retrieved 2008-05-06.
225. ^ Wu, HM; Tang, JL; Lin, XP; Lau, J; Leung, PC; Woo, J; Li, YP; Wu, Hong Mei (2006). Wu, Hong Mei. ed. "Acupuncture for stroke rehabilitation". Cochrane Database of Systematic Reviews 2006 (3): CD004131. doi:10.1002/14651858.CD004131.pub2. PMID 16856031. http://www.cochrane.org/reviews/en/ab004131.html. Retrieved 2008-05-06.
226. ^ Green, S; Buchbinder, R; Barnsley, L; Hall, S; White, M; Smidt, N; Assendelft, W; Green, Sally (2002). Green, Sally. ed. "Acupuncture for lateral elbow pain". Cochrane Database of Systematic Reviews 2002 (1): CD003527. doi:10.1002/14651858.CD003527. PMID 11869671. http://www.cochrane.org/reviews/en/ab003527.html. Retrieved 2008-05-06.
227. ^ Peng, WN; Zhao, H; Liu, ZS; Wang, S; Weina, Peng (2008). Weina, Peng. ed. "Acupuncture for vascular dementia". Cochrane Database of Systematic Reviews 2007 (2): CD004987. doi:10.1002/14651858.CD004987.pub2. PMID 17443563. http://www.cochrane.org/reviews/en/ab004987.html. Retrieved 2008-05-06.
228. Helms, Acupuncture for the management of primary dysmenorrhea. Obstet Gynecol. 1987 Jan;69(1):51-6.
229. ^ "Cochrane and Alternative Medicine – Acupuncture". Danish Knowledge and Research Center for Alternative Medicines. 2011-09-28. http://www.vifab.dk/uk/cochrane+and+alternative+medicine/acupuncture? Retrieved 2011-10-19. Online Wellness Network Information Resource: Acupuncture ..,

http://www.onlinewellnessnetwork.com/resource_descriptions.asp?mdid=136 (accessed July 21, 2013).

230. ^ Proctor, ML; Smith, CA; Farquhar, CM; Stones, RW; Zhu, Xiaoshu; Brown, Julie; Zhu, Xiaoshu (2002). Zhu, Xiaoshu. ed. "Transcutaneous electrical nerve stimulation and acupuncture for primary dysmenorrhoea". Cochrane Database of Systematic Reviews 2002 (1): CD002123. doi:10.1002/14651858.CD002123. PMID 11869624. http://www.cochrane.org/reviews/en/ab002123.html. Retrieved 2008-05-02.

231. ^ Isaacs, Lyndsey; West, Zita (2008). Acupuncture in pregnancy and childbirth. Philadelphia: Churchill Livingstone/Elsevier. ISBN 0-443-10371-2. http://books.google.ca/books?id=BhVvDfLypxIC&printsec=frontcover#v=onepage&q&f=false.Online Wellness Network Information Resource: Acupuncture .., http://www.onlinewellnessnetwork.com/resource_descriptions.asp?mdid=136 (accessed July 21, 2013).

232. Tandon, Soh, and Wood, Acupuncture for bronchial asthma?

233. Aldridge and Pietroni, Clinical assessment of acupuncture in asthma therapy.

234. Jerner B, Skogh M, Vahlquist A. A controlled trial of acupuncture in psoriasis: no convincing effect. Acta Derm Venereol (Stockh). 1997;77:154-156.

235. White AR, Rampes H, Liu JP, Stead LF, Campbell J. Acupuncture and related interventions for smoking cessation. Cochrane Database of Systematic Reviews 2011. Issue 1. Art. No.: CD000009. DOI: 10.1002/14651858.CD000009.pub3. Acupuncture and related therapies do not appear to help .., http://summaries.cochrane.org/CD000009/acupuncture-and-related-therapies-do-not-appear-to-help-smokers-who-are-trying-to-quit. (accessed July 21, 2013).

236. Acupuncture and related therapies do not appear to help .., http://summaries.cochrane.org/CD000009/acupuncture-and-related-therapies-do-not-appear-to-help-smokers-who-are-trying-to-quit. (accessed July 21, 2013).

237. Ibid.

238. Acupuncture may not help relieve birth pains - News - BJOG .., http://www.bjog.org/details/news/688257/Acupuncture_may_not_help_relieve_birth_pains.html (accessed July 21, 2013).

239. MacKenzie, I., Xu, J., Cusick, C., Midwinter-Morten, H., Meacher, H., Mollison, J. and Brock, M. (2011), Acupuncture for pain relief during induced labour in nulliparae: a randomised controlled study. BJOG: An International Journal of Obstetrics & Gynaecology, 2011. 118: 440–447. doi: 10.1111/j.1471-0528.2010.02825.x Posted online. January 18, 2011.

240. Cho SH, Lee H, Ernst E. Acupuncture for pain relief in labour: a systematic review and meta-analysis. BJOG. 2010 Jul;117(8):907-20. Epub 2010 Apr 28. DOI: 10.1111/j.1471-0528.2010.02570.x. Acupuncture may not help relieve birth pains - News - BJOG .., http://www.bjog.org/details/news/688257/Acupuncture_may_not_help_relieve_birth_pains.html (accessed July 21, 2013).

241. Acupuncture may not help relieve birth pains - News - BJOG .., http://www.bjog.org/details/news/688257/Acupuncture_may_not_help_relieve_birth_pains.html (accessed July 21, 2013).

242. Ibid.

243. Ibid.

244. Ramnero A, Hanson U, Kihlgren M., Department of Obstetrics and Gynaecology, Orebro University Hospital, Sweden. Acupuncture treatment during labour--a randomised controlled trial. Published on Acubalance Wellness Centre -

Acupuncture Infertility Clinic - IVF Support - Pregnancy (Vancouver Langley Surrey) (http://www.acubalance.ca). Acupuncture Treatment During Labour: A Randomised Controlled ..,
http://www.chiro.org/acupuncture/ABSTRACTS/Acupuncture_Treatment_During_Labour.shtml (accessed July 21, 2013).
245. Gorski T, Does Acupuncture Affect Labor and Delivery? Sci Rev Alt Med 3(1):42-45, 1999. (c) 1999 Prometheus Books. Alternative methods of childbirth pain relief-acupunture, http://www.painfreebirthing.com/english/acupuncture.htm (accessed July 21, 2013).
246. Eappen S, Robbins D., Nonpharmacological means of pain relief for labor and delivery, Int Anesthesiol Clini. 2002 Fall; 40(4): 103-14, Review. Alternative methods of childbirth pain relief-acupunture,
http://www.painfreebirthing.com/english/acupuncture.htm (accessed July 21, 2013).
247. Linde, K et al. Acupuncture for Patients With Migraine. Journal of the American Medical Association. (JAMA) 2005. 293. (17) 2118-2125. doi: 10.1001/jama.293.17.2118. The quack page, http://www.ucl.ac.uk/pharmacology/dc-bits-old/quack4.html (accessed July 21, 2013).
248. The quack page, http://www.ucl.ac.uk/pharmacology/dc-bits-old/quack4.html (accessed July 21, 2013).
249. Melchart, D et al. Acupuncture in patients with tension-type headache: randomised controlled trial. BMJ 2005;331:376. BMJ 2005; 331 doi: 10.1136/bmj.38512.405440.8F (Published 11 August 2005).The quack page, http://www.ucl.ac.uk/pharmacology/dc-bits-old/quack4.html (accessed July 21, 2013).
250. Tavola T, Gala C, Conte G, Invernizzi G. Traditional Chinese acupuncture in tension-type headache: a controlled study. Pain. 1992 Mar;48(3):325-9. http://www.ncbi.nlm.nih.gov/pubmed/1594255 (accessed July 21, 2013).
251. Traditional Chinese acupuncture in tension-type headache: a ..,
http://www.ncbi.nlm.nih.gov/pubmed/1594255 (accessed July 21, 2013).
252. ^ White A, Foster NE, Cummings M, Barlas P (2007). "Acupuncture treatment for chronic knee pain: a systematic review". Rheumatology 46 (3): 384–90. doi:10.1093/rheumatology/kel413. PMID 17215263.
253. ^ Selfe TK, Taylor AG (2008 Jul–Sep). "Acupuncture and osteoarthritis of the knee: a review of randomized, controlled trials". Fam Community Health 31 (3): 247–54. doi:10.1097/01.FCH.0000324482.78577.0f (inactive 2009-11-14). PMC 2810544. PMID 18552606.
254. ^ a b Manheimer, E; Linde, K; Lao, L; Bouter, LM; Berman, BM (2007). "Meta-analysis: acupuncture for osteoarthritis of the knee.". Annals of internal medicine 146 (12): 868–77. PMID 17577006.
255. Albert C. Gaw, M.D., Lennig W. Chang, M.D., and Lein-Chun Shaw, M.D. Efficacy of Acupuncture on Osteoarthritic Pain — A Controlled, Double-Blind Study. N Engl J Med 1975; 293:375-378August 21, 1975
256. Richardson PH, Vincent CA. Acupuncture for the treatment of pain: a review of the evaluative research. Pain. 1986;23: 15-40.
257. ^ Zhang, W; Moskowitz, RW; Nuki, G; Abramson, S; Altman, RD; Arden, N; Bierma-Zeinstra, S; Brandt, KD et al. (2008). "OARSI recommendations for the management of hip and knee osteoarthritis, Part II: OARSI evidence-based, expert consensus guidelines" (pdf). Osteoarthritis and Cartilage 16 (2): 137–162. doi:10.1016/j.joca.2007.12.013. PMID 18279766.

http://www.oarsi.org/pdfs/oarsi_recommendations_for_management_of_hip_and_knee_oa.pdf.
258. ^ Manheimer, E.; Cheng, K.; Linde, K.; Lao, L.; Yoo, J.; Wieland, S.; Van Der Windt, D. L. A. M.; Berman, B. M. et al. (2010). Acupuncture for peripheral joint osteoarthritis. In Manheimer, Eric. "Acupuncture for peripheral joint osteoarthritis". Cochrane database of systematic reviews (Online) (1): CD001977.
doi:10.1002/14651858.CD001977.pub2. PMC 3169099. PMID 20091527. edit
259. The Scientific Review of Alternative Medicine and Aberrant Medical Practices. Fall/Winter 1999.
260. Editorial. Does acupuncture relieve pain? BMJ 2009;338:a2760 doi: 10.1136/bmj.a2760.
261. J. David, S. Townsend, R. Sathanathan, S. Kriss and C. J. Dorél The effect of acupuncture on patients with rheumatoid arthritis: a randomized, placebo-controlled cross-over study. Rheumatology (1999) 38 (9): 864-869. doi:
10.1093/rheumatology/38.9.864.
262. Ernst E. Acupuncture as a symptomatic treatment of osteoarthritis. Scand J Rheumatol 1997;26:444–7.
263.^ a b c d e f g h i j k l m n o p q r s NIH Consensus Development Program (November 3–5, 1997). "Acupuncture --Consensus Development Conference Statement". National Institutes of Health.
http://consensus.nih.gov/1997/1997Acupuncture107html.htm. Retrieved 2007-07-17.
264.^ a b c d e f Ernst, G; Strzyz, H; Hagmeister, H (2003). "Incidence of adverse effects during acupuncture therapy—a multicentre survey". Complementary Therapies in Medicine 11 (2): 93–7. doi:10.1016/S0965-2299(03)00004-9. PMID 12801494.
265. Ibid.
266. ^ a b c d e f Lao L, Hamilton GR, Fu J, Berman BM (2003). "Is acupuncture safe? A systematic review of case reports". Alternative therapies in health and medicine 9 (1): 72–83. PMID 12564354.
267. ^ a b Lewith, G; Field, J; MacHin, D (1983). "Acupuncture compared with placebo in post-herpetic pain". Pain 17 (4): 361–8. doi:10.1016/0304-3959(83)90167-7. PMID 6664681.
University of San Clemente - Courses, Programs, Degrees ..,
http://corporatefitnessorangecounty.com/ (accessed July 21, 2013).
268. ^ a b Flachskampf, F. A.; Gallasch, J.; Gefeller, O.; Gan, J.; Mao, J.; Pfahlberg, A. B.; Wortmann, A.; Klinghammer, L. et al. (2007). "Randomized Trial of Acupuncture to Lower Blood Pressure". Circulation 115 (24): 3121–9.
doi:10.1161/CIRCULATIONAHA.106.661140. PMID 17548730. Acupuncture - Wikipedia, the free encyclopedia, http://en.wikipedia.org/wiki/Acu_detox (accessed July 21, 2013).
269. ^ a b c d e f Lao L, Hamilton GR, Fu J, Berman BM (2003). "Is acupuncture safe? A systematic review of case reports". Alternative therapies in health and medicine 9 (1): 72–83. PMID 12564354.
270. ^ Norheim, Arne Johan (1996). "Adverse Effects of Acupuncture: A Study of the Literature for the Years 1981–1994". The Journal of Alternative and Complementary Medicine 2 (2): 291–7. doi:10.1089/acm.1996.2.291. PMID 9395661. The Use of Acupuncture in Addiction Treatment Programs ..,
http://article.wn.com/view/2012/07/16/The_Use_of_Acupuncture_in_Addiction_Treatment_Programs/ (accessed July 21, 2013).

271. ^ a b Woo, P. C Y; Lin, A. W C; Lau, S. K P; Yuen, K.-Y. (2010). "Acupuncture transmitted infections". BMJ 340: c1268. doi:10.1136/bmj.c1268. PMID 20299695. http://www.bmj.com/content/340/bmj.c1268.full. Acupuncture - Wikipedia, the free encyclopedia, http://en.wikipedia.org/wiki/Acu_detox (accessed July 21, 2013).
272. ^ White, A.; Hayhoe, S.; Hart, A.; Ernst, E. (2001). "Adverse events following acupuncture: prospective survey of 32 000 consultations with doctors and physiotherapists". BMJ 323 (7311): 485–6. doi:10.1136/bmj.323.7311.485. PMC 48133. PMID 11532840. The Use of Acupuncture in Addiction Treatment Programs .., http://article.wn.com/view/2012/07/16/The_Use_of_Acupuncture_in_Addiction_Treatment_Programs/ (accessed July 21, 2013).
273. ^ a b c d e f Ernst, G; Strzyz, H; Hagmeister, H (2003). "Incidence of adverse effects during acupuncture therapy—a multicentre survey". Complementary Therapies in Medicine 11 (2): 93–7. doi:10.1016/S0965-2299(03)00004-9. PMID 12801494.
274. ^ a b c d e f Ernst, E.; Lee, M. S.; Choi, T. Y. (2011). "Acupuncture: Does it alleviate pain and are there serious risks? A review of reviews" (pdf). PAIN 152 (4): 755–764. doi:10.1016/j.pain.2010.11.004. PMID 21440191. http://www.dieutridau.com/thongtin/detai/acupuncture-does-it.pdf. edit
275. ^ Ernst, E (2010). "Deaths after acupuncture: A systematic review". The International Journal of Risk and Safety in Medicine 22 (3): 131–6. doi:10.3233/JRS-2010-0503. Acupuncture - Wikipedia, the free encyclopedia, http://en.wikipedia.org/wiki/Acu_detox (accessed July 21, 2013).
276. ^ a b c d e f Ernst, E.; Lee, M. S.; Choi, T. Y. (2011). "Acupuncture: Does it alleviate pain and are there serious risks? A review of reviews" (pdf). PAIN 152 (4): 755–764. doi:10.1016/j.pain.2010.11.004. PMID 21440191. http://www.dieutridau.com/thongtin/dctai/acupuncture-does-it.pdf. edit. The Use of Acupuncture in Addiction Treatment Programs .., http://article.wn.com/view/2012/07/16/The_Use_of_Acupuncture_in_Addiction_Treatment_Programs/ (accessed July 21, 2013).
277 a b Woo, P. C Y; Lin, A. W C; Lau, S. K P; Yuen, K.-Y. (2010). "Acupuncture transmitted infections". BMJ 340: c1268. doi:10.1136/bmj.c1268. PMID 20299695. http://www.bmj.com/content/340/bmj.c1268.full.
278. ^ Leavy, Benjamin R. (2002). "Apparent adverse outcome of acupuncture.". The Journal of the American Board of Family Practice / American Board of Family Practice 15 (3): 246–8. PMID 12038734. http://www.jabfm.org/cgi/pmidlookup?view=long&pmid=12038734. The Use of Acupuncture in Addiction Treatment Programs .., http://article.wn.com/view/2012/07/16/The_Use_of_Acupuncture_in_Addiction_Treatment_Programs/ (accessed July 21, 2013).
279. ^ Leow TK (2001). "Pneumothorax Using Bladder 14". Medical Acupuncture 16 (2). http://www.medicalacupuncture.org/aama_marf/journal/vol16_2/case_2.html. The Use of Acupuncture in Addiction Treatment Programs .., http://article.wn.com/view/2012/07/16/The_Use_of_Acupuncture_in_Addiction_Treatment_Programs/ (accessed July 21, 2013).
280. ^ Yekeler, E.; Tunaci, M; Tunaci, A; Dursun, M; Acunas, G (2006). "Frequency of Sternal Variations and Anomalies Evaluated by MDCT". American Journal of Roentgenology 186 (4): 956–60. doi:10.2214/AJR.04.1779. PMID 16554563. http://www.ajronline.org/content/186/4/956.full. Safety and risks of Acupuncture -

Health and Wellbeing .., http://www.wellbeingspot.com/flex/safety-and-risks-of-acupuncture/73/1 (accessed July 21, 2013).
281. The Use of Acupuncture in Addiction Treatment Programs .., http://article.wn.com/view/2012/07/16/The_Use_of_Acupuncture_in_Addiction_Treatment_Programs/ (accessed July 21, 2013).
282. ^ Barret, S (2007-12-30). "Be Wary of Acupuncture, Qigong, and "Chinese Medicine"". Quackwatch. http://www.quackwatch.org/01QuackeryRelatedTopics/acu.html. Retrieved 2010-11-03.
283. ^ "Final Report, Report into Traditional Chinese Medicine" (pdf). Parliament of New South Wales. 2005-11-09. http://www.parliament.nsw.gov.au/prod/parlment/committee.nsf/0/ca78e168ce1b6fa2ca2570b400200a34/$FILE/reportversion2.pdf. Retrieved 2010-11-03.
284. Carron H, Epstein BS, Grand B. Complications of acupuncture. JAMA. 1974;228(12):1552-1554.
285. Blanchard BM. Letter. Deep vein thrombophlebitis after acupuncture. Annals of Internal Medicine. 1991;115(9):748.
286 Goldberg I. Pneumothorax associated with acupuncture. Medical Journal of Australia. 1973;1:941-942.
287. Ritter HG, Tarala R. Pneumothorax after acupuncture. British Medical Journal. 1978;2(6137):602-603.
288. Scheel O, et al. Letter. Endocarditis after acupuncture and injection treatment by a natural healer. JAMA. 1992;267(1):56.
289. Vilke GM, Wulferrt EA. Case reports of two patients with pneumothorax following acupuncture. Journal of Emergency Medicine. 1997;15(2):155-157.
290. Abumi K, Anbo H, Kaneda K. Migration of an acupuncture needle into the medulla oblongata. European Spine Journal. 1996;5(2):137-139.
291. National Health and Medical Research Council, Report of Working Party on Acupuncture, p. 15
292. Acupuncture: Past and Present, http://www.acuwatch.org/hx/basser.shtml (accessed July 21, 2013).
293. Acupuncture - Through the Maze, Christian Apologetics Ministry, http://www.mazeministry.com/resources/books/doombook/graphpix/quackwatch.htm (accessed July 21, 2013).
294. ^ a b c d e f g Ernst, E.; Pittler, MH; Wider, B; Boddy, K (2007). "Acupuncture: its evidence-base is changing.". The American Journal of Chinese Medicine 35 (1): 21–5. doi:10.1142/S0192415X07004588. PMID 17265547. Acupuncture - Acupuncture & Alternative Medicine Crentre For .., http://www.drkulkarnis.in/acupuncture.html (accessed July 21, 2013).
295. ^ Napadow, Vitaly; Ahn, Andrew; Longhurst, John; Lao, Lixing; Stener-Victorin, Elisabet; Harris, Richard; Langevin, Helene M. (2008). "The Status and Future of Acupuncture Mechanism Research". The Journal of Alternative and Complementary Medicine 14 (7): 861–9. doi:10.1089/acm.2008.SAR-3. PMID 18803495.
296.^ a b c d e f g h i j k l m n o p q r s NIH Consensus Development Program (November 3–5, 1997). "Acupuncture --Consensus Development Conference Statement". National Institutes of Health. http://consensus.nih.gov/1997/1997Acupuncture107html.htm. Retrieved 2007-07-17.

297. ^ a b c d e f g Ernst, E.; Pittler, MH; Wider, B; Boddy, K (2007). "Acupuncture: its evidence-base is changing.". The American Journal of Chinese Medicine 35 (1): 21–5. doi:10.1142/S0192415X07004588. PMID 17265547.
298. ^ a b c White, A.R.; Filshie, J.; Cummings, T.M.; International Acupuncture Research Forum (2001). "Clinical trials of acupuncture: consensus recommendations for optimal treatment, sham controls and blinding". Complementary Therapies in Medicine 9 (4): 237–245. doi:10.1054/ctim.2001.0489. PMID 12184353.
299. ^ a b c Johnson, M. I (2006). "The clinical effectiveness of acupuncture for pain relief – you can be certain of uncertainty". Acupuncture in Medicine 24 (2): 71–9. doi:10.1136/aim.24.2.71. PMID 16783282.
300. ^ a b c Committee on the Use of Complementary and Alternative Medicine by the American Public (2005). Complementary and Alternative Medicine in the United States. National Academies Press. http://www.nap.edu/catalog.php?record_id=11182
301.^ a b c d e f g h i j k l m n o p q r s NIH Consensus Development Program (November 3–5, 1997). "Acupuncture --Consensus Development Conference Statement". National Institutes of Health. http://consensus.nih.gov/1997/1997Acupuncture107html.htm. Retrieved 2007-07-17.
302. ^ a b c d e f g "Acupuncture". US National Center for Complementary and Alternative Medicine. 2006. http://nccam.nih.gov/health/acupuncture/. Retrieved 2006-03-02.
303. ^ a b c d e f Ernst, G; Strzyz, H; Hagmeister, H (2003). "Incidence of adverse effects during acupuncture therapy—a multicentre survey". Complementary Therapies in Medicine 11 (2): 93–7. doi:10.1016/S0965-2299(03)00004-9. PMID 12801494.
304. ^ a b c d e f Lao L, Hamilton GR, Fu J, Berman BM (2003). "Is acupuncture safe? A systematic review of case reports". Alternative therapies in health and medicine 9 (1): 72–83. PMID 12564354.
305. ^ a b c Lee A, Copas JB, Henmi M, Gin T, Chung RC (2006). "Publication bias affected the estimate of postoperative nausea in an acupoint stimulation systematic review". J Clin Epidemiol. 59 (9): 980–3. doi:10.1016/j.jclinepi.2006.02.003. PMID 16895822.
306. ^ a b Tang, JL; Zhan, SY; Ernst, E (1999). "Review of randomised controlled trials of traditional Chinese medicine.". BMJ (Clinical research ed.) 319 (7203): 160–1. PMC 28166. PMID 10406751.
307. ^ a b Vickers, A; Goyal, N; Harland, R; Rees, R (1998). "Do Certain Countries Produce Only Positive Results? A Systematic Review of Controlled Trials". Controlled Clinical Trials 19 (2): 159–66. doi:10.1016/S0197-2456(97)00150-5. PMID 9551280.
308. Acupuncture - Acupuncture & Alternative Medicine Crentre For .., http://www.drkulkarnis.in/acupuncture.html (accessed July 21, 2013).
309. ^ Vickers, A.; Goyal, N.; Harland, R.; Rees, R. (1998). "Do certain countries produce only positive results? A systematic review of controlled trials" (pdf). Controlled clinical trials 19 (2): 159–166. doi:10.1016/S0197-2456(97)00150-5. PMID 9551280. http://www.dcscience.net/Vickers_1998_Controlled-Clinical-Trials.pdf. edit
Retrieved 2011-06-15. Acupuncture - Wikipedia, the free encyclopedia, http://en.wikipedia.org/wiki/Acu_detox (accessed July 21, 2013).
310.^ a b c d e f g h i Goddard B (2008). 2. "The Truth about Acupuncture". In Singh S, Ernst E. Trick or Treatment: The Undeniable Facts about Alternative Medicine. pp. 39–90.

http://books.google.com/books?id=TnDHoXyi388C&pg=PA39#v=onepage&q&f=false. Acupuncture - Acupuncture & Alternative Medicine Crentre For .., http://www.drkulkarnis.in/acupuncture.html (accessed July 21, 2013).
311. ^ a b c d e f g h Braverman S (2004). "Medical Acupuncture Review: Safety, Efficacy, And Treatment Practices". Medical Acupuncture 15 (3). http://www.medicalacupuncture.org/aama_marf/journal/vol15_3/article1.html.
312.^ a b c d e f g h i j k l m n o p q r s NIH Consensus Development Program (November 3–5, 1997). "Acupuncture --Consensus Development Conference Statement". National Institutes of Health. http://consensus.nih.gov/1997/1997Acupuncture107html.htm. Retrieved 2007-07-17.
313. ^ a b c d e f g "Acupuncture". US National Center for Complementary and Alternative Medicine. 2006. http://nccam.nih.gov/health/acupuncture/. Retrieved 2006-03-02.
314. ^ a b c d e f Ernst, G; Strzyz, H; Hagmeister, H (2003). "Incidence of adverse effects during acupuncture therapy—a multicentre survey". Complementary Therapies in Medicine 11 (2): 93–7. doi:10.1016/S0965-2299(03)00004-9. PMID 12801494.
315. ^ a b c d e f Lao L, Hamilton GR, Fu J, Berman BM (2003). "Is acupuncture safe? A systematic review of case reports". Alternative therapies in health and medicine 9 (1): 72–83. PMID 12564354.
316. ^ a b c Furlan, Andrea D.; Van Tulder, Maurits; Cherkin, Dan; Tsukayama, Hiroshi; Lao, Lixing; Koes, Bart; Berman, Brian (2005). "Acupuncture and Dry-Needling for Low Back Pain: An Updated Systematic Review Within the Framework of the Cochrane Collaboration". Spine 30 (8): 944–63. doi:10.1097/01.brs.0000158941.21571.01. PMID 15834340.
317.^ a b c d e f g h i j k l m n o p q r s NIH Consensus Development Program (November 3–5, 1997). "Acupuncture --Consensus Development Conference Statement". National Institutes of Health. http://consensus.nih.gov/1997/1997Acupuncture107html.htm. Retrieved 2007-07-17. Phys.org - acupressure, http://phys.org/tags/acupressure/ (accessed July 21, 2013).
318.^ a b c d e f Ernst, G; Strzyz, H; Hagmeister, H (2003). "Incidence of adverse effects during acupuncture therapy—a multicentre survey". Complementary Therapies in Medicine 11 (2): 93–7. doi:10.1016/S0965-2299(03)00004-9. PMID 12801494.
319. ^ a b "Acupuncture: Evidence for its effectiveness". National Health Service. 2010-03-18. http://www.nhs.uk/Conditions/Acupuncture/Pages/Evidence.aspx. Retrieved 2010-08-10.
320. ^ a b c World Health Organization (2003). "Acupuncture: Review and Analysis of Reports on Controlled Clinical Trials". In Zhang X. World Health Organization. http://www.who.int/medicinedocs/en/d/Js4926e/#Js4926e.5.
321. ^ a b Sampson, W (2005-03-23). "Critique of the NIH Consensus Conference on Acupuncture". Quackwatch. http://www.acuwatch.org/general/nihcritique.shtml. Retrieved 2009-06-05.
322. ^ a b c d McCarthy, Michael (2005). "Critics slam draft WHO report on homoeopathy". The Lancet 366: 705–6. doi:10.1016/S0140-6736(05)67159-0.
323. ^ a b Singh & Ernst, 2008. In Singh S, Ernst E. Trick or Treatment: The Undeniable Facts about Alternative Medicine. p. 277-8
324. ^ a b c d e f g h Braverman S (2004). "Medical Acupuncture Review: Safety, Efficacy, And Treatment Practices". Medical Acupuncture 15 (3). http://www.medicalacupuncture.org/aama_marf/journal/vol15_3/article1.html

325. ^ a b c d e f g h i j k l m n o p q r s NIH Consensus Development Program (November 3–5, 1997). "Acupuncture --Consensus Development Conference Statement". National Institutes of Health. http://consensus.nih.gov/1997/1997Acupuncture107html.htm. Retrieved 2007-07-17.
326. ^ a b c d e f g "Acupuncture". US National Center for Complementary and Alternative Medicine. 2006. http://nccam.nih.gov/health/acupuncture/. Retrieved 2006-03-02.
327. ^ a b c d e f Ernst, G; Strzyz, H; Hagmeister, H (2003). "Incidence of adverse effects during acupuncture therapy—a multicentre survey". Complementary Therapies in Medicine 11 (2): 93–7. doi:10.1016/S0965-2299(03)00004-9. PMID 12801494.
328. ^ a b c d e f Lao L, Hamilton GR, Fu J, Berman BM (2003). "Is acupuncture safe? A systematic review of case reports". Alternative therapies in health and medicine 9 (1): 72–83. PMID 12564354.
329. ^ a b c Furlan, Andrea D.; Van Tulder, Maurits; Cherkin, Dan; Tsukayama, Hiroshi; Lao, Lixing; Koes, Bart; Berman, Brian (2005). "Acupuncture and Dry-Needling for Low Back Pain: An Updated Systematic Review Within the Framework of the Cochrane Collaboration". Spine 30 (8): 944–63. doi:10.1097/01.brs.0000158941.21571.01. PMID 15834340.
330. ^ "Position Paper on Acupuncture". National Council Against Health Fraud. 1990. http://www.ncahf.org/pp/acu.html. Retrieved 2011-01-27. Acupuncture - Wikipedia, the free encyclopedia, http://en.wikipedia.org/wiki/Acu_detox (accessed July 21, 2013).
331. ^ Arthur Taub (1993). Acupuncture: Nonsense with Needles. http://www.acuwatch.org/general/taub.shtml.
332. ^ Stephen Barrett, M.D.. "Be Wary of Acupuncture, Qigong, and "Chinese Medicine"". http://www.quackwatch.org/01QuackeryRelatedTopics/acu.html. Retrieved 2010-05-31.
Acupuncture | Mission Holistic , http://missionholistic.ca/traditional-chinese-medicine/acupuncture/ (accessed July 21, 2013).
333. ^ John P. Jackson. "What is acupuncture?". http://www.ukskeptics.com/acupuncture.php. University of San Clemente - Courses, Programs, Degrees .., http://corporatefitnessorangecounty.com/ (accessed July 21, 2013).
334. ^ Steven Salzberg (2008). "Acupuncture infiltrates the University of Maryland and NEJM". http://genome.fieldofscience.com/2010/08/acupuncture-infiltrates-university-of.html.
335. ^ Steven Novella. "Acupuncture Pseudoscience in the New England Journal of Medicine". http://www.sciencebasedmedicine.org/?p=6391. Acupuncture - Wikipedia, the free encyclopedia, http://en.wikipedia.org/wiki/Acu_detox (accessed July 21, 2013).
336. Acupuncture - Wikipedia, the free encyclopedia, http://en.wikipedia.org/wiki/Acu_detox (accessed July 21, 2013).
337. ^ Sampson WI (2005). "Critique of the NIH Consensus Conference on Acupuncture". Acuwatch. http://www.acuwatch.org/general/nihcritique.shtml.
338. ^ Sampson WI, Atwood K (5/19 December 2005). "Propagation of the Absurd: demarcation of the Absurd revisited". Med J Aust 183 (11/12): Viewpoint. https://www.mja.com.au/public/issues/183_11_051205/sam10986_fm.pdf.
339.^ a b c Mann, F (2000). Reinventing acupuncture: a new concept of ancient medicine. Elsevier. pp. 14; 31. ISBN 0750648570. The Use of Acupuncture in

Addiction Treatment Programs ..,
http://article.wn.com/view/2012/07/16/The_Use_of_Acupuncture_in_Addiction_Treatment_Programs/ (accessed July 21, 2013).
340. The Use of Acupuncture in Addiction Treatment Programs ..,
http://article.wn.com/view/2012/07/16/The_Use_of_Acupuncture_in_Addiction_Treatment_Programs/ (accessed July 21, 2013).
341. ^ a b c d e f Madsen, M. V.; Gotzsche, P. C; Hrobjartsson, A. (2009). "Acupuncture treatment for pain: systematic review of randomised clinical trials with acupuncture, placebo acupuncture, and no acupuncture groups". BMJ 338: a3115. doi:10.1136/bmj.a3115. PMC 2769056. PMID 19174438.
342. ^ a b c White, A.R.; Filshie, J.; Cummings, T.M.; International Acupuncture Research Forum (2001). "Clinical trials of acupuncture: consensus recommendations for optimal treatment, sham controls and blinding". Complementary Therapies in Medicine 9 (4): 237–245. doi:10.1054/ctim.2001.0489. PMID 12184353.
343. ^ a b c d e f g h Ernst, E. (2006). "Acupuncture - a critical analysis". Journal of Internal Medicine 259 (2): 125–137. doi:10.1111/j.1365-2796.2005.01584.x. PMID 16420542. edit
344. ^ a b c O'Connell, NE; Wand, BM; Goldacre, B (2009). "Interpretive bias in acupuncture research?: A case study.". Evaluation & the health professions 32 (4): 393–409. doi:10.1177/0163278709353394. PMID 19942631.
345. Acupuncture - Wikipedia, the free encyclopedia, http://en.wikipedia.org/wiki/Acu_detox (accessed July 21, 2013).
346. ^ "Report 12 of the Council on Scientific Affairs (A-97) – Alternative Medicine". American Medical Association. 1997. http://www.ama-assn.org/ama/no-index/about-ama/13638.shtml. Retrieved 2009-10-07.
347. Stephen Barrett, M.D. Be Wary of Acupuncture, Qigong, and "Chinese Medicine". Quackwatch. 2007 Dec 30. This article was revised on December 30, 2007. scienceinmedicine.org/fellows/Barrett.html . Acupuncture - Wikipedia, the free encyclopedia, http://en.wikipedia.org/wiki/Acu_detox (accessed July 21, 2013).
348. Acupuncture - Through the Maze, Christian Apologetics Ministry, http://www.mazeministry.com/resources/books/doombook/graphpix/quackwatch.htm (accessed July 21, 2013).
349. Acupuncture: Past and Present, http://www.acuwatch.org/hx/basser.shtml (accessed July 21, 2013).
350. Ibid.
351. Stephen Basser, M.D. The Skeptical Guide to Acupuncture History, Theories, and Practices . The Scientific Review of Alternative Medicine. Spring/Summer 1999 issue. Originally posted on February 22, 2005.

CHAPTER SIX - QUACKERY - MIRACLE CURES

Goldacre, in his book, mentions "miracle cures" a much-loved term amongst "quacks" and he quotes research undertaken by a team of Australian oncologists. Over the course of many years they followed 2,337 terminal cancer patients in palliative care. They died, on average, after five months but around one per cent of them were still alive after five years. This study was reported in *The Independent* in January 2006. According to Goldacre,[1] the researchers made clear that claims for miracle cures should be treated with caution, because "miracles" do occur routinely and maybe without any specific intervention. The British mathematician J. E. Littlewood suggested that individuals should statistically expect one-in-a-million events ("miracles") to happen to them at the rate of about one per month. By Littlewood's definition, seemingly miraculous events are actually commonplace. Therefore the so-called miracle cures may well be attributed to any form of treatment conventional or otherwise including, as Goldacre says, "special diets, herbal potions and faith healing".

Oxygen, Ozone and Hydrogen peroxide therapy

In a hilarious chapter on Dr. Gillian McKeith a "clinical nutritionist", Goldacre[2] describes how he managed to purchase the same certified membership of the American Association of Nutritional Consultants that Gillian McKeith has for US$60.00. He purchased this in the name of his dead cat Hettie and he has the certificate hanging in his toilet. This in spite of McKeith's spokeswoman stating that to gain professional membership, Dr. McKeith had to provide proof of her degree and three professional references. It is certainly true that one can purchase degrees in different parts of the world.

Dr McKeith was quoted as recommending the eating of spinach, and the darker leaves on plants, because they contain more chlorophyll. According to her these were "high in oxygen" and would "really oxygenate one's blood". Chlorophyll is used to convert carbon dioxide and water into sugar and oxygen. This we know from schooldays but we also know that it only takes place in the presence of sunlight. As Goldacre points out there is no sunlight in the bowel and even if there was, and oxygen was manufactured in this way, it could not be absorbed through the bowel. Oxygen is absorbed through the lungs!

Ben Goldacre wrote of her[3]: Dr Gillian McKeith PhD.: "is an empire, a prime-time TV celebrity, a bestselling author. She has her own range of foods and mysterious powders, she has pills to give you an erection, and her face is in every health food store in the country. Scottish Conservative politicians want her to advise the government. The Soil Association gave her a prize for educating the public. But to anyone who knows the slightest bit about science, she is a joke".

On November 21st 2006 The Medicine and Healthcare products Regulators Agency (MHRA) issued a press release. The MHRA discovered that McKeith's organisation was advertising and selling goods without legal authorisation whilst making medicinal claims about their efficacy.[4] Dr McKeith's products were determined by the MHRA to be medicines because of the presence of some well-known medicinal herbs and because of the claims being made by Dr McKeith's organisation.[5] The MHRA, said: "The Wild Pink Yam and Horny Goat Weed products marketed by McKeith Research Ltd. were never legal for sale in the UK."[6] She was ordered to remove the products from sale immediately. She complied. The alternative would have been prosecution. *The Guardian* printed this story under the heading "A Menace to Science."

For years, "Dr" Gillian McKeith used the title of doctor until the Advertising Standards Authority recently stopped this. She had previously been described as a "clinical nutritionist" regarded as "Dr" Gillian McKeith PhD usually seen on television in a laboratory setting and dressed in a white coat. Owen Gibson reporting in *The Guardian* of Monday February 12, 2007 said "Gillian McKeith, the You Are What You Eat presenter, has agreed to drop the title Dr from her company's advertising after a complaint to the industry watchdog.[7] She has made millions from book and health food spin-offs, but her credentials have been questioned by some experts. After the Advertising Standards Authority came to the provisional conclusion that the honorific was likely to mislead the public, McKeith Research said it planned to drop it from its advertising, obviating the need for a full investigation. The complaint was brought by a *Guardian* reader. The self-styled health guru has consistently argued she is entitled to call herself a doctor because of her distance learning PhD in holistic nutrition from the American Holistic College of Nutrition.[8]

The ASA was minded to rule that the adverts were misleading, because the college was not accredited by any recognised educational authority at the time she took the course, and she does not hold a general medical qualification.[9] While the adverts usually stated somewhere in the text Ms McKeith was not a medical doctor, the initial impression given was that she was, it said. According to documents seen by *The Guardian,* the agreement prevents Ms McKeith calling herself a doctor in any advertising or mailshots relating to her company and its products. They include a Dr Gillian McKeith-branded range of health foods and the Dr Gillian Club, which offers online health plans. She told *The Guardian* she understood the offending ad was a leaflet without the usual disclaimer she was not a medical doctor. She said she understood the honorific had to go from leaflets, but not from all adverts. "As far as I'm concerned, because of the hard work I have done, I'll continue to put PhD after my name; I'm entitled to use the word Dr as and when I choose. Her PR representative, Max Clifford, said her degree had not played a part in her career. "Personally, I wish it had never been mentioned. She never needed it, and it's done nothing but cause her embarrassment."[10]

Humans need oxygen but there are extraordinary claims that oxygenation therapy in various forms may cure cancer, AIDS and other illnesses. Various theories have been used to explain how this might happen. The administrations of hydrogen peroxide or ozone are two of the methods that have been suggested as means by which the tissues may become more highly oxygenated. One of my golfing friends consumes large amounts of hydrogen peroxide orally on a daily basis.

Dr. Saul Green, a biochemist at Memorial Sloan-Kettering Cancer Centre for 23 years described in detail how hydrogen peroxide and ozone have been used in the treatment of cancer, AIDS and other illnesses[11]. The idea that infusion of ozone-treated blood can cure AIDS patients is being marketed despite its lack of efficacy. Green's conclusions were that ingestion, infusion, or injection of hydrogen peroxide cannot re-oxygenate the tissues of the body and that ozone-treated blood infused during autohemotherapy does not kill the AIDS virus in vivo.

Antioxidants

In human cell metabolism, the mitochondria convert glucose and oxygen into energy. Oxygen radicals are formed as a normal by-product. These highly reactive oxygen radicals can damage cell proteins and membranes. The DNA molecules in the mitochondria themselves are especially susceptible. The body's own antioxidant defences neutralise most but not all free radicals. An enzyme, superoxide dismutase (SOD) helps to convert the free radicals into hydrogen peroxide which is then converted into oxygen and water. As free radicals are mostly considered to be harmful this is a protective mechanism. Not widely known however is that free radicals are also beneficial in that they help to protect the body against bacteria. The proponents of antioxidant therapy claim that the administration of antioxidants enhances the action of the superoxide dismutase in neutralising the free radicals. This may be true but the administration of antioxidants to humans by means of oral supplements, despite huge advertising campaigns, has not been proven to be beneficial.

Lisa Melton[12] in her book "The antioxidant myth" made some interesting statements. "Cranberry capsules. Green tea extract. Effervescent vitamin C. Pomegranate concentrate. Beta carotene pills. Selenium. Grape seed extract. High-dose vitamin E. Pine bark extract. Bee spit. You name it, if it's an antioxidant, we'll swallow it" she said. "According to some estimates around half of United States adults take antioxidant pills daily in the belief that they promote good health and stave off disease."

Beta carotene and Vitamin E are two of the most well known and popular antioxidants. In 1992 researchers at the US National Cancer Institute tested beta carotene. Two-thirds of the way through, the trial which was set to run for six years, was stopped because the researchers discovered that those participants taking supplements had developed 28 per cent more cases of lung cancer than the controls and their overall death rate was 17 per cent higher.

In the early 1990s two large studies involving more than 127,000 people in total found that those with a diet high in vitamin E were significantly less likely to suffer cardiovascular disease. Use of vitamin E supplements soared and by the end of the decade an estimated 23 million US citizens were taking regular daily doses but Cochrane reviews have now shown that antioxidant supplements are either "ineffective, or perhaps even actively harmful". The Cochrane review[13] on preventing lung cancer found no benefit from antioxidants, and indeed an increase in the risk of lung cancer in participants taking ß-carotene, an antioxidant, and retinol together. The Cochrane systematic review and meta-analysis on the use of antioxidants to reduce heart attacks[14] and stroke looked at vitamin E, and separately carotene, in fifteen trials, and found no benefit for either. For carotene, there was a small but significant increase in death. Although the review found no significant detrimental effect caused by vitamin C, it found no evidence that it helped ward off disease.[15] It also found no evidence to support taking antioxidant supplements to reduce the risk of dying earlier in healthy people or patients with various diseases.[16] The authors stated that: "If anything, people in trial groups given the antioxidants beta-carotene, vitamin A, and vitamin E showed increased rates of mortality".[17]

Researchers at Copenhagen University[18] carried out a review of 67 studies on 230,000 healthy people and found "no convincing evidence" that any of the antioxidants helped to prolong life expectancy. But some "increased mortality". They warned that healthy people who take popular antioxidant supplements, including vitamins A and E,[19] to try to keep diseases such as cancer at bay are interfering with their natural body defences and may be increasing their risk of an early death by up to 16 per cent.[20]

As stated previously antioxidants, including vitamins A, E, C and beta-carotene and selenium, are said to mop up free radicals, a process which may cause harm.[21] It is this action that the researchers believed may cause problems with the defence system.[22]

The Danish research, released by the influential Cochrane Library, applied only to synthetic supplements and not to vitamins that occur naturally in vegetables and fruit. It found that vitamin A supplements increased the risk of death in healthy people by 16 per cent.[23] Taking beta-carotene was linked to a seven per cent increased risk, while regular users of vitamin E supplements increased the risk of an early death by four per cent.[24]

Although the review found no significant detrimental effect caused by vitamin C, it found no evidence that it helped ward off disease. Following Linus Pauling's "cherry-picking" millions of people take this vitamin in the unproven hope of avoiding a common cold. Goran Bjelakovic, who led the Danish review, said: "We could find no evidence to support taking antioxidant supplements to reduce the risk of dying earlier in healthy people or patients with various diseases.[25] If anything, people in trial groups given the antioxidants beta carotene, vitamin A, and vitamin E showed increased rates of mortality."

Nevertheless and in spite of the Cochrane reviews the biscuits I buy for my cat contain antioxidants. On the packet it states that "A healthy cat is a happy cat. Strong immune system. Did you know that WHISKAS contains a blend of antioxidants that boosts your cat's natural defence system against disease? For every bowl of WHISKAS you are assured of a healthy, happy cat." If this advertising is to be believed and antioxidants do not help humans they may at least help cats!

The Australasian Society of Clinical Immunology and Allergy (ACAI) has issued an analysis of about 30 allergy-related tests and treatments that "have been promoted in the absence of any scientific rationale."[26] Among the many things they found to be useless or dangerous were: *for diagnosis;* cytotoxic testing (Bryans' test), oral provocation and neutralisation, Vega testing (electrodermal testing), kinesiology, radionics (psionic medicine, dowsing), iridology and tests for "dysbiosis". *For treatment*; homeopathy, acupuncture, reflexology (zone therapy) and autogenous urine therapy. Physical therapies: chiropractic therapy, osteopathy, cranial therapy allergy elimination techniques (also known as "Advanced Allergy Elimination", "Nambudripad's Allergy Elimination"), Vega MRT (Matrix Regeneration Therapy) and clinical ecology/ environmental illness. These tests and therapies are not regulated in Australia or New Zealand.

Regarding the infamous Vega test, they concluded: "Results are not reproducible in blinded studies, and do not correlate with results from conventional testing." And "substitution of homeopathic 'vaccines' for those with proven effectiveness has both individual and public health implications."

A letter in the "readers write"' section of *The Independent* on 1st August, 2006 stated that "I know homeopathy has taken a bit of a bashing recently but homeopathic remedies for travel sickness have a long and excellent reputation for working. The most important ones are cocculus, petroleum and tabacum. A reply by the same David Colquhoun mentioned above, agreed that homeopathy had taken a bashing but that it should have done so, as selling pills that contained nothing whatsoever but sugar, as medicines was not just delusional, it was fraud. He went on to say that one of the recommendations for travel sickness was for cocculus, a plant that contains the poisonous alkaloid, picrotoxin. Luckily, he said, the label on the bottle was untrue and that the pills contained none. Travel sickness was known to be influenced by expectations. That made it a good candidate for placebo effects and also good for the income of charlatans."

Anyone who suffers from cancer, or knows someone else who does understands the fear and desperation of cancer sufferers. When so-called orthodox or Western medicine is no longer effective or fails there can be a great temptation to accept any alternative form of hope. People accept anything that appears to offer a chance for cure. No blame can be attached for this. Medicinal products and devices used in the treatment of cancer must be approved by the Food and Drug Administration before they are marketed. This helps to ensure that these products are safe and effective. Other forms of cancer treatment, not regulated by the Food and Drug Administration, may not be safe or effective.

Health fraud is a cruel form of greed at the best of times but fraud involving cancer treatments can be particularly heartless. There are many companies selling bogus cancer "treatments." They may cause harm on their own but they may also cause indirect harm by delaying or interfering with proven beneficial treatments. These fraudulent "cancer treatments" are frequently sold as natural treatments or dietary supplements. They are widely advertised but are now offered on the internet as well. Fraudulent information regarding these products can be provided in an instant and obtained immediately by accessing the Web, day or night. Many of these websites provide false hope for cancer sufferers.

An article in the *British Sunday Tribune* of 8th August 2004 by Kate Devlin quotes Professor Ernst, who warned [27]that the lives of thousands of cancer patients were at risk due to internet websites promoting bogus cures. He said that a flood of so-called "miracle cures" were available on the internet which were not clinically proven to be effective. These varied from powdered shark fin to a cyanide compound, laetrile, found in apricot kernels. The study found that not one of the multitudes of treatments or medications advocated could be proven to cure or prevent the onset of cancer and three sites were found to offer advice that was potentially harmful to cancer sufferers. A further 16 per cent of sites actively discouraged patients from continuing with conventional treatment as opposed to complementary therapies which implied a significant risk to cancer patients. "This was to us quite an eye-opener and pretty scary stuff," said Ernst.[28] "Our conclusion was that a significant proportion of these websites was actually a risk to cancer patients" he added. "Not everything that is natural is risk free. People should use their common sense and think twice about the motives of these websites."[29]

One of the "misleading" cures featured on the internet was Gerson's diet. It was this therapy which sparked an outcry in the scientific world when Prince Charles controversially praised it during a speech. "I think Prince Charles is doing a very good job in raising awareness of complementary medicines, but I very much regret his mention of Gerson's diet," said Professor Ernst. "There's no evidence at all to show that it helps anybody". Offering advice to patients, Profesor Ernst said, "If it sounds too good to be true, it probably is. Don't believe ridiculous promises and claims. Use your brain; take some reasonable and responsible advice." This, remember is from a Professor of "Alternative Medicine".

Richard Dawkins[30] quotes the results of a 2008 Gallup Poll showing that 44 per cent of Americans deny evolution totally. In Britain the figure is slightly less. Partly as a result of Charles Darwin's work, in Britain today, more people attend museums than attend church.[31] In the United Kingdom 1.6 million people are regular churchgoers and there are 47,000 churches. There are about 1,500 mosques.[32]

Faith has been described as a "valuable ally in achieving a 'cure' and a dangerous enemy in assessing it."[33] No wonder then that a large proportion of people believe in "so-called" alternative medicine. The tooth fairy is alive and well.

The question of where delusion ends and fraud begins is an interesting one. A book by Robert Park of the American Physical Society[34] discusses the question particularly well. Park deals with everything from perpetual motion machines to homeopathy and his thoughts are that those who propagate these delusional ideas often start with a genuine belief that what they say is true. Rejection of the ideas by sensible people just makes them more determined. Eventually, though, many of them probably realise that they have made a mistake. At this point they may recant, but very often they have so much reputation to defend, and frequently "too much income to protect", that they will continue to propagate their ideas. This occurs after they have realised that they are wrong and this is when, according to Park, foolishness or delusion becomes fraud. Park also states that "Alas, to wear the mantle of Galileo it is not enough that you be persecuted by an unkind establishment; you must also be right."

References:

1. Ben Goldacre. "Bad Science". Fourth Estate. London. 2009. p 41. Miracle - Wikipedia, the free encyclopedia, http://en.wikipedia.org/wiki/Miricle (accessed July 21, 2013).
2. Ben Goldacre. "Bad Science". Fourth Estate. London. 2009. p .124.
3. Ibid. p 112.
4. The quack page - UCL - London's Global University, http://www.ucl.ac.uk/pharmacology/dc-bits-old/quack-01-06-07.html (accessed July 21, 2013).
5. Ibid.
6. What's wrong with Dr Gillian McKeith PhD? – Bad Science, http://www.badscience.net/2007/02/ms-gillian-mckeith-banned-from-calling-herself-a-doctor/ (accessed July 21, 2013).
7. Ibid.
8. Ibid.
9. Ibid.
10. Ibid.
11. Oxygenation Therapy: Unproven Treatments for Cancer and AIDS. Saul Green, Ph.D. The Scientific Review of Alternative Medicine. Prometheus Books, 1997. Quackwatch Home Page. This article was posted on June 17, 2001.
12. Lisa Melton. The Antoxidant Myth: a medical fairy tale. New Scientist. 5 August 2006. Issue 2563, p.40-43. www.bogrees.com/Articles/TheAntioxidantMyth.pdf
13. Caraballoso, M., Sacristan, M., Serra, C., and Bonfill, X. Drugs for preventing lung cancer in healthy people. Cochrane Database of Systematic Reviews (2003); 2. The Nonsense du Jour for [Ben Goldacre] Bad Science, http://www.scribd.com/doc/145552156/6/The-Nonsense-du-Jour (accessed July 21, 2013).
14. DP Vivekananthan Use of antioxidant vitamins for the prevention of cardiovascular disease: meta analysis of randomised trials. Lancet (Jun 14th 2003); 361(9374): 2017 23. www.ncbi.nlm.nih.gov/pubmed/12814711. 2004 Feb 21;363(9409):662. Comment in Lancet. 2003 Sep 13;362(9387):920; author reply 921. ACP J Club. The Nonsense du Jour for [Ben Goldacre] Bad Science, http://www.scribd.com/doc/145552156/6/The-Nonsense-du-Jour (accessed July 21, 2013).
15. The Libertarian: Vitamins Will Kill You, Have .., http://2164th.blogspot.com/2008/04/vitamins-will-kill-you-have-apple.html (accessed July 21, 2013).
16. Research: Vitamins may increase risk of death - CNN.com, http://www.cnn.com/2008/HEALTH/diet.fitness/04/16/vitamins.health/index.html (accessed July 21, 2013).
17. The Libertarian: Vitamins Will Kill You, Have .., http://2164th.blogspot.com/2008/04/vitamins-will-kill-you-have-apple.html (accessed July 21, 2013).

18. Bjelakovic, G., Nikolova, D., Gluud, L. L., Simonetti, R. G., Gluud, C. Antioxidant supplements for prevention of mortality in health participants and patients with various diseases. Cochrane Database of Systematic Reviews (2008); 2. T h e L i b e r t a r i a n: Vitamins Will Kill You, Have .., http://2164th.blogspot.com/2008/04/vitamins-will-kill-you-have-apple.html (accessed July 21, 2013).

19. T h e L i b e r t a r i a n: Vitamins Will Kill You, Have .., http://2164th.blogspot.com/2008/04/vitamins-will-kill-you-have-apple.html (accessed July 21, 2013).

20. Ibid.
21. Ibid.
22. Ibid.
23. Ibid.
24. Ibid.
25. Ibid.

26. Mullins, R. J. Unorthodox techniques for the diagnosis and treatment of allergy, asthma and immune disorders. The Australasian Society of Clinical Immunology and Allergy. (ASCIA) Position statement. Oct 2004.

27. "Bogus Cancer Remedies Cost Lives". Annals of Oncology.
Refs?? Schmidt and Ernst

28. Cancer patients at risk from websites | Mail Online, http://www.dailymail.co.uk/health/article-312505/Cancer-patients-risk-websites.html (accessed July 21, 2013).

29. Cancer patients at risk from websites | Mail Online, http://www.dailymail.co.uk/health/article-312505/Cancer-patients-risk-websites.html (accessed July 21, 2013).

30. Richard Dawkins. "The Greatest Show on Earth". The Evidence for Evolution. Transworld Publishers. London. Bantam Press. 2009.p 429.

31. Fifty things you need to know SKY News. 11.01.12.

32. www.MuslimsInBritain.org

33. Michael O'Donnell. A Sceptic's Medical Dictionary. BMJ publishing. 1997.

34. Park, Robert L (2000), Voodoo Science: The road from foolishness to fraud, Oxford, U.K. & New York: Oxford University Press, ISBN 0-19-860443-2, http://books.google.com/books?id=xzCK6-Kqs6QC&printsec=frontcover&dq=%22voodoo+science%22&src=bmrr#v=onepage&q&f=false

Chapter seven - Quackery - Medical Quackery

While a student at the University of Cape Town I learned a few little tricks in obstetrics the first of which I still use regularly. Obstetricians routinely use a round plastic object with the dates of the year on it. One looks up the date of the first day of the patient's last menstrual period and, from that, one can work out the expected date of delivery. This can look a little clumsy when doing it in front of the patient. A much faster method is to add seven days on to the date given and subtract three months. For example if the first day of the patient's last menstrual period is on the 10th of July adding on seven days and subtracting three months gives the expected date of delivery of 17th of April. Working the date out in this way in front of the patient is much faster and much more impressive. The second trick was always to add on seven days to the expected date of delivery as patients always like to be early. In the days prior to ultrasonic scanning I was also taught by one consultant to prophesy the sex and then write the opposite down in the patient's notes. One would write "boy" in the notes and tell the patient that her baby was going to be a girl. If the patient had a girl one was praised for being correct. If she had a boy one could deny saying the baby would be a girl and point out where you had written down "boy" in the notes. Either way the patient's opinion of you as a doctor was enhanced. I do not use the latter two tricks and would deem them to be a form of deceit but, as it is not done for profit, it is probably not quackery.

On the subject of dates, it is amazing when a doctor asks a lady patient the date of her last menstrual period how often they reply giving the date when the period stopped. Having practised gynaecology for many years now I still do not know how this originated. We always want to know the date when the menstrual period started. All ladies please note.

"Free lunches" and conflicts of interest

Stories are legion of doctors demanding to use a certain specific company's products and insisting that these be available in the clinics in which the doctor works. Orthopaedics, especially, seems to have a poor reputation in this connection. This may be because of the cost of prostheses, which is very high. This demand by the doctor may have been occasioned by a lunch or dinner to which the doctor had been invited by a representative of the company concerned. The doctor's demand might also have been occasioned by a gift from the company. Financial inducements have also been used. In South Africa until fairly recently many companies held their own sponsored golf tournaments to which, of course, doctors were invited. The prizes at some of these tournaments were often excessive taking no notice of the limits in value of prizes set by the Royal and Ancient golf club of St. Andrews. Most reputable companies have now stopped this practice. The saying that "there is no such thing as a free lunch" is a good saying and worth remembering.

The *New York Times* business section recently reported on "free" lunches provided by drug companies in the USA. A few universities have now banned them. "It's an issue of professionalism and integrity" the article read. Healthwatch was invited to a "free" lunch[1] presentation of "exclusive insights" into an exciting double-blind trial on the effect of ginkgo biloba on short-term memory. The investigator who was to present his research findings at the lunch was Ian Hindmarch, Professor of Human Psychopharmacology at the University of Surrey. The host was Pegasus Publications, on behalf of LichtwerPharma who market Ginkyo, a concentrated extract of ginkgo. The venue was the Ivy Restaurant in London WC2, which is highly rated by gastronomic cognoscenti. The event was billed as an "expert lunch". Not all the journalists present were very expert, though, A features editor who worked for the Women's' Institute asked what was meant by a "double-blind trial". The proceedings were opened by Mr Peter Josling of the Ginkgo Information Centre who emphasised the antiquity of the ginkgo tree, and the importance of using the correct commercial preparation to obtain the greatest benefit. Professor Hindmarch assured those present that subjects given ginkgo extract for 48 hours performed much better than controls. Lunch followed, with liberal quantities of very acceptable red or white wine. Healthcare journalists may be exposed to the potential for conflict of interest when pharmaceutical firms provide lavish entertainment.

Journalists have rightly exposed the similar danger medical practitioners face. They may prescribe their sponsor's products. Doctors are often invited to lunches of this nature. The lunches may often be in the faint disguise of presentations of the sponsor's drugs. In many countries doctors, in addition to prescribing them, dispense their own drugs. Lavish free lunches may influence the doctor in his prescribing or dispensing habits. It has also been known for pharmaceutical and medical equipment companies to offer very good discounts and other inducements for the doctors to use their products.

When I was in Bahrain I was informed proudly by one of the doctors that a "special deal" had been arranged with the company providing the drugs needed for in vitro fertilisation. These are very expensive drugs and the doctor was very pleased with himself for making this arrangement. He did not disclose what the deal was nor did he say how he personally had benefited.

Deaths

Paul Mason[2] reported a scheme by a British company called CARD to test a totally unproven "cure" for AIDS on patients in the African kingdom of Swaziland. The "cure" is based on goat serum. CARD claimed that "antiretrovirals are regarded more as poisons than therapies and are mostly unavailable to the masses."[3]

In this way they attempted to "rubbish" anti-retroviral drugs, which are being used effectively on a daily basis all round the world, and have them replaced by their own products. On their business plan, CARD stated that "The trials have now to this date gone through three phases, all of which have proved totally reliable in the cure of Aids."[4]

The background to the goat serum cure for AIDS, according to Paul Mason, is that it was literally dreamed up by a United States doctor called Gary Davis.[5]

He saw himself in a dream injecting goats and concluded, as anyone would, that this was a revelation from God that goats can cure HIV. He developed a serum, injecting HIV into goats to produce antibodies that, if HIV were any old virus, would fight the disease. But it is not: the point about the AIDS virus is that antibodies do not kill it. Davis applied to the US government for a licence to trial the serum on humans, but this was refused.[6,7] Then in 2000 he came back into the limelight claiming that his business partner, Steve Migliaccio, had stolen 80 litres of the serum. The FDA issued a safety notice about this, warning that it may turn up in the Third World. Gary Davis was apparently trying to test the serum in Ghana. To their embarrassment the Swaziland Health Ministry became involved in the scheme.

Approximately 25 million people have already died from AIDS around the world. The adverse influence that people like Matthias Rath. Thabo Mbeki, Manto Tshabalala-Msimang, a previous Minister of Health in South Africa, and others have had on the AIDS epidemic has been well documented. Rath advocated the use of vitamins to cure AIDS and cancer and advocated that AIDS sufferers stop their anti-retroviral treatments. Naturally he also sold vitamins. It is of interest to note that Rath had previously been ordered by a court in Germany to stop claiming that his vitamins could cure cancer, or face a fine of €250,000.[8] The South African government at one stage argued that HIV was not the cause of AIDS and that anti-retroviral drugs were not useful in the treatment of AIDS.

According to an item on Sky News on 8th January, 2012 at the time of the centenary celebrations of the African National Congress it is estimated that this policy of denial of the correct aetiology of AIDS resulted in over 355,000 avoidable and unnecessary deaths. The same item mentioned that 2.1 billion US dollars was apparently paid in the "arms deal" scandal. The poorer people of South Africa could have done with this money. Financial scandals of this nature occur all round the world. It seems to be that it occurs when people come to power or when they have been in power too long. Someone once told me that it is to be expected when "rabbits are put in charge of lettuce!"

Another cause of totally unnecessary deaths was the advice given by Dr. Benjamin Spock in his book "Baby and Child Care". In this book and without any evidence for it, he advised that babies should sleep face down. This advice was incorrect and led to thousands of, otherwise avoidable, cot deaths.[9] This was not medical quackery but was equally disastrous. Every day there are numerous advertisements in the press and elsewhere advertising cures for AIDS, cancers and other illnesses. Many of these are without any scientific basis whatsoever.

Real "medical" quacks

A "Dr." J Buba, with no letters of qualification after his name, advertises openly in a local paper in Zimbabwe. His is one of many similar quack advertisements. He is not shy proclaiming himself as "The famous and legendary Dr. J Buba with all natural medicine practitioners legal registered healers" alongside a picture of a hand, spreading stardust. He advertises medicine to protect marriages, family, homes, business, cars, jobs and girlfriends. He offers "muti", the local word for medicine, for lucky charms to win casino, lotto, gambling and to "pay after you win". He does not say what happens if one loses. The "muti" allegedly attracts business and customers. It wins court and divorce cases, enables one to pass examinations, helps with job recruitment and promotions, to be liked at work and to be loved by a "straight" boyfriend. The advertisement offers to help debt, repayment of bonds, credit cards and personal loans. In the field of gynaecology Dr Buba offers to help fertility problems, "period menstruation problems", love problems ("make him to love you alone"), women who cannot reach orgasm (enjoy sex) and to get a baby fast. He apparently does this through light and a mirror! His extraordinary talents do not stop there. He offers to stop people taking drugs, smoking and drinking. He counsels HIV patients although he stops short of offering a cure for this condition. He offers to prolong life, to treat sugar diabetes and both high or low blood pressure. It is his offer to men which is outstanding. He offers to increase the size of one's penis by four inches. He claims expertise in making the penis big and strong. He increases libido and controls early ejaculation. He can stop smoking drinking and drugs, unblock blocked blood vessels and render inactive blood cells active. All of this with no side effects or allergies. His treatment is cheaper than others. All services are by appointment. Diabetics are welcome and the real ultimate selling point, the treatment is 100 per cent natural. People of all races are welcome and he gives his telephone numbers. How can orthodox medicine possibly compete?

Although this advertisement is preposterous it is no worse than Gillian McKeith or any of the other purveyors of unnecessary vitamins, supplements and the like. Where is the evidence for colonic irrigation or coffee enemas? These are procedures recently introduced into Harare by a qualified medical doctor. Where does quackery begin and end?

Zimbabwe medical doctors are not immune to quackery. One particular patient who complained of subfertility was attended to by a well known Zimbabwe gynaecologist. The patient had one child born 22 years previously. A laparoscopy and dye studies was done in 1996. This was accompanied by a dilatation and curettage of the uterus. Extensive pelvic adhesions were found with both fallopian tubes being blocked. In October 1996 she had a tuboplasty and a ventral suspension was also performed at the same time. Ventral suspensions are seldom done these days but, in Zimbabwe, additional charges may be raised by the surgeon for these additional procedures. A tuboplasty, better known as a salpingoplasty, is surgery to "unblock" the fallopian tubes and render them patent. This operation is successful in some cases but very often because of intra abdominal scarring the fallopian tubes rapidly become blocked again. In a letter to me after I enquired about this particular patient, the surgeon explained that the patient "started having recurrent pelvic inflammatory disease, which resulted in her tubes getting blocked again". This may well have been due to unsuccessful surgery which is very common in these cases and not due to "recurrent pelvic inflammatory disease". A repeat laparoscopy and dye studies was done in June 1997 together with the, by then, mandatory dilatation and curettage. Indeed, in the particular operating theatre register used by this gynaecologist, I cannot find any gynaecological procedure performed by him without an accompanying dilatation and curettage. Again an additional charge may be raised for this procedure. At this repeat operation the patient was found to have extensive pelvic adhesions and both fallopian tubes were again found to be blocked. Repeat tuboplasty and removal of adhesions was performed in August 1997. The patient was seen "regularly due to recurrent pelvic inflammatory disease" and yet another laparoscopy and dye studies, together with the now routine accompanying dilatation and curettage was performed on the 26th of October 1998. Not surprisingly both fallopian tubes were again found to be blocked and extensive pelvic adhesions were again present. This poor lady had a total of one "out of date" operation, three laparoscopy and dye studies all with accompanying dilatation and curettage procedures and two tuboplasty and removal of adhesions operations before being referred for in vitro fertilisation as, according to the referral letter "the tubes are blocked". No semen analysis had ever been requested. This is quackery. This patient should not have had all these unnecessary operations.

This same surgeon wanted to operate on an 89 year old lady who had noticed, in passing, that she had a small amount of prolapse. She was sent to me for a second opinion and was much relieved to hear that, as her symptoms did not worry her in any way whatsoever, she did not need major surgery. In the operating theatre register I found one entry where the patient had a laparoscopy and dye studies which is done for subfertility and at the same time had an insertion of an intrauterine contraceptive device. I cannot understand this. Another patient had a laparoscopy and dye studies and removal of Norplant. Norplant is a progesterone pellet which is inserted under the skin usually of the upper arm. This means that she was being investigated for subfertility at the same time that her chosen method of contraception was being removed. I cannot understand this either.

Another patient was referred to me in 1999 by a fellow consultant because of primary subfertility. The patient had been trying to conceive for 10 years. She had nine laparoscopies and dye studies between 1990 and 1992. Every one of the nine procedures had shown patent fallopian tubes and normal ovaries! Again no semen analysis had been requested. According to the referral letter "the male factor has been excluded (husband has three children from previous marriage)".

In another case a patient had two fallopian tube operations before her husband had his semen tested. This showed poor quality and on examination he was found to have bilateral varicoceles. These are varicose veins in the scrotum and can easily be corrected by simple surgery. Semen analyses should always be done prior to investigative surgery on the female.

The in vitro fertilisation department in the International Hospital of Bahrain was reported in the local "Gulf News" to have been "very successful" over the last 15 years. The truth was that there had been six pregnancies out of a total of 242 attempts. The number of live births resulting from the six pregnancies was not mentioned but assuming that all six pregnancies resulted in live births that would give a figure of less than 2.5 per cent. That is hardly "very successful". Most in vitro fertilisation units have live birth rates of approximately 20 to even 40 per cent per embryo transfer. With a 2.5 per cent chance of a live birth one is not offering patients a fair chance. Another example of medical quackery.

We even meet quackery among patients although this example was not done for pecuniary reasons. One particular husband was referred to a consultant urologist for subfertility as no sperm were found to be present on a semen analysis. The urologist reported back that the man had fathered three children in the past before undergoing a vasectomy after the birth of the third child. He went on to say that "unfortunately that marriage did not last and he moved to South Africa where he re-married in 1997 to a 23 year old wife". The husband did not want his wife to be examined by anyone and "further, she does not know that he has had a vasectomy".

Caesarean sections

A Caesarean section is usually performed when a vaginal delivery would put the baby's or mother's life or health at risk although in recent times it has also been performed upon request for childbirths that could otherwise have been normal.[10,11,12]

The earliest recorded case of maternal survival following caesarean section dates to 1500 AD.[13] The first modern Caesarean section was performed by a German gynecologist Ferdinand Adolf Kehrer in 1881 but successful caesarean sections had been performed by indigenous healers in Kahura, Uganda as observed by R. W. Felkin in 1879. The law in Ancient Rome, the Lex Regia, of 715–673 BC, required that the dead child of a mother in childbirth be "cut from her womb".[14]

Being "cut from the womb" seems to have begun as a religious requirement that mothers not be buried pregnant[15] and to have evolved into a way of saving the fetus. On March 5, 2000, Inés Ramírez performed a caesarean section on herself and survived, as did her son, Orlando Ruiz Ramírez.[16] She is believed to be the only woman to have performed a successful caesarean section on herself.

Caesarean section is the most common major surgical procedure performed on women and over the past years the rate of caesarean sections has dramatically increased. The 2005 World Health Organization global survey which was done in 24 geographic areas and eight countries in Latin America showed a median caesarean section rate of 33 per cent. In the United Kingdom in 2004, the caesarean section rate was about 20 per cent. In a private clinic in Harare the average figure is approximately 37 per cent.

In Italy the incidence of caesarean sections is particularly high, although it varies from region to region.[17] In Campania, 60 per cent of 2008 births reportedly occurred via caesarean sections.[18] In the Rome region, the mean incidence is around 44 per cent, but can reach as high as 85 per cent in some private clinics.[19,20] In the United States the caesarean rate has risen 48 per cent since 1996, reaching a level of 31.8 per cent in 2007.[21] China has been cited as having the highest national rates of caesarean sections in the world at 46 per cent as of 2008.[22]

The US National Institutes of Health says that rises in rates of caesarean sections are not, in isolation, a cause for concern, but may reflect changing reproductive patterns.[23] The most quoted optimal caesarean section rate is the World Health Organizations' 10 to 15 per cent.[24] This figure was arrived at during a WHO consensus conference attended by 62 participants from over 20 countries.[25] Following a thorough review of published work participants were aware of all the risks of caesarean sections. They then studied variations in caesarean section rates and found several countries with very low maternal and perinatal mortality rates had caesarean section rates close to ten percent. There was no evidence that caesarean section rates above this level lowered mortality rates. The final consensus recommendation was modified to 10 to15 percent (10 percent for general populations, 15 percent for high-risk populations). This recommendation was anything but arbitrary. In Sweden, Denmark, and the Netherlands the caesarean section rate is close to 10 percent with some of the world's lowest maternal and perinatal mortality rates and there is no evidence that those women's babies are smaller or their women's hips bigger than they are in the USA, Canada or Brazil.

The increase in the caesarean section rates may be accredited to the improved technology in detecting pre-birth fetal distress or "non-reassuring fetal status" but a key distinction should be made between hospital or doctor-centric reasons and mother-centric reasons. Critics of doctor-ordered caesareans worry that the operations are in some cases performed because they are profitable for the hospital, because a quick caesarean section is more convenient for an obstetrician than a lengthy vaginal birth or because it is easier to perform surgery at a scheduled time than to respond to nature's schedule and deliver a baby at an hour that is not predetermined.[26]

In China, doctors are compensated based on the monetary value of medical treatments offered.[27] As a result, doctors have an incentive to persuade mothers to choosing the more expensive caesarean section.

Another contributing factor for doctor-ordered procedures may be fear of medical malpractice lawsuits.[28] Doctors have turned to defensive medicine. If a pregnant woman is facing an even minimal risk, a caesarean section may be recommended.[29] For this reason too if a caesarean section is anticipated to be likely to be needed for a woman, it may be preferable to perform this electively or pre-emptively during daylight operating hours, rather than wait for it to become an emergency with the increased risk of surgical and anaesthetic complications that can follow from emergency surgery. While there may be medical reasons for this increase, non-medical factors are at least partly responsible. Caesarean sections are in some cases performed for reasons other than medical necessity.[30]

Patients may request them. This may be partly due to considerations of pain during labour and preservation of vaginal tone for later in life.[31] It is well-known that parous women have excess risk for pelvic floor disorders, including prolapse and incontinence. Vaginal birth, particularly when vacuum- or forceps-assisted, is associated with a substantially higher risk for prolapse. This has prompted the question of whether caesarean delivery should be performed to prevent prolapse? Most women with prolapse discovered on routine examination in later life are asymptomatic and do not require surgical treatment. Pelvic floor disorders occurring soon after delivery often improve over time without treatment. These points should be considered before concluding that elective caesarean sections for the sole purpose of protecting the pelvic floor should become routine. Preservation of vaginal tone for sexual purposes is something that has recently been considered. I do not know if this has been studied. It would be difficult to prove either way.

On 30th October 2011 it was reported by a political journalist, David Wooding, talking on Sky News and quoting the Sunday Times that the United Kingdom based National Institute for Clinical Excellence (NICE) recommended the availability of caesarean sections on the National Health Service for all patients on their request. This will add considerably to the National Health Service budget. It is estimated that it would cost the NHS 800 pounds more for each caesarean section birth. There has been pressure to reduce the number of caesarean sections performed on the NHS and if this figure could be reduced from 25 to 24 per cent of all deliveries the NHS would save 5.6 billion pounds per year. There is also operating theatre time to be considered as well. Wooding then went on to say that he had always felt that childbirth was the most natural thing in the world. I wonder how he would fare in labour. The idiotic expression that a patient is "too posh to push" should not be used by men. Adequate pain relief during labour will be discussed later but this alone would go a long way to reducing the caesarean section rate. Although childbirth is natural so are kidney stones and pain relief may be required for both. On the 23rd November, 2011 it was announced that patients would be able to have caesarean sections on request on the National Health Service in Britain.

A study published in the 13 February 2007 issue of the *Canadian Medical Association Journal* found that the absolute differences in severe maternal morbidity and mortality was small, but that the additional risk over vaginal delivery should be considered by women contemplating an elective caesarean delivery and by their physicians.[32] An elective caesarean section with no emergency present has a 2.84-fold greater chance of the woman's death than if she had a vaginal birth.[33] Although small, the patient's choice is therefore not without added risk. There is also the risk of iatrogenic prematurity to the baby.

Even with repeated ultrasound scans, there are errors in judging when to do an elective caesarean section. It may be done too early resulting in neonatal prematurity and consequent respiratory distress syndrome both of which are major causes of morbidity and mortality.

Some authors feel that due to the comparative risks of caesarean section with an uncomplicated vaginal delivery, patients should be discouraged or even forbidden from choosing it.[34] I agree with the former but not with the latter. Patient choice is important.

Some 42 per cent of obstetricians believe the media and women are responsible for the rising caesarean section rates[35] but some studies conclude that relatively few women wish to be delivered by caesarean section.[36]

Caesarean section. Who chooses?

Marsden Wagner[37] quotes Al-Mufti and colleagues[38] who surveyed 282 obstetric consultants in London to find out the method of delivery they personally would prefer if they or their partners were pregnant for the first time in an otherwise uncomplicated pregnancy. They found that, overall, 17 per cent would choose an elective caesarean delivery. Thirty one per cent of those questioned were female and eight per cent were male. Their choice was based on concern about perineal damage from vaginal delivery, risk of injury to the baby, and the desire for an electively timed delivery. Sixty eight per cent preferred a caesarean delivery for a cephalic presentation with an estimated weight of more than 4·5 kg. and 39 per cent for an estimated weight of 4·0 to 4·5 kg. Al-Mufti and colleagues concluded that feelings of obstetricians might influence the way they counsel their patients. The same authors found, in a survey of female obstetricians, that 31 percent would choose caesarean section[39] if they had an uncomplicated singleton pregnancy at term.

Members of the audience at the American College of Obstetricians and Gynecologists (ACOG) District VIII and IX Meeting held in August, 2000 were asked if they would personally prefer to be delivered by caesarean section.[40] Of 117 participants, 46·2 per cent said they would choose caesarean delivery. 56.5 per cent male and 32·6 per cent of female obstetricians said they would prefer a caesarean section. When asked what route of delivery they would personally select for an infant weighing four to four and a half kilograms, 70 per cent said they would prefer a caesarean section, and for an estimated weight of 4·6 kg or more, 88 per cent would desire a caesarean section.

This survey of obstetricians supported the findings of Al-Mufti and colleagues. Of those surveyed nearly half would prefer a caesarean delivery and, surprisingly, more of the male obstetricians would have opted for a caesarean delivery. With birth weights of four kilograms or more, at least 70 per cent would request a caesarean section. W Benson Harer Jr., President of the ACOG wrote "… a woman's right to participate in the decision and to choose to deliver her child by caesarean delivery will be respected"[41] thereby showing the support of the patient's right of choice.

Two Australian studies provided evidence that women request caesarean sections.[42] More than 20 per cent of women who had had caesarean sections in a large South Australian hospital said that they had insisted on or were keen to have this procedure.[43] In Western Australia, in 633 women, 27per cent had caesarean sections solely because of maternal request, even when vaginal birth was judged safe.[44] Doctors seem to be more ready to accept the right of women to choose caesarean section but they sometimes commit insurance fraud by finding a medical reason for the operation, when there is none that will suit the insurance company.[45]

Society also appears to condone or even advocate the woman's choice of a caesarean section. A professor of English was quoted in the *British Medical Journal* (BMJ) as saying; "medical and social prejudices against women sidestepping their biblical sentence to painful childbirth are still with us"[46] and in the *New England Journal of Medicine* (NEJM)[47] a consumer advocate stated, "I do not believe that anyone has the right to demand women give birth vaginally."[48]

A woman who chooses caesarean section as a means of avoiding the "biblical sentence to a painful childbirth" is badly misinformed.[49] By choosing a caesarean section, she exchanges some hours of labour pain for severe post-operative pain and debility and a longer recovery period with maybe a few weeks of pain. These days there is no need whatsoever to have pain with labour. Epidural analgesia is extremely effective in providing total pain relief.

A caesarean section, which is done because a woman chooses it, requires a surgeon, possibly a second doctor to assist, an anaesthetist, nurses, equipment, an operating theatre, blood ready for transfusion and a longer post-operative hospital stay.[50] If a woman receives an elective caesarean section simply because she prefers it, there will be fewer resources for the rest of health care.[51]

In Brazil there are hospitals with 100 percent caesarean section rates, health districts with 85 percent caesarean section rates, and an entire state with a caesarean section rate of 47.7 percent.[52] This is a huge drain on the limited resources of that country. Worse, maternal mortality rates have risen in those areas of Brazil with these high caesarean section rates.[53] Caesarean section on demand is an expensive and dangerous luxury.

Another ethical issue is the right to equal access in health care. If wealthy women can choose caesarean section, should not all women have this right?

There are many benefits for the doctor in doing elective caesarean sections. It is more convenient. It allows for more "daylight obstetrics." Studies have shown not only that births occur much more commonly during daylight hours, Monday to Friday but also that emergency caesarean sections are more often done at those times as well.[54]

A caesarean section takes about 20 minutes while with a vaginal birth the doctor is in the hospital or on call sometimes for 12 hours or more.[55] In those countries where doctors attend normal births the convenience of a caesarean section may be vital to their practice.[56]

Doctors and hospitals nearly always earn much more money from a caesarean section than from a vaginal delivery. US studies show that women most likely to receive a caesarean section are white, married, have private health insurance, and give birth in private hospitals.[57] These are the women one might expect to be at lowest risk of complications that might necessitate a caesarean section, a rare example of wealthy women receiving less safe care than poor women. The World Health Organisation reported that in the United States the profit motive explained hospital-specific caesarean section rates that were high even by United States standards.[58]

A woman's basis for choosing a caesarean section may be fear and lack of confidence as a result of doctors who may themselves fear vaginal delivery and so fuel their patients' anxieties.[59] There are reasons for this fear on the part of the doctor. In one survey 82 percent of physicians employed "defensive obstetrics" to avoid negligence claims.[60] Ireland saw a 450 percent rise from 1990 to 1998 in medical negligence claims, with obstetrics and gynecology cases accounting for nearly half of the payouts.[61]

With a bad birth outcome doctors are often sued and find themselves criticised for not performing interventions such as caesarean sections. Doctors are rarely criticised for performing unnecessary interventions but if a doctor does a caesarean section solely because he or she is afraid of being sued or the fear of rising insurance costs, that doctor is not practicing good medicine.

In private health care, caesarean section is one of the most common major surgical procedures, filling beds and operating rooms and providing important income.[62] High caesarean section rates profit doctors, hospitals and industry.

In the light of these many ethical issues, the Committee for the Ethical Aspects of Human Reproduction and Women's Health of FIGO (the international umbrella organisation of national obstetric organisations) stated in a 1999 report: "Performing cesarean section for non-medical reasons is ethically not justified."[63]

To decrease the caesarean section rate Khunpradit and others[64] have suggested that prevention efforts should target clinicians. Mandatory second opinions, peer review feedback, post-caesarean surveillance to prevent repeat caesarean deliveries, and guidelines endorsed and supported by local opinion leaders were among the most effective interventions identified in the analysis. The authors state that antenatal education and support programs, computer patient decision-aids, decision-aid booklets and intensive group therapy to women have not been shown to decrease caesarean sections effectively.

The same is true of insurance reform, legislative changes, external feedback to doctors on their performance and training of public health nurses to provide information in childbirth classes. The authors said that the strategies that had clearest evidence of reducing the incidence of caesarean sections were those that focused on the clinicians. If the caesarean section rate is to be reduced, as Khunpradit says, this is who we should be targeting.

Quackery by medical academics

Since the deregulation of industry that started around 1979 with Ronald Reagan and Margaret Thatcher, one has become accustomed to dishonesty by big business. But academics and doctors are involved too. Tales of scientific conflict of interest have become all too familiar. Recently, two top medical journals have been in the news for failing to disclose the financial ties of the academic authors of published papers. But nondisclosure is only part of the story. Companies hire medical academics or other doctors to do research to help keep businesses scientifically honest. They also, however, trade on the researchers' names.

Charles B. Nemeroff,[66] the editor in chief of *Neuropsychopharmacology*, whose name obviously carried considerable weight, resigned a few years ago after a paper he co-authored about a specific device used in treatment for depression had been published in his journal[67] without disclosing that eight of the nine authors, including himself, had financial ties to the company that made the device. The journal carried a positive review of a vagus nerve stimulation (VNS) device, a $15,000 chest implant that sends pulses of electricity to the brain, and which was approved for depression in 2005 after intense debate over its effectiveness. It was manufactured by Cyberonics, Inc, of Houston, Texas.[68]

Nemeroff was the lead author for the paper, which described VNS as a "promising and well-tolerated intervention that is effective in a subset of patients with treatment-resistant depression." The article acknowledged funding from Cyberonics, and listed coauthor Stephen Brannan as an employee of Cyberonics. But it did not reveal that the eight other academic co-authors were all consultants for the firm. In 2003, Nemeroff had co-authored a review in *Nature Neuroscience* in which he had neglected to mention significant financial interests in three therapies that were reviewed favourably (including owning the patent on one of the treatments). As a result the Nature Publishing Group widened its disclosure policies. Nemeroff and his co-author Michael Owens said at the time that in the future they intended to provide all financial disclosure information "even if it is not requested by the journal editor."[69]

Clare Stanford, past president of the British Association for Psychopharmacology and an editor at several journals in the field, said Nemeroff was an influential researcher in his field who was unlikely to have been swayed by the Cyberonics money. "I don't believe for a minute that the fact the paper was funded by a company would have influenced his conclusions," she told The Scientist. "It is unfortunate that he has had to stand down over this incident which is largely a reflection of the scientific community's paranoia rather than any failing of his professional integrity." Nemeroff, told *The Scientist* in an Email that the financial disclosures of all authors were submitted to the journal, but due to an "oversight," were not included in the print version. "There was absolutely no intent to withhold any information concerning financial disclosures."[70]

Neuropsychopharmacology printed a correction but, at least as important as the failure to disclose financial ties were the authors themselves and other consultants that Cyberonics had hired. Other very influential psychiatrists were involved, all helping to give respectability to Cyberonic's device. Apparently more than 20 experts at the Food and Drug Administration opposed the approval of this device for the treatment of depression before being overruled by a senior official, according to a Senate Finance Committee investigation.

Companies give top researchers large grants for research, or to consult, because they know their names attached to reports make them look more legitimate. The very presence of those names on papers reviewing the treatment is a big part of the salesmanship that comes after obtaining approval. Harold Sackeim, a professor of psychiatry and radiology at Columbia University, said that if device makers could not hire the field's top experts, effective new devices would never be approved.

Food and Drug Administration (FDA) rules in the USA allow doctors to prescribe federally approved drugs for any purpose, even if it is not indicated on the medicine's label.[71] But drug companies are tightly constrained in what they can say about their medicines. Companies can promote drugs only for their federally approved purposes, their so-called "on label" use. "Off label" promotion by drug companies is illegal, and since 2000, drug makers have paid large fines to settle Federal criminal cases over off-label prescriptions.[72] Pfizer, for example, paid $430 million in 2004 to settle allegations that it had promoted Neurontin, an anti-epilepsy medicine, for pain and bipolar disorder.

Some companies circumvent the FDA rules by hiring independent doctors to talk to other physicians about their medicines.[73] Companies can also sponsor "continuing medical education" sessions, ranging from lunches to weeklong conferences, where specialist doctors tell other physicians about the latest developments in their fields, including off-label uses for drugs already on the market. For such speaking engagements, doctors can receive $3,000 or more a day from the companies. In other words, the FDA rules allow drug makers to pay independent doctors to discuss medicines in ways that might be illegal for the companies themselves to do so.

A Maryland psychiatrist Dr. John Gleason[74] was arrested, and later charged for promoting a drug for purposes other than those approved by the federal government. Dr. Gleason freely acknowledged that in meetings with other doctors he had advised that Xyrem, a powerful drug for narcolepsy could also be prescribed for depression and fibromyalgia, a poorly understood pain disorder. He did the same at hundreds of speeches and seminars where he was rewarded with generous fees. The prosecutors claimed that he had conspired with the drug's manufacturer to recommend it for potentially dangerous uses. The indictment also charged that Dr. Gleason committed fraud against insurance companies by advising doctors to leave blank an area on the Xyrem prescription form that asked for a disease diagnosis.[75] Dr. Gleason acknowledged that he told doctors not to offer a diagnosis but says he never told them to lie if they were asked for one.[76]

Dr. Gleason received more than US$100,000 in one year alone from Jazz Pharmaceuticals, which made Xyrem. He received $450 to visit a doctor in the office, $750 for speaking at a luncheon and $1,500 for a dinner speech.[77] He said that he made as much as $3,000 a day. Although he continued to see some patients, the Xyrem talks gradually became his primary source of income.[78]

Orphan Medical superceded Jazz Pharmaceuticals and in 2007, Jazz and its Orphan Medical unit pled guilty to one felony count of introducing a misbranded drug into interstate commerce.[79] Both Jazz and Orphan settled with the government for US$20 million in civil and criminal payments and entered a corporate integrity agreement. A former Orphan Medical sales manager also pleaded guilty for encouraging doctors to engage in off-label usage.[80]

The active ingredient in Xyrem is gamma hydroxybutyrate, or GHB, an illegal street drug with a history of use in date rape and of overdose hazards. Xyrem is listed as a federally controlled substance, with distribution tightly monitored.[81] This fact may have influenced the prosecutors in selecting Dr. Gleason from among the countless other doctors who act in the same way.

Through it all, Gleason maintained he did nothing wrong.[82] Rather, he repeatedly insisted that he disseminated truthful information about the drug and, moreover, was entitled to discuss off-label use since physicians are allowed to prescribe medications for uses that were not approved by the FDA. In doing so, he also cited his right to free speech. Dr Gleason's sister said that, in her view, her brother spoke truthfully at meetings and promotional talks.[83]

He believed he was doing this correctly and he had a company overseeing his talks and they never indicated that he was doing something inappropriate. She felt that the government had hounded her brother in order to make a case and collect a fine. She said that she believed the entire investigation by the department of justice and prosecutor was in excess; "In the end, they just wore him down."[84]

The 57-year-old Dr Gleason recently saw his medical licenses suspended in Pennsylvania and California and the accumulated weight of all the events apparently led him to commit suicide.

Dr. Steven Nissen, the interim chairman of cardiovascular medicine at the Cleveland Clinic, said the case could "have a chilling effect on physicians, because when we give lectures, we assume that giving an opinion about the use of a drug is not going to get us into legal difficulty."[85] The FDA and federal lawyers, he said, need to restrict criminal prosecutions to especially egregious cases of off-label promotion.[86]

In February 1994, the BBC Channel 4 program, *Preying on Hope* broadcast a secretly filmed and recorded consultation[87] between Dr Peter Nixon and an AIDs patient, Ian Hughes, who subsequently died in 1996. Hughes was told by Dr Nixon that his fatigue was caused, not by AIDS, but by hyperventilation and an antihistamine and the sedative diazepam (Valium) were prescribed for this. Dr Nixon had recommended the course of diazepam and "two weeks of sleeping" as a cure for hyperventilation. The program claimed that Dr. Nixon had "rigged" tests and misdiagnosed a terminally ill AIDs patient. Dr. Nixon, in a two million pounds libel case, claimed that Channel Four had branded him as a charlatan unfit to practice medicine.[88]

Dr. Nixon, who had a turnover of more than £100,000 a year until his retirement from Charing Cross Hospital six years previously, had claimed that illnesses such as heart attacks, the Gulf War Syndrome, premenstrual tension and the chronic fatigue syndrome could be caused by hyperventilation. Dr Nixon's views were promoted in *The Sunday Times* by the then medical correspondent, Neville Hodgkinson, who wrote a front page article in 1988 claiming that Dr Nixon had found a 100 percent effective treatment for chronic fatigue syndrome.

The libel case against Channel 4, at the Royal Courts of Justice in London, collapsed after five weeks when Dr Nixon was compelled to admit[89] that a series of papers co-authored by him and published in the *Journal of the Royal Society of Medicine* contained a number of errors that appeared to be, he conceded in the trial, "more than an honest slip of the pen".[90] Dr Nixon agreed to pay £765,520 in costs.

Dr Nixon, aged 71 at the time, had outlined his theories in a series of articles in medical journals. He admitted in court that the articles contained a number of errors and said he had not written or in some cases even read all the papers which bore his name. He acknowledged that it "looked rather suspicious" that three patients of 27 reported on in a *Journal of the Royal Society of Medicine* paper had been removed when he later reported the same study in the *American Journal of Clinical Hypnosis*. He conceded that this invalidated the results published in the latter journal which had not been told about the earlier paper. He also admitted that at Charing Cross and in private practice, he had carried out exercise tests and other diagnostic tests, which could in some circumstances be fatal, without explaining the risks and obtaining patients' informed consent, and had not sought the approval of Charing Cross Hospital ethics committee.

The settlement left the Medical Defence Union, which backed Dr Nixon, facing a bill estimated at nearly £2 million, including its own costs. In October 1997, Dr Nixon's name was removed from the Medical Register by the General Medical Council. This action removes legal entitlement to practice medicine.

In his award-winning investigation for *The Sunday Times* of London, reporter Brian Deer[91] exposed fraudulent research, published in *The Lancet* medical journal, which had caused "global epidemics of fear, guilt and infectious disease". When the investigation concluded in January 2011, a poll found that in the USA alone nearly 145 million people knew of his key finding.

Deer reported that, according to a Doctor Andrew Wakefield, the measles virus in the measles, mumps and rubella (MMR) vaccine attacked the gut, which in turn led to brain damage. This theory led Wakefield and the Royal Free Hospital in London to make the astounding claim that an anti-measles treatment would prevent the brain damage, possibly allowing autistic children to be cured by their product, a "safer" measles vaccine produced using the same technology. This "safer" measles vaccine would presumably be used in place of the MMR vaccine. Nine months before the publication of his article in *The Lancet*, Wakefield and the Royal Free Hospital Medical School filed patent claims for their products which could only succeed if MMR's reputation was damaged. Their products would theoretically be vastly profitable. They were purported to be a safer measles vaccine as well as potential treatment for bowel disease and autism. All were based on claims that the attenuated measles virus contained in the MMR vaccine was at fault.

Wakefield's claims that the MMR vaccination could be related to autism, Crohn's disease and inflammatory bowel disease[92] caused widespread alarm. As a consequence, rates of MMR vaccination fell from 92 per cent in 1996–1997 to 88 per cent in 1998.[93] In a survey for BBC Radio 5 Live, more than half of GPs surgeries reported that the uptake of the MMR vaccine had fallen [94.] Anti-vaccination groups and campaigns are gaining support, particularly in the USA and Western Europe.[95] Wakefield irresponsibly started a panic with tragic repercussions. Vaccination rates fell so low that childhood diseases once all but eradicated re-emerged endangering young lives. There is no doubt that this caused the deaths of children who were not vaccinated. One such tragic case was reported in the *Weekly Telegraph*[96] Eliza-Mae Benson was five weeks old when she died of whooping cough, three weeks before she would have been old enough for the vaccination. Dawn and David Benson had to bury their daughter but Mrs Benson, 36, a nurse, said: "Young babies waiting to be vaccinated would normally be protected by older children being vaccinated against whooping cough, but if people are refusing to have their children vaccinated, then it can let the infection in. When parents decide not to vaccinate their children it is not just a personal decision it has an impact on other families." The couple appealed to parents to have their babies vaccinated against whooping cough at the earliest opportunity to give all children what is known as "herd immunity." They also urged parents to ensure their pre-school children have a booster jab to help protect babies by building up the "herd immunity." National immunisation figures are still below the levels that existed before the scare over the measles, mumps and rubella (MMR) vaccine.[97] Hundreds of thousands of parents have refused to have their children immunised because of the alleged link to autism claimed by Dr Andrew Wakefield.

On 28th January 2010, a five-member panel of the General Medical Council in the United Kingdom handed down rulings vindicating Brian Deer's investigation and dubbing Andrew Wakefield "dishonest", "unethical" and "callous". They revoked Wakefield's medical license after a lengthy hearing, citing numerous ethical violations that tainted his work.[98] These included failing to disclose financing from lawyers who were mounting a case against the vaccine manufacturers,[99] subjecting developmentally disabled children to unnecessary invasive procedures such as venesection , mishandling funds and failing to disclose conflicts of interest. The General Medical Council, in its ruling against Wakefield, said that he displayed conduct that "fell seriously short of the standards expected of a doctor and which was a breach of the trust that the public is entitled to have in members of the medical profession" and they deemed his actions "serious professional misconduct."

The Lancet retracted the original Wakefield paper. The *British Medical Journal* concluded that the research was not just unethically financed but also "fraudulent" in that timelines were misrepresented, for example, to suggest direct culpability of the vaccine.[100] Wakefield also claimed, for example, that a "safer" measles vaccine was not, in fact, a rival to the MMR vaccine which would have been a clear conflict of interest.[101] It was instead an immune-boosting vaccine for those with compromised immune systems; an unfortunate semantic mix-up.[102]

Wakefield apparently still has an unshakeable belief in his theory and Susan Dominus[103] having interviewed Wakefield, wrote that Peter Medawar, a British scientist who wrote a famous critique of a book of specious ideas about evolution, came to mind. Medawar said that "Its author can be excused of dishonesty only on the grounds that before deceiving others he has taken great pains to deceive himself."

In August 1996 in one of Britain's most dramatic cases of medical fraud Malcolm Pearce, a senior lecturer at St George's Hospital Medical School in South London and a world famous expert on ultrasonography in obstetrics, claimed a major breakthrough.

The story was reported in the *British Journal of Obstetrics and Gynaecology* of which Pearce was an assistant editor under the title "Term delivery after intrauterine relocation of an ectopic pregnancy".[104] The case report was said to concern a 29 year old African woman who had previously had two ectopic pregnancies. It described a procedure whereby the fetus in her third ectopic pregnancy was removed and replaced into her uterus. Doctors had been trying for many years to successfully implant an ectopic pregnancy obtained from an unruptured fallopian tube into the uterus with a resultant birth of a live baby. Pearce claimed to have accomplished this. The report, which received wide publicity in the mass media, claimed that the pregnancy reached term with no further problems. It was a huge achievement with attendant worldwide media coverage

A second author of the case report was Geoffrey Chamberlain, editor of the journal, President of the Royal College of Obstetricians and Gynaecologists and professor and head of department at St George's Hospital. The same issue also contained another article "Randomised controlled trial of the use of human chorionic gonadotrophin in recurrent miscarriage associated with polycystic ovaries." by Malcolm Pearce and others. A front page story in The *Daily Mail* exposed the two papers as fraudulent. Chamberlain said that he had not known the work to be fraudulent and that it was common in medicine for people to have their name on papers when they had not done much work on the project. This was indeed common practice at that time. For many heads of departments this was usual. The "whistle-blower" in this case was a young doctor at St George's Hospital Medical School who had raised questions about the two papers.

A prompt investigation showed that the patient did not exist, the patients supposedly in the second trial could not be found and among other studies by Pearce dating back to 1989 three others were found to be fraudulent, two of them published in the *British Medical Journal.*

All the papers were retracted. Pearce was fired and subsequently struck off the medical register by the General Medical Council.[105] Chamberlain retired or resigned from all his positions, a terrible end to a very distinguished career. His crime was gift authorship of a fraudulent article. Gift authorship was normal and acceptable at the beginning of his career but scandalous by the end. Professor Peter Rubin, head of the department of medicine at the University of Nottingham, said: "The practice of heads of department putting their names on papers with which they have had no involvement other than to create the environment in which the research took place is still more widespread than might be imagined."

References:

1. John Garrow.
HealthWatch
Newsletter no 33: April 1999.
2. Paul Mason. 1st Dec 2006. BBC NEWS | Talk about Newsnight | AIDS: We expose the "goat ...
www.bbc.co.uk/.../ newsnight/2006. BBC NEWS | Talk about Newsnight | AIDS: We expose the "goat ..,
http://www.bbc.co.uk/blogs/newsnight/2006/12/aids_we_expose_the_goat_cure_sales men_1.html (accessed July 21, 2013).
3. CARD Business Proposal, November 2006. BBC NEWS | Talk about Newsnight | AIDS: We expose the "goat ..www.bbc.co.uk/.../2006.
http://www.bbc.co.uk/blogs/newsnight/2006/12/aids_we_expose_the_goat_cure_sales men_1.html (accessed July 21, 2013).
4. BBC NEWS | Talk about Newsnight | AIDS: We expose the "goat ..,
http://www.bbc.co.uk/blogs/newsnight/2006/12/aids_we_expose_the_goat_cure_sales men_1.html (accessed July 21, 2013).
5. Ibid.
6. Ibid.
7. Ibid.
8. Ben Goldacre. "Bad Science". Fourth Estate. London. 2009. p 183.
9. Ibid. p 108.

10. "Fear a factor in surgical births". The Sydney Morning Herald. 2007-10-07. http://www.smh. com.au/news/ national/fear-a-factor-in-surgical-births/2007/10/06/ 1191091421081.html
11. "Kiwi caesarean rate continues to rise". Stuff.co.nz. 12 September 2007. http://www.stuff.co.nz/stuff/4198257a11.html. Retrieved 22 September 2011.
12. Finger, C. (2003). "Caesarean section rates skyrocket in Brazil. Many women are opting for Caesareans in the belief that it is a practical solution." Lancet 362 (9384): 628. doi:10.1016/S0140-6736(03)14204-3. PMID 12947949. Caesarean section - Wikipedia, the free encyclopedia, http://en.wikipedia.org/wiki/C%C2%A7 (accessed July 21, 2013).
13. "Cesarean Section – A Brief History: Part 1". US National Institutes of Health. 2009-06-25. http://www.nlm.nih.gov/exhibition/cesarean/part1.html. Retrieved 2010-11-27.
14. Caesarean section: etymology and early history South African Journal of Obstetrics and Gynaecology, August, 2009 by Pieter W.J. van Dongen.
15. "As there was a cultural taboo against burying an undelivered woman in Roman and German societies, according to Lex Caesarea..." U Högberg, E Iregren, CH Siven, "Maternal deaths in medieval sweden: an osteological and life table analysis", Journal of Biosocial Science, 1987, 19: 495–503 Cambridge University Press. Answerit - So where did the word/act Caesarean section come .., http://answerit.news24.com/Question/Question.aspx?QuestionID=89397 (accessed July 21, 2013).
16. Caesarean section - Headache Research - Diseases Research, http://www.diseases-diagnosis.com/virtual/Caesarean_section (accessed July 21, 2013).
17. "La clinica dei record: 9 neonati su 10 nati con il parto cesareo". Corriere della Sera. January 14, 2009. Caesarean section - Wikipedia, the free encyclopedia, http://en.wikipedia.org/wiki/C%C2%A7 (accessed July 21, 2013).
18. "Sagliocco denuncia boom di parti cesarei in Campania". Pupia informazione Campania. January 31, 2009.
19. http://www.asplazio.it/asp_online/tut_soggetti_deb/files/files_cesareo/09/TC_tot08_ 09.pdf
20. "Cesarei, alla Mater Dei il record". TgCOM Mediaset www.tgcom.mediaset.it. January 14th, 2009. http://www.tgcom.mediaset.it/cronaca/articoli/articolo438555.shtml=.
21. "Births: Preliminary Data for 2007". National Center for Health Statistics. http://www.cdc.gov/nchs/data/nvsr/nvsr57/nvsr57_12.pdf. Retrieved 2006-11-23.
22. "China's C-Section Rate Highest Worldwide, WHO Study Says," Medical News Today, January 15, 2010. Caesarean section - Wikipedia, the free encyclopedia, http://en.wikipedia.org/wiki/C%C2%A7 (accessed July 21, 2013).
23. Caesarean section - Headache Research - Diseases Research, http://www.diseases-diagnosis.com/virtual/Caesarean_section (accessed July 21, 2013).
24. World Health Organization. 1985. Appropriate technology for birth. Lancet ii: 436–37.
25. Wagner, M. 1994. Pursuing the Birth Machine: The Search for Appropriate Birth Technology. Sydney: ACE Graphics.
26. Goldstick O, Weissman A, Drugan A (2003). "The circadian rhythm of 'urgent' operative deliveries". Isr Med Assoc J 5 (8): 564–6. Ca esarean section - Wikipedia, the free encyclopedia, http://en.wikipedia.org/wiki/C%C2%A7 (accessed July 21, 2013).

27. Caesarean section - Headache Research - Diseases Research, http://www.diseases-diagnosis.com/virtual/Caesarean_section (accessed July 21, 2013).
28. Caesarean section - Wikipedia, the free encyclopedia, http://en.wikipedia.org/wiki/C%C2%A7 (accessed July 21, 2013).
29. "La clinica dei record: 9 neonati su 10 nati con il parto cesareo". Corriere della Sera. January 14, 2009. Caesarean section - Wikipedia, the free encyclopedia, http://en.wikipedia.org/wiki/C%C2%A7 (accessed July 21, 2013).
30. Caesarean section - Wikipedia, the free encyclopedia, http://en.wikipedia.org/wiki/C%C2%A7 (accessed July 21, 2013).
31. Wagner, Marsden. Born in the USA: How a Broken Maternity System Must Be Fixed to Put Women and Children First. p. 42. ISBN 0520245962.
32. Liu S, Liston RM, Joseph KS, Heaman M, Sauve R, Kramer MS (2007). "Maternal mortality and severe morbidity associated with low-risk planned cesarean delivery versus planned vaginal delivery at term". CMAJ 176 (4): 455–60. Caesarean section - Headache Research - Diseases Research, http://www.diseases-diagnosis.com/virtual/Caesarean_section (accessed July 21, 2013).
33. Hall, M.H. & Brewley, S. 1999. Maternal mortality and mode of delivery. Lancet 354: 776.
34. Bewley S, Cockburn J. (2002). "The unfacts of 'request' Caesarean section". BCOG 109 (6): 597–605. Caesarean section - Headache Research - Diseases Research, http://www.diseases-diagnosis.com/virtual/Caesarean_section (accessed July 21, 2013).
35. Usha Kiran TS, Jayawickrama NS (2002). "Who is responsible for the rising Caesarean section rate?" J Obstet Gynaecol 22 (4): 363–5.
36. Hildingsson I, Rådestad I, Rubertsson C, Waldenström U (2002). "Few women wish to be delivered by Caesarean section." BJOG 109 (6): 618–23. Caesarean section - Headache Research - Diseases Research, http://www.diseases-diagnosis.com/virtual/Caesarean_section (accessed July 21, 2013).
37. Wagner M. Choosing caesarean section. Lancet. November 11, 2000; 356: 1677-1680. Full Text | PDF(75KB) | CrossRef | PubMed
38. Al-Mufti R, McCarthy A, Fisk NM. Obstetrician's personal choice and mode of delivery. Lancet 1996; 347: 544. CrossRef | PubMed
39. Al-Mufti, R., McCarthy, A. & Fisk, N.M. 1997. Survey of obstetricians' personal preference and discretionary practice. Eur J Obstet Gynecol Reprod Biol 73: 1–4.
40. SG Gabbe and GB Holzman. Obstetricians' choice of delivery. 3 March 2001. The Lancet, Volume 357, Issue 9257, Page 722, www.thelancet.com/.../lancet/article/PIIS0140-6736(05)7148.doi:10.1016/S0140-6736(05)71484-7
41. Harer WB. Patient choice cesarean. AOCG Clin Rev 2000; 5: 1-15. PubMed
42. Ruth Walker, Eleni Golois, Deborah Turnbull, Chris Wilkinson. Why choose caesarean section? 24 February 2001. The Lancet Volume 357, Issue 9256, Pages 635 - 636, doi:10.1016/S0140-6736(05)71426-4.
43. Turnbull DA, Wilkinson C, Yaser A, Carty V, Svigos JM, Robinson JS. Women's role and satisfaction in the decision to have a caesarean section. Med J Aust 1999; 170: 580-583. PubMed.
44. Quinlivan JA, Petersen RW, Nichols CN. Patient preference the leading indication for elective caesarean section in public patients: results of a 2 year prospective audit in a teaching hospital. Aust NZ J Obstet Gynaecol 1999; 174: 199-205. PubMed
45. M. Wagner. "Choosing caesarean section" November 11, 2000.The Lancet, 356:1677–80.

46. 1998. Controversies: should doctors perform an elective caesarean section on request? BMJ 317: 463. Choosing Caesarean Section - by Marsden Wagner, MD, http://www.midwiferytoday.com/articles/ChoosingCaesarean.asp (accessed July 21, 2013).

47. Sachs, B.P., Kobelin, C., Castro, M.A. & Frigoletto, F. 1999. The risks of lowering the cesarean-delivery rate. N Engl J Med 340: 54–57.

48. Showalter, E. & Griffen, A. 1999. All women should have a choice; and Bastien, H. Health has become secondary to a sexually attractive body. BMJ 319: 1397. Choosing Caesarean Section - by Marsden Wagner, MD, http://www.midwiferytoday.com/articles/ChoosingCaesarean.asp (accessed July 21, 2013).

49. Choosing Caesarean Section - by Marsden Wagner, MD, http://www.midwiferytoday.com/articles/ChoosingCaesarean.asp (accessed July 21, 2013).

50. Ibid.

51. Ibid.

52. Ratmer, D. 1996. Sobre a hipotese de establizacao das taxas de cesarea do Estado de Sao Paulo, Brasil. Rev Saude Publ 30: 19–33. Choosing Caesarean Section - by Marsden Wagner, MD, http://www.midwiferytoday.com/articles/ChoosingCaesarean.asp (accessed July 21, 2013).

53. Secretariat of Health. Sao Paulo State, Brazil, 1999. Choosing Caesarean Section - by Marsden Wagner, MD, http://www.midwiferytoday.com/articles/ChoosingCaesarean.asp (accessed July 21, 2013).

54. Wagner, M. 1994. Pursuing the Birth Machine: The Search for Appropriate Birth Technology. Sydney: ACE Graphics.

55. Choosing Caesarean Section - by Marsden Wagner, MD, http://www.midwiferytoday.com/articles/ChoosingCaesarean.asp (accessed July 21, 2013).

56. Ibid.

57. Wagner, M. 1994. Pursuing the Birth Machine: The Search for Appropriate Birth Technology. Sydney: ACE Graphics. Choosing Caesarean Section - by Marsden Wagner, MD, http://www.midwiferytoday.com/articles/ChoosingCaesarean.asp (accessed July 21, 2013).

58. FIGO Committee for the Ethical Aspects of Human Reproduction and Women's Health. 1999. Ethical aspects regarding cesarean delivery for non-medical reasons. Int J Obst Gynecol 64: 317–22.

59. Choosing Caesarean Section - by Marsden Wagner, MD, http://www.midwiferytoday.com/articles/ChoosingCaesarean.asp (accessed July 21, 2013).

60. Birchard, K. 1999. Defence union suggest new approach to handling litigation costs in Ireland. Lancet 354: 1710.

61. Ibid. Choosing Caesarean Section - by Marsden Wagner, MD, http://www.midwiferytoday.com/articles/ChoosingCaesarean.asp (accessed July 21, 2013).

62. Choosing Caesarean Section - by Marsden Wagner, MD, http://www.midwiferytoday.com/articles/ChoosingCaesarean.asp (accessed July 21, 2013).

63. FIGO Committee for the Ethical Aspects of Human Reproduction and Women's Health. 1999. Ethical aspects regarding cesarean delivery for non-medical reasons. Int J Obst Gynecol 64: 317–22. Choosing Caesarean Section - by Marsden Wagner, MD, http://www.midwiferytoday.com/articles/ChoosingCaesarean.asp (accessed July 21, 2013).
64. Suthit Khunpradit, Emma Tavender, Pisake Lumbiganon, Malinee Laopaiboon, Jason Wasiak, Russell L Gruen. Non-clinical interventions for reducing unnecessary caesarean section. The Cochrane Database of Systematic Reviews. Published online June 15, 2011. Issue 6. Art. No.: CD005528 DOI: 10.1002/14651858.CD005528.pub2 Local efforts can stem the increasing unnecessary cesarean .., http://www.eurekalert.org/pub_releases/2011-07/w-lec072611.php (accessed July 21, 2013).
65. Local efforts can stem the increasing unnecessary cesarean .., http://www.eurekalert.org/pub_releases/2011-07/w-lec072611.php (accessed July 21, 2013).
66. Stephen Pincock "Journal editor quits in conflict scandal" - The Scientist - Magazine of the Life Sciences http://www.the-scientist.com/news/display/24445/#ixzz1ewCHev89. July24, 2006.
67. Nemeroff C., et al, "VNS Therapy in Treatment-Resistant Depression: Clinical Evidence and Putative Neurobiological Mechanisms," Neuropsychopharmacology (2006) 31, 1345-1355. PM_ID: 16880768. Alliance for Human Research Protection - THE SCIENTIST .., http://www.ahrp.org/cms/content/view/330/149/ (accessed July 21, 2013).
68. Alliance for Human Research Protection - THE SCIENTIST .., http://www.ahrp.org/cms/content/view/330/149/ (accessed July 21, 2013).
69. Ibid.
70. Ibid.
71. Indictment of Doctor Tests Drug Marketing Rules, http://archive.truthout.org/article/indictment-doctor-tests-drug-marketing-rules (accessed July 21, 2013).
72. Ibid.
73. Ibid.
74. David Colquhoun's Improbable Science page. http://dcscience.net/. Indictment of Doctor Tests Drug Marketing Rules, http://archive.truthout.org/article/indictment-doctor-tests-drug-marketing-rules (accessed July 21, 2013).
75. Indictment of Doctor Tests Drug Marketing Rules, http://archive.truthout.org/article/indictment-doctor-tests-drug-marketing-rules (accessed July 21, 2013).
76. Ibid.
77. Ibid.
78. Ibid.
79. Florida Goes After Dead Doc For Off-Label Marketing | Pharmalot, http://www.pharmalive.com/florida-goes-after-dead-doc-label-marketing (accessed July 21, 2013).
80. Dr. Gleason - Page 3 - Cafepharma Message Boards, http://www.cafepharma.com/boards/showthread.php?goto=newpost&t=408887 (accessed July 21, 2013).
81. Indictment of Doctor Tests Drug Marketing Rules, http://archive.truthout.org/article/indictment-doctor-tests-drug-marketing-rules (accessed July 21, 2013).

82. Florida Goes After Dead Doc For Off-Label Marketing | Pharmalot, http://www.pharmalive.com/florida-goes-after-dead-doc-label-marketing (accessed July 21, 2013).
83. Ibid.
84. Ibid.
85. Doctor indicted for off-label drug promotion: NY Times .., http://www.mmm-online.com/doctor-indicted-for-off-label-drug-promotion-ny-times/article/23453/ (accessed July 21, 2013).
86. Indictment of Doctor Tests Drug Marketing Rules, http://archive.truthout.org/article/indictment-doctor-tests-drug-marketing-rules (accessed July 21, 2013).
87. Paul McCann. BBC Channel 4 program1994. Preying on hope. Cardiologist admits research misconduct. Independent (UK), 16 May 1997, page 2. Also Guardian (UK), 27 May 1997, G2 supplement. http://news.bbc.co.uk/hi/english/health/newsid 1897000/1897261.stm .
88. Clare Dyer. Legal correspondent. British Medical Journal. 24 MAY 1997 BMJ. 314 p1501.
89. HealthWatch Newsletter no 26, http://www.healthwatch-uk.org/newsletters/nlett26.html (accessed July 21, 2013).
90. Ibid.
91. Brian Deer. http://briandeer.com/mmr-lancet.htm
92. Wakefield AJ, Murch SH, Anthony A, et al. Ileal-lymphoid-nodular hyperplasia, non-specific colitis, and pervasive developmental disorder in children. Lancet 1998;351:637–41.
93. Anderson P. Another media scare about the MMR vaccine hits Britain. BMJ 1999;318:1578..
94. http://news.bbc.co.uk/hi/english/health/newsid 1897000/1897261.stm
95. Douglas Jr RG. The Jeremiah Metzger Lecture. Vaccine prophylaxis today: its science, application and politics. Trans Am Clin Climatol Assoc 1998;109:185–96.
96. The Weekly Telegraph. Dec 28th 2011 to Jan 3rd 2012.p 8 Kantar Media Intelligence Health News, http://presswatch.com/health/?limit=101&searchterm=separately (accessed July 21, 2013).
97. Kantar Media Intelligence Health News, http://presswatch.com/health/?limit=101&searchterm=separately (accessed July 21, 2013).
98. Andrew Wakefield: Exiled in Texas | thAutcast.com, http://thautcast.com/drupal5/content/andrew-wakefield-exiled-texas (accessed July 21, 2013).
99. Ibid.
100. Ibid.
101. Autism Guru Fights for His Reputation and Theory .., http://www.heraldtribune.com/article/20110424/ZNYT04/104243000 (accessed July 21, 2013).
102. Ibid.
103. Susan Dominus. The New York Times Magazine. April 20th 2011. Autism Guru Fights for His Reputation and Theory .., http://www.heraldtribune.com/article/20110424/ZNYT04/104243000 (accessed July 21, 2013).
104. Research misconduct and biomedical journals Richard Smith Editor, BMJ
www.bmj.com/talks. www.iupap.org/wg/communications/ethics/speakers/smith.ppt
105. Ibid.

CHAPTER EIGHT - QUACKERY - RESEARCH MISCONDUCT

In the USA, at Congressional hearings into scientific misconduct, the President of the National Academy of Sciences said: "Problems of scientific misconduct are rare and the product of psychopathic behaviour' originating in temporarily deranged minds." How rare is "rare"? Al Gore, the chairman of the hearing said that "one reason for the persistence of this type of problem is the reluctance of people high in the science field to take these matters very seriously."[1]

Misconduct jeopardizes the good name of medicine and any institution in which it originates. The way in which research misconduct is policed and corrected reflects the integrity of the whole of science. People "high in the science field" are now beginning to take these matters very seriously but misconduct is not always easy to detect and may be difficult to counter. How common is misconduct in medicine?

Titus et al[2] in a survey of 2,212 researchers in the United States found that a large number of potential misconduct cases may go unreported to the Office of Research Integrity every year. They discuss why this is so and suggest ways that institutions can encourage researchers to speak out if they feel that misconduct has occurred.

The incidence of scientific misconduct and fraud depends on the definitions used. The US Commission on Research Integrity in 1996 defined research misconduct as "significant misbehaviour that improperly appropriates the intellectual property or contributions of others, that intentionally impedes the progress of research, or that risks corrupting the scientific record or compromising the integrity of scientific practices.[3] Such behaviours are unethical and unacceptable in proposing, conducting, or reporting research, or in reviewing the proposals or research reports of others."[4]

The U.S. Office of Research Integrity (ORI)[5] defines research misconduct as fabrication, falsification, or plagiarism in proposing, performing, or reviewing research, or in reporting research results.[6]

Fabrication is making up data or results and recording or reporting them. Falsification is manipulating research materials, equipment, or processes, or changing or omitting data or results such that the research is not accurately represented in the research record. Plagiarism is the appropriation of another person's ideas, processes, results, or words without giving appropriate credit but they add that research misconduct does not include honest error or differences of opinion.

A consensus statement[7] proposed by a British consensus panel in 1999 agreed that there was a problem and the statement suggested a broad definition of research misconduct. They said that research misconduct was: "Behaviour by a researcher, intentional or not, that falls short of good ethical and scientific standards." United Kingdom bodies were working together to set up a panel on misconduct.

Richard Smith, listed research misconduct which he ranked by "seriousness" starting with fabrication of data and including falsification or wilful distortion of data, plagiarism, failing to obtain ethics committee consent and progressing all the way down to failure to perform an adequate search of existing research before beginning new research. Rather than list a full taxonomy of fraud he recommended that more attention be given to codes of good research practice.

Redundant publication, one facet of research misconduct, occurs in around a fifth of published papers and about a fifth of authors of studies in medical journals have contributed little or nothing to the article itself. The finding that most current members of guideline panels and half of chairs of panels have conflicts of interest[8] is concerning and suggests that a risk of considerable influence of industry on guideline recommendations exists. The prevalence and under-reporting of conflicts of interest are high and transparency is incomplete among a wide range of guideline producing organisations

How common is fraud? Like misconduct the incidence of research fraud also obviously relates to the different definitions used. Stephen Lock[9] asked 80 researchers mostly British and mostly professors of medicine who were friends and he therefore obtained an 100 per cent response rate. This was obviously not a random sample but over half of the researchers knew of cases involving research misconduct or fraud. Over half of the "the dubious results" had been published and there had only been six "retractions". All of these were worded vaguely and none used the actual term "retraction".

The incidence of scientific misconduct is worryingly high in the UK.[10] A survey was emailed to 9,036 academics and clinicians who had submitted articles to the *British Medical Journal* or acted as peer reviewers for the journal. Only 2,700 researchers responded, a disappointingly low response rate of only 31per cent. One wonders why. Of these researchers, 13 per cent admitted knowledge of colleagues "inappropriately adjusting, excluding, altering, or fabricating data" for the purpose of publication. Just over one in 20 (six per cent) said they were aware of cases of possible misconduct within their own institutions that remained insufficiently investigated.

Dr Fiona Godlee, *British Medical Journal* editor in chief, said: "UK science and medicine deserve better. Doing nothing is not an option." According to her the survey could not show a true estimate of how much research misconduct there is in the UK. It did show that there were a substantial number of cases and that UK institutions were failing to investigate adequately, if at all.[11]

She said that the BMJ had been told of junior academics being advised to keep concerns to themselves to protect their careers, being bullied into not publishing their findings, or having their contracts terminated when they spoke out.[12]

This view was echoed by Committee on Publication Ethics (COPE), a forum for editors and publishers, Chair, Elizabeth Wager, who noted that the survey was consistent with the experience of COPE where there were many cases of institutions that were not cooperating with journals and were failing to investigate research misconduct properly.

The results of the BMJ survey mirrored those of a 2001 study[13] conducted among newly appointed hospital consultants in Merseyside, which found about ten per cent had witnessed their peers altering or fabricating data for the purpose of publication, and nearly six per cent admitted they had personally been involved in research fraud

The prevailing attitude that such instances were rare and anomalous was countered by Dr Godlee and Dr Wager in a recent BMJ editorial. They said: "There are enough known or emerging cases to suggest that the United Kingdom's apparent shortage of publicly investigated examples has more to do with a closed, competitive, and fearful academic culture than with Britain's researchers being uniquely honest."[14]

Clive Cookson[15] the Science Editor of the *Financial Times* said that speaker after speaker at a meeting he attended said that Britain should not be complacent just because the most publicised cases of fraud in recent years had taken place in other countries. "The British public does not know what is going on," said Dr Godlee.[16] "People need to realise that misconduct is affecting patients every day and it is a misappropriation of public funds." Journal editors were often the first to come across cases of misconduct, when they spotted inconsistencies in scientific or medical papers, said Elizabeth Wager . "But they are not the right people to investigate misconduct," she said;[17] "that responsibility lies with the researchers' institutions" and she criticised the institutions for "not co-operating with journals and failing to investigate research misconduct properly." She said that one United States editor had told her that UK institutions were the worst to deal with in cases of suspected misconduct and that "Our reputation in the world is not looking good."[18] Research institutions or universities who should be responsible for investigating allegations of misconduct by their staff have a conflict of interest as they may wish to suppress such allegations to preserve their reputations.

Ginny Barbour, a senior editor with the Public Library of Science (PloS) group of journals, said that one-third of authors could not find the original data to back up figures in scientific papers when these were questioned.[19]

Unlike some other countries, the UK has no official national body to deal with research misconduct. The closest equivalent is the UK Research Integrity Office (UKRIO), established in 2006 as a voluntary body funded mainly by universities. Vice-chair Mike Farthing, vice-chancellor of Sussex University said that UKRIO was a fairly modest organisation and that becoming established was a "bumpy ride" as some players "wanted us to die a death."

Research-integrity issues in the United Kingdom have long been fretted over.[20] In 2011 the House of Commons Science and Technology Select Committee found "the general oversight of research integrity in the UK to be unsatisfactory". According to Daniel Cressey, a journalist for Nature News and Comment, Peter Wilmshurst, a cardiologist who is well known for exposing research misconduct had said that the gains are high and the risks low for would-be cheats as long as institutions refuse to deal with such problems.[21]

"Dishonesty is common and institutionalized in medicine and medical research," he said. He mentioned a joke about the three 'F's in research integrity: Fabrication, Falsification and Honesty. There is, he said, "no 'F'-in honesty."[22]

Dr Ram B Singh published many papers in many journals between 1989 and 1993. He had been the first author on 28 full articles and on a further 25 clinical research trials or case-control studies. In April 1992 the *British Medical Journal* (BMJ) published yet another article by Singh[23] but he later became the focus of an international investigation into suspicions of scientific misconduct and data fabrication. The BMJ concluded that the data from the trial were "either fabricated or falsified."[24]

Jon Sudbø, a respected Norwegian oral cancer researcher, admitted in 2006 that he had fabricated data for 900 patients in a study published in *The Lancet*. The article has since been retracted. He also "fundamentally mishandled" data for a 2001 article in *The New England Journal of Medicine and a 2005 article in Journal of Clinical Oncology*. Sudbø was set to receive $312,000 per year from a grant for his research. The editor of *The Lancet* described this as the biggest scientific fraud ever conducted by a single researcher.[25]

The Hospital appointed a special commission to investigate all of Sudbø's previous research. The commission found evidence of falsified and fabricated data dating back to Sudbø's Ph.D. project.[26] As a result of the scandal, Sudbø resigned from his position as consultant oncologist at The Radium Hospital and as an associate professor at the University of Oslo in 2006. His licenses to practice medicine and dentistry were revoked. He is now on indefinite leave from the Norwegian Radium Hospital.[27,28]

The Norwegian government established a national office chaired by a judge to investigate cases of alleged scientific misconduct, and new legislation on ethics and integrity in research was put into effect. They also formed a national research ethics committee tasked with proactive, preventive education on research integrity.

The journal *Nature Chemical Biology* retracted a paper[29] by Won et al. entitled "Small molecule–based reversible reprogramming of cellular lifespan."[30] which appeared in their July 2006 issue describing the discovery of a small molecule that was reported to modulate the "senescence clock" in human cells. The paper included several misrepresentations and data fabrications that undermined the scientific integrity of the study. The editor stated that the retraction of a paper is "a step toward a full accounting of a case of scientific misconduct."

The *Journal of the American Medical Association* (JAMA) retracted an article[31] by Cheng et al.[32] The title of the paper included the statement that it was "a randomized controlled trial" it was neither randomised nor controlled. It was also not well designed and it was found that the authors had not submitted their protocol or ethics of the study to the Academic Committee of Shandong University for approval.

The Dean at Shandong University School of Medicine, Yun Zhang, who investigated the work of Cheng, was thanked by the editor of JAMA for the thorough and detailed way his group had investigated the case together with their professional response to JAMA's concerns. They had recommended that the article by Dr Cheng should be withdrawn from JAMA.

In 1974 William Summerlin from the Sloan-Kettering Institute in New York claimed to have transplanted human corneas into the eyes of rabbits.[33] He also faked transplantation experiments in white mice by blackening patches of their skin with a pen! This is difficult to believe. For a long time his misconduct was ignored but eventually it was attributed to a mental health problem. A form of scientific denial according to Richard Smith.[34]

Smith also listed other examples of fraudulent medical writings. Vijay Soman of Yale University was exposed in 1980. He was a diabetologist and the author of 12 papers where data were either missing or fraudulent. All were eventually retracted. A paper co-authored with Philip Felig, a senior researcher, was stolen from another author when Felig was sent a paper to review and passed it on to Soman. Felig was forced to resign. Senior figures putting their names on papers which eventually prove to be fraudulent is a recurrent problem.

John Darsee, of the department of cardiology at Harvard University was observed to be falsifying data in1981. His superior, Eugene Braunwald decided that this misconduct was an isolated incident and allowed Darsee to retain his position. A few months later it became clear that results he had obtained in a multicentre study were very different from those of others. An investigation showed that many of his more than a 100 studies dating back to when he was an undergraduate and which included the names of many distinguished authors were fraudulent. These had to be retracted. Darsee's case led to congressional hearings. The first witness, the president of the National Academy of Sciences, "asserted that problems of misconduct were rare—the product of 'psychopathic behaviour' originating in 'temporarily deranged' minds."[35] Accumulating evidence shows otherwise.[36,37]

Robert Slutsky, a cardiological radiologist at the University of California published 137 papers between 1978 and 1985; sometimes one every 10 days. A reviewer raised anxieties about some of Slutsky's work and an investigation decided that 12 of Slutsky's studies were definitely fraudulent and a further 49 were questionable. Many were retracted.

Anjan Banerjee and Tim Peters' paper in Gut on drug induced enteropathy in inflammatory bowel disease in 1990 contained falsified data. The same issue contained an abstract due to be presented at the British Society of Gastroenterology. This was withdrawn but still published in *Gut* and both papers were retracted in March 2001. Banerjee was awarded a Master of Surgery degree by the University of London for work that included the fraudulent paper. In December 2000 he was found guilty of serious professional misconduct for falsifying data and he was suspended. In March 2001 Tim Peters, the professor who supervised Banerjee, was found guilty of serious professional misconduct for failing to take action over the falsified research. Banerjee was later found guilty of serious professional misconduct for financial fraud and he was struck off the medical register. According to Richard Smith the General Medical Council hearings were hampered by notebooks being "selectively shredded" by King's

College Medical School. Authorities at King's had conducted an inquiry in 1991 but did not inform the General Medical Council or *Gut*.

Smith[38] also described a study by a Canadian researcher R K Chandra published by the journal *Nutrition* and later retracted in 2001.[39, 40] Chandra had resigned before the Memorial University of Newfoundland could investigate his previous studies. Smith quoted Stephen Lock's "imperfect history" of research misconduct in medicine showing how cases of fraud are likely to be seen as isolated incidents but how investigations often eventually showed a history of previous fraud.[41] Smith questioned whose responsibility it should be to investigate the previous work of a researcher found to have published fraudulent work. If necessary how and by whom the researcher should be punished? How should the scientific record be corrected?

The Memorial University of Newfoundland said that it could not investigate Chandra further as he had resigned and left and that the responsibility for the investigation lay with the journals that had published more than 200 of Chandra's articles. The Canadian Institutes of Health Research had tried to investigate, but Chandra refused to provide his research data.[42] According to Smith the "safe and right thing to do" was to assume that the author had been the author of other fraudulent papers in the past and start an investigation. It was clearly dangerous to assume that there were no problems with all previous work.

The process of investigation must be effective, fair, and efficient, and it must be conducted by a body that has the legal legitimacy to do so and the means to administer suitable punishment. Who should do this? Smith argues that it could be the accuser's employer, usually a university, a medical school, or a hospital, in the case of a medical researcher. It could also be the funders of the research or a professional regulatory body such as the General Medical Council in the United Kingdom. A drawback to this idea is that bodies such as the General Medical Council can only investigate people who are registered with them and most medical research is done by people who are not medically qualified. Smith points out that the journal in which the article is published cannot investigate. It does not have the legal legitimacy to investigate even the particular study. A journal making a judgment on whether a paper was fraudulent would be nothing more than "trial by media."

Ideally, Smith argues, there would be an international body to take the lead on cases that are left unaddressed and the editors of journals may need a means of marking studies that are under suspicion. This could prevent them being cited.

An interesting suggestion is that the criminal law might be used to manage research misconduct.[43] Misuse of funds such as grants from public bodies may be involved making research fraud an example of financial fraud. Alexander or "Sandy" McCall Smith, who suggested this, was, incidentally born in Rhodesia (now Zimbabwe) in 1948. He is an Emeritus Professor of Medical Law at the University of Edinburgh[44] and is a respected expert on medical law and bioethics.

His other significant "claim to fame" is that he is an internationally known writer of fiction. He is most widely known as the creator of The No. 1 Ladies' Detective Agency series set in Botswana where he lived for a time.

Some institutions and Universities in other parts of the world have taken action to stop scientific misconduct.[45] In early October 2008, the editor of the

International Journal of Cardiology discovered that figures in a manuscript by He Haibo, a scientist researching traditional Chinese medicine who had been hired by the Zhejiang University (ZJU) in Hangzhou, China, only months before, were suspiciously similar to those in an article that He (the capital is correct. It his correct name. He is not a deity!) had published elsewhere. Confronted, He quickly owned up, submitting a 12-page confession to Yang Wei, president of (ZJU) "There was plagiarism, fabrication and falsification.[46] It was a showcase of every kind of problem," said Yang. The case, which eventually led to the retraction of eight papers, became an international media catastrophe for the ZJU, one of China's oldest and largest universities, as well as one of the most successful in publishing science.

In March 2009, the ZJU fired He but Yang did not stop there: he launched a campaign to make the ZJU more responsive to misconduct.[47] With a companion named Yuehong and assistance from a group of university administrators who shared his determination and commitment to a zero-tolerance policy for misconduct, Yang hoped to make the ZJU into a role model that could help to clean up China's reputation for rife scientific misconduct. That reputation had been exacerbated in the previous five years by a string of high-profile cases[48] that had made observers and journal editors increasingly critical of the ability of Chinese research institutions to ensure trustworthy science.

Yang Wei's companion, Yuehong Zhang became the first journal editor in China to introduce CrossCheck,[49] a tool that compares text against published articles to flag up plagiarism. Two years later, she had found that 31 per cent of the 2,233 submissions over that time to the Journal of Zhejiang University — Science, contained unoriginal material.[50] After reporting the number in *Nature* Zhang was harassed. She said[51] "Many people criticized me. They say I am unpatriotic. I don't care. I think I'm doing the right thing. I think it could make science stronger in China." It has. Only 15 per cent of submissions in the first half of 2011 contained unoriginal content.

Zhang's journal, unlike many Chinese journals, insisted on peer review. In December 2010, she became the first Chinese person to win a grant from the International Committee on Publication Ethics, for using CrossCheck to analyse types of plagiarism.[52] There are 5,000 science and technology journals in China, but only 200 are in English and are able to use CrossCheck.[53] Zhang says that some 20 do so. A separate effort is under way to police Chinese-language journals. In 2009, the China National Knowledge Infrastructure (CNKI) in Beijing launched a system called the Academic Misconduct Literature Check (AMLC).[54]

Sun Xiongyong, director of the CNKI Academic Integrity Research Centre, said that the organisation was pushed by publishers and universities to develop the AMLC, which now includes about 80 million Chinese articles, conference proceedings and doctoral theses.[55] Its subscribers include some 4,500 publishers and 600 universities. Sun said that a crucial component of the system was the ability to check Chinese articles against the 30 million or so English articles in the database, and vice versa. "It's the only multi-language check system," noted Sun.[56]

The systems can be cheated. Students could, and do, use the AMLC to check their theses before submission.[57] They might find passages that trigger the plagiarism warning and then tweak their manuscripts until the text scrapes through.[58] In response, the CNKI has established a monitoring system that can check, for example, whether the AMLC was being used before submission.[59] But "the arms race continues;" Sun's latest headache is the use of software available outside China, such as Turnitin, to defeat the check system. The human mind can be so devious it has the ability to beat any system.

Mark Frankel, director of the Scientific Freedom, Responsibility and Law Program at the American Association for the Advancement of Science (AAAS) in Washington DC is working with Yang to improve research ethics.[60] Frankel says that efforts such as Yang's are driving change. "What is most impressive is how open and willing the people with whom I work in China are to admit that a serious problem exists, and that they are committed to turning things around for the younger generation of scientists," he said.

David Cyranoski has a different opinion.[61] According to him; surveys and anecdotal evidence in China suggest that students are learning unethical behaviour alongside their science. In an unpublished 2008 survey of 1,641 students at 10 universities, Cao Nanyan, a research-integrity specialist at Tsinghua University in Beijing, found that more than 20 per cent of students admitted to changing data that did not match their expectations. Some 60 per cent of PhD students said that they sometimes witnessed misconduct, yet only five per cent would report it.

Yang said that he had dealt with another 40 or so misconduct cases at the ZJU and more than 20 researchers had been found guilty of wrongdoing. Of ten cases involving recent graduates, more than half lost their degrees.[62] One of these sued the ZJU to overturn the ruling of plagiarism.[63] She lost the case. According to Cyranoski, three faculty members had their employment terminated, four faced disciplinary action including a pay cut, and the rest were issued with public or internal warnings.[64]

Yang also realised the importance of prevention of misconduct. A system for mentoring young faculty members on research ethics was established and seminars and lectures on research integrity have been held at the ZJU with attendance at some surpassing 1,000.[65]

A very good sign of the will to improve the standard of Chinese scientific research was a recent full page advertisement in Scientific American.[66] As part of a major strategic move into China, Nature Publishing Group (NPG), publisher of the science journal *Nature* and part of the Macmillan group, advertised for a "Country Head" to lead the group's future business and editorial activities in China. This was part of a broader initiative by the Macmillan Group (to which NPG belongs) that aims to establish a strong presence for Macmillan in China, with particular emphasis on science and education.[67] Within the first half of 2012, The Country Head and four editors of the new online multidisciplinary science journal *Nature Communications* will be based in Shanghai.[68]

This initiative was in response to the "rapidly growing output of high-quality research from China." The Country Head will co-operate with colleagues in Tokyo and Melbourne to continue the rapid expansion of the Asian

Academic Journal program of NPG in China, which will have expanded to seven journals by July 2012.[69] One of the aims is to assist scientists in their writing and presentation of research articles and also to help institutions in China promote their best research to the world. One of the requirements was "a keen understanding of the rapidly evolving research sector in China, including its goals and challenges."[70]

A United States congressional inquiry heard over 700 cases, the British General Medical Council has dealt with over 30 cases and the Committee on Publication Ethics has discussed over 150 cases.[71]

Does conflict of interest matter? Financial benefit makes doctors more likely to refer patients for tests, operations, hospital admission, or to ask that drugs be stocked by a hospital pharmacy.[72][1] I was once offered a position in a private clinic in Houston, Texas. The stipulation was that I had to admit virtually every patient I saw. Income for the clinic.

Reviews that acknowledge sponsorship by the pharmaceutical or tobacco industry are more likely to draw conclusions that are favourable to the industry. Barnes and others looked at 106 review articles to do with passive smoking.[73] With all the correct statistical safeguards in place they found that the only factor associated with the review's conclusion was whether the author was affiliated with the tobacco industry. Thirty seven per cent of the reviews concluded that passive smoking was not harmful. The remainder said that it was. Interestingly only 23 per cent of the reviews disclosed the sources of funding for their research.

Competing or conflicting interests are common. In reviewing 75 articles Stelfox and others[74] found that 45 (63 per cent) of these had financial conflicts of interest yet in only two of the articles was a conflict of interest disclosed. Why do authors not declare conflicts of interest? Some journals do not require disclosure. The culture is one of not disclosing. Many authors are confident that they are not affected by conflicts of interest.

At the end of 1998 three major studies found a higher risk of venous thrombosis for third generation contraceptive pills.[75] These studies were not sponsored by the industry. Three other studies sponsored by the pharmaceutical companies did not find this increased risk to patients. Of nine studies of this subject which were not sponsored by pharmaceutical companies, one study found no difference and the other eight found increased relative risks ranging from 1.5 to 4.0. Four sponsored studies found relative risks between 0.8 and 1.5. The one sponsored study with a higher relative risk of 1.5 was re-analysed several times attempting to achieve a lower figure but after this failed to convince, a new reanalysis was sponsored by another different company. One sponsored study finding an increased risk has not been published.

Does medicine have a culture that turns a blind eye to research misconduct? Why does scientific fraud happen? Was Al Gore correct when he said that there was a reluctance of people high in the science field to take these matters seriously? Richard Smith[76] has an interesting and different point of view in relation to the question of why does scientific fraud happens. He asks why it would not happen, it happens in all other human activities. In addition there is considerable pressure for scientists or physicians "climbing the ladder" to publish. He says that there is inadequate training. Doctors are not taught good writing practice and indeed are sometimes taught the opposite. In addition doctors can get away with fraud because the system works on trust. Maybe sloppy behaviour may spill over to fraud?

In the United States there is a commonly followed motto of "publish or perish". To "climb the ladder" one must publish. The frequency with which scientists fabricate and falsify data, or commit other forms of scientific misconduct is a matter of controversy.[77]

Accepting the definitions of fraud mentioned previously, how common is it? A recent study conducted at the University of Edinburgh in the United Kingdom found that while only 1.97 per cent of respondents admitted to committing research misconduct, one third of respondents admitted to "other questionable research practices."

Fanelli,[78] in a meta-analysis of the relevant surveys quoting scandals like Hwang Woo-Suk's cloning scandal using fake stem-cell lines[79] or Jan Hendrik Schön's duplicated graphs[80] showed how easy it was for a scientist to publish fabricated data in the most prestigious of journals, how this caused a waste of financial and human resources that might pose a risk to human health and what the true incidence of scientific fraud was. This question of incidence is obviously crucial, yet, as Fanelli says, the answer is a matter of great debate.[81, 82]

A popular view propagated by the media[83] and by many scientists[84] and following the line expressed by the President of the National Academy of Sciences, mentioned previously, sees fraudsters as just a "few bad apples."[85]

Increasing evidence, however, suggests that known frauds are just the "tip of the iceberg", and that many cases are never discovered. Fanelli pointed out that all the estimates of the number of frauds depend on the cases that have been discovered and have reached the public domain.[86]

This significantly underestimates the real frequency of misconduct which is estimated to be roughly between 0.2 and two per cent. Fanelli's study was the first systematic review and meta-analysis of survey data on scientific misconduct and, from this study, it is estimated that about two per cent of scientists admitted to have fabricated, falsified or modified data or results at least once, "a serious form of misconduct by any standard."[87,88,89] Berk, Korenman and Wenger based their findings on survey results from 606 scientists who received funding in 1993 and 1994.[90]

By means of a questionnaire 1005 postdoctoral fellows at the University of California San Francisco were sampled. The response rate was only 33 per cent but 3.4 per cent of the responders said that they had modified data in the past. A staggering 17 per cent said they were "willing to select or omit data to improve their results."[91] Among 2,010 clinical and biomedical science trainees at the University of California, San Diego surveyed regarding their perceptions about unethical practices in research and the extent of their training exposure to the ethics of scientific investigation; 549 responded., 4.9 per cent said they had modified research results in the past[92] but 81 per cent were "willing to select, omit or fabricate data to win a grant or publish a paper." [93]

It is likely that, if on average two per cent of scientists admit to have falsified research at least once and up to 34 per cent admit other questionable research practices, the actual frequencies of misconduct could be higher than this.[94] "Publish or perish" seems to have gone too far or is it that the large financial interests that often drive medical research are severely biasing it?[95,96,97]

Marcia Angell, in a superb editorial,[98] questions whether academic medicine is for sale? She does not believe that disclosure of conflict of interest is enough to deal with the problem of possible bias. She likens this policy to the requirement that judges recuse themselves from hearing cases if they have financial ties to a litigant.

One problem is that many potential authors, experts in their fields, have financial ties to drug companies. This may not only be in the form of grant support, but also many other financial arrangements. Angell says that "Researchers serve as consultants to companies whose products they are studying, join advisory boards and speakers' bureaus, enter into patent and royalty arrangements, agree to be the listed authors of articles ghostwritten by interested companies, promote drugs and devices at company-sponsored symposiums, and allow themselves to be plied with expensive gifts and trips to luxurious settings. Many also have equity interest in the companies."[99] She has been quoted as saying "To buy a distinguished, senior academic researcher, the kind of person who speaks at meetings, who writes textbooks, who writes journal articles – that is worth 100,000 salespeople".

In the book *Rescuing Science from Politics*,[100] edited by Wendy Wagner, Professor Thomas O. McGarrity shows how interested parties have abused the legal system to "threaten scientific independence, undermine the objectivity and therefore the integrity of research, and, in some cases, threaten the careers of individual scientists." These intrusions, according to Professor McGarrity[101] violate several basic, non controversial principles of scientific independence which he lists; Scientists must be able to conduct research without unjustified restrictions, including undue influence by research sponsors, sponsors must never place restrictions or otherwise influence the designer or conduct of a study in an attempt to obtain results favourable to their interests, research must never be suppressed because it produces results that are adverse to a sponsor or other interested parties and no publication or summary of research should be influenced, in tone or content, by the sponsoring entity.[102]

If vested interests used the legal system to harass scientists whose research or expert testimony calls into question the safety of their practices or products, the harassers must be held accountable with sanctions and must compensate injured scientists for the resulting interference with their research and potential damage to their reputations.[103]

Some academic institutions have entered into partnerships with drug companies to set up research centers and teaching programs in which students and faculty members essentially carry out industry research.[104] Both sides see great benefit in this arrangement. The researchers, sponsored by the pharmaceutical company may produce a drug that the company can then market.

Drug companies used to give small gifts to junior doctors.[105] They now receive free meals and many other substantial favors from drug companies virtually daily, and they are often invited to opulent dinners and other quasi-social events to hear lectures on various medical topics.

In 1980, the Bayh–Dole Act, in the USA encouraged academic institutions supported by federal grants to patent and license new products developed by their faculty members and to share royalties with the researchers.[106] This act is now frequently invoked to justify the ubiquitous ties between academia and industry.[107] It is argued that the more contacts there are between academia and industry, the better it is for clinical medicine; the fact that money changes hands is considered merely the way of the world but there is now considerable evidence that researchers with ties to drug companies are indeed more likely to report results that are favourable to the products of those companies than researchers without such ties.[108]

It is well to remember that the costs of the industry-sponsored trips, meals, gifts, conferences, and symposiums and the honorariums, consulting fees, and research grants are often simply added to the prices of drugs and devices.[109]

Lisa Schwartz[110] and others also warned that doctors should be wary of the increasing entanglement of medical journalists and the drug industry. Financial ties between medical journalists and for-profit pharmaceutical companies warrant scrutiny as the public often first learn about new treatments from the news media. Industry sponsorship of training and further education of journalists now occurs in a variety of contexts; universities, conferences, and professional associations, raising similar concerns to those that apply to education of doctors.[111] For example, the University of North Carolina's post of Glaxo Wellcome chair of medical journalism is an endowed position created by a grant from the company worth $333,000[112] Pfizer also offers a medical journalism scholarship at the university that is worth $28,000 a year and also offers healthcare benefits.[113]

A Glaxo Wellcome professor, Tom Linden, told the *BMJ* that he was grateful for support from the industry. "As long as the funding has no strings attached," he said. Although there was no suggestion that this sponsorship influenced the university's curriculum, the authors of the article considered that it could send a symbolic message to students and engender a subtle sense of loyalty to the industry. The American Medical Writers Association receives sponsorship from the drug industry.[114] but sponsorship of speakers must be approved by the association's executive committee, "to maintain balance and reduce bias."

One of the more astonishing forms of financial ties between journalists and drug companies is the sponsored award.[115] For example, Eli Lilly and Boehringer Ingelheim[116] both offer opportunities for international travel or prizes worth from €5,000 to €7,500.[117] Sometimes awards are sponsored by organisations that are themselves heavily funded by industry.

The non-profit Mental Health America obtained half of its funds from drug companies, including more than $1m each from Bristol Myers Squibb, Lilly, and Wyeth.[118] Interactions between the industry and medical journalists can affect prescribing judgments[119] and journalists who accept such prizes may be engendering conflicts of interest for themselves.[120] Two thirds of charities and patients' groups receive funding from drug or device manufacturers[121] but when experts or studies with industry ties were quoted, these ties were disclosed in less than 40 per cent of the stories.[122]

To enhance the credibility of medical journalism Schwartz and colleagues suggest "that journalism educators should not accept funding from the healthcare and drug industries, that journalists should not accept gifts, awards, or any financial support from the industries they cover, and that journalists should routinely disclose their conflicts of interest and those of their sources."

Guest and ghost authorship

The editor of *Science,* Donald Kennedy recently stated that he would consider adding new requirements that authors "detail their specific contributions to the research submitted," and sign statements that they agree with the conclusions of their article. This followed the two fraudulent articles on embryonic stem cells published in *Science* by Hwang Woo Suk. A statement of authors' contributions has long been required by many medical journals. This could help to prevent traditional scientific practices, such as honorary authorship.

Elizabeth Wager [123] wrote a superb piece about medical authorship. She is a medical writer and trainer for a variety of organisations, including pharmaceutical companies. She is a coauthor of the European Medical Writers Association Guidelines for Medical Writers and Good Publication Practice for pharmaceutical companies,[124] and occasionally receives payment for speaking about or providing training on publication ethics. She was paid a commission by the Public Library of Science (PLoS) for writing the article. There is nothing wrong with that. I was paid by the Namibian Medical Association for giving a talk on "Change". I did not publicise any drug or device. Professional medical writers are often involved in writing protocols and in preparing manuscripts for publication.[125,126]

Original scientific findings are usually published in the form of a "paper". Papers are normally prepared by a group of researchers who did the research and are then listed at the top of the article. The authors are accountable and responsible for the article. They also receive the credit for the publication of their paper. "Guest authorship has been defined as the designation of an individual who does not meet authorship criteria as an author."[127, 128, 129] Ghost authorship is different.

"Ghostwriting has been defined as the failure to designate an individual (as an author) who has made a substantial contribution to the research or writing of a manuscript."[130] The bioscience literature has been haunted by ghost and guest authors. Ghost writing is present if individuals who wrote the trial protocol, performed the statistical analyses, or wrote the manuscript are not listed as authors of the publication, or as members of a study group or writing committee, or in an acknowledgment. It is commonplace. A study may be more credible if the names of the true authors for example, company employees or freelance medical writers are not revealed. This practice might also hide competing interests that readers should be aware of, and for this reason it has been condemned by academics, groups of editors, and some pharmaceutical companies.

Wyeth employed ghostwriters to write articles favourable to hormone-replacement therapy and downplaying their side effects. The written articles were forwarded by eminent physicians who appeared to be the authors.[131] The drug company involvement in the production of these articles is therefore hidden from the reader. This lack of authorship transparency with advertising being portrayed as research medical articles may influence physicians and patients unfairly.

Newspaper articles on medical topics are sometimes forced to signify that they are indeed advertisements. They are then labelled as such.

Considerable controversy arose in 2001when it was claimed that pain pills Celebrex, Bextra and Vioxx could cause more harm than good. They were shown in some cases to have deleterious effects on the heart and brain in the form of heart attacks and strokes. The journal *Circulation* published an article denying that rofecoxib (Vioxx) was associated with these adverse cardiovascular events[132] The *Circulation* article quite correctly identified that the two principal authors Konstam and Weir were paid consultants of Merck and Pharmacia, and that Dr. Konstam was a paid consultant to Pfizer. A total of five of the seven named authors were Merck employees. These authors received income and had stock interests in the company.

By 2004, there was increasing evidence that rofecoxib was associated with cardiovascular events and Merck voluntary withdrew Vioxx from the market. During the course of ensuing litigation it was alleged that the article in *Circulation* had been ghostwritten by Merck. Merck acknowledged that it sometimes hired outside medical writers to draft research reports before handing them over to doctors whose names would eventually appear on the publication. This was confirmed in a 2008 paper published in JAMA.[133] Financial support from Merck was also not always disclosed.

The Food and Drug Administration advisory panel held meetings to decide whether to allow continued marketing of Celebrex, Bextra and Vioxx.[134] The panel consisted of 32 government drug advisers of whom ten, amazingly, according to disclosures in medical journals and other public records, had consulted in recent years for the manufacturers of the products involved. Eight of these 10 members said in interviews later that their past relationships with the drug companies had not influenced their votes. The two others did not respond to phone or e-mail messages. The endorsement of continued marketing of Celebrex, Bextra and Vioxx was deeply important to the three companies, Merck, Pfizer and Novartis. Shares of Merck and Pfizer soared after the panel's votes. If the ten advisers had not cast their votes the results would have been very different. Bextra and Vioxx would have been withdrawn from the market.

Researchers with ties to industry commonly serve on Food and Drug Administration advisory panels. The agency has said it tries to balance expertise, often found among those who have conducted clinical trials of the drugs in question or otherwise studied them, with potential conflicts of interest. Merck eventually settled lawsuits concerning Vioxx for $4.85 billion!

Ross and others have reported that guest authorship was identified in 16 per cent of research articles, 26 per cent of review articles, 21 per cent of editorials and in 41 per cent of Cochrane reviews.[135,136,137] They also reported that ghostwriting was identified in 13 per cent of research articles, ten per cent of review articles, six per cent of editorials, and 11 per cent of Cochrane reviews.[138] In Ross' pivotal article, many prestigious journals (including *Pharmacotherapy*) were identified as having been victims of guest or ghost authorship.

The *Pharmacotherapy* Board of Directors and Scientific Editor Council conducted their own intensive investigation of ghost writing and could not refute any of the findings reached in Ross' article. As a direct result, they created a policy on authorship, ghost writing, and guest authorship. They also carefully redesigned the mandatory questions that all authors had to answer when submitting papers for publication in their journal to ensure that ghost and guest authorship were eliminated and that all real and potential conflicts of interest were clearly revealed.[139]

The Editor-in-Chief of the journal, Richard T Schiefe, stated that "the integrity of a scientific journal is 'job one.' We all strive to attain the highest quality and impact in scientific publication, but without integrity, those attributes are worthless. By shining a light on these practices and instituting clear, unambiguous, and uniform game rules, with severe and sure penalties (much like the current Draconian rules and penalties exacted for plagiarism or scientific fraud), we will take a giant step toward exorcising these ghosts (and guests) from the scientific literature." The *Pharmacotherapy* Board, on December 17th 2008, did just that. They ensured that a person designated as an author must have contributed to the conception and design, or analysed and interpreted the data; drafted the article or revised it critically for important intellectual content; and approved the final version to be published. They said that supporting the study or collecting data did not constitute authorship and that authorship based solely on position (e.g., research supervisor, department chair) was not permitted. Any person not meeting all three criteria above should instead be listed in an acknowledgment. Application of this principle may have saved Geoffrey Chamberlain's embarrassment.

Manuscripts submitted for publication had to list all authors, including the person who drafted the original manuscript. This included paid or unpaid medical writers ("ghost writers"). "Ghost" authorship was most common when a commercial entity (e.g., a medical writer acting on behalf of a pharmaceutical manufacturer) actually created the first or subsequent drafts of a manuscript. The ethical breach was that an actual author was missing from the list of authors. The remedy was to reveal all "real" authors to the readers, as well as their affiliations. "Guest" authorship occurred when a "ghost" author created a manuscript, and invited the "guest" author to be named as the author, with little or no intellectual input to the manuscript from the guest author. Guest authorship in this context was never ethical.

Pharmacotherapy also required that all authors reveal all potential conflicts of interest in a "conflict of interest" statement that had to be completed prior to submitting papers. Significant conflicts of interest would be revealed in the opening footnote of the published paper. All authors had to declare that they met the qualifications to be considered an author and that everyone who had contributed to the manuscript as a qualified author had been named as an author.

Great care must be taken in the submission of papers for publication. Attempting to follow the correct guidelines and publish in the most appropriate journal may often be difficult. One example potential authors must be aware of is that editors have a policy of considering a manuscript for publication only if its substance has not been submitted or reported elsewhere. This policy was promulgated in 1969 by Franz J. Ingelfinger, then the editor of *The New England Journal of Medicine*. Called the Ingelfinger rule the aim is to protect a journal from publishing material that has already been published elsewhere and thus had lost its originality. It attempts to prevent duplicate publications of the same study.

Another aspect of author misconduct is the practice of publishing many papers in different journals with minor differences drawn from the same study. This is termed "salami publishing".

Larry Claxton[140,141] provided a historical overview of commonly encountered scientific authorship issues. He showed that although a number of organisations provided guidelines for author allocation, a comparison showed that these guidelines differed on who should be an author, rules for ordering authors, and the level of responsibility for coauthors.[142] He recommended "a need for more controlled studies on authorship issues, an increased awareness
and a buy-in to consensus views by non-editor groups, e.g., managers, authors, reviewers, and scientific societies, and a need for editors to express a greater understanding of authors' dilemmas and to exhibit greater flexibility."[143]

He suggested occasions such as international congresses where editors and others such as managers and authors could directly exchange views, develop consensus approaches and solutions, and seek agreement on how to resolve authorship issues.[144]

Al-Marzouki and others[145, 146] showed that fraudulent data have particular statistical features that are not evident in data containing accidental errors and that statistical methods could be applied to detect large scale fabrication of data in a randomised trial where data are available.

In Elizabeth Wager's 2007article[147] she wrote that since the earliest peer-reviewed publications of the late 17th century, conventions about the authorship of scientific papers have evolved considerably[148].These earlier papers were generally anonymous and attributed to the sponsor (in those days, usually the church or the king). Readers now want to know not only who paid for the research but also who did the work.[149]

Transparency (i.e., full disclosure) is now considered a moral responsibility, and many medical journals have introduced mechanisms for increasing transparency.[150] The International Committee of Medical Journal Editors (ICMJE) has also issued guidance on who qualifies for authorship[151] and their criteria have been updated and augmented several times in response to several authorship scandals.[152] Yet problems with authorship still persist. Peter Gøtzsche and colleagues[153] showed that 75 per cent of the publications they investigated had ghost authors. The ICMJE criteria state that all authors should have made a substantial contribution not only to developing the manuscript but also to other aspects such as collecting, analysing, or interpreting the data.[154]

The authorship of the memorable quote that "there are three types of lie: lies, damned lies, and statistics" is uncertain [155] although it has been attributed to Benjamin Disraeli and was used by Mark Twain.[156] Whoever the author was, Elizabeth Wager suggests that perhaps it should now be admitted that there are four types of lie: "lies, damned lies, statistics, and the authorship lists of scientific papers."

Richard Smith[157] suggested that in order to respond to the issues of scientific misconduct and fraud a country needed a recognition of the problem by the medical community and its leaders, an independent body to lead with investigations, prevention, teaching and research, an agreement on what fraud is, protection for whistleblowers, a body to investigate allegations, a fair system for reaching judgements, systems for teaching good practice and a code for the latter.

A Committee on Publication Ethics (COPE) was founded in 1997 by British medical editors,[158] including those of the *BMJ, Gut,* and *Lancet,* as a response to growing anxiety about the integrity of authors submitting studies to medical journals. According to Smith, COPE's five aims were to advise on cases brought by editors, publish an annual report describing those cases, produce guidance on good practice, encourage research, offer teaching and training and last but not least to shame the British establishment into mounting a proper response to publication misconduct and fraud.

Guidelines on good publication practice were described in the COPE report of 2000.[159] The guidelines in the report are aimed at authors, editors, editorial board members, readers, owners of journals, and publishers. Intellectual honesty was stressed. Good research should be well justified, well planned, appropriately designed, and ethically approved.[160] To conduct research to a lower standard might constitute misconduct. Data should be appropriately analysed, but inappropriate analysis would not necessarily amount to misconduct; fabrication and falsification of data would. All authors would have to take public responsibility for the content of their papers.

Conflicts of interest were defined as "those which, when revealed later, would make a reasonable reader feel misled or deceived."[161] They might be personal, commercial, political, academic or financial. Such interests, where relevant, would have to be declared to editors by researchers, authors, and reviewers. Redundant publication would occur when two or more papers, without full cross reference, share the same hypothesis, data, discussion points, or conclusions.[162]

Plagiarism ranged from the unreferenced use of others' published and unpublished ideas, including research grant applications to submission under "new" authorship of a complete paper, sometimes in a different language.[163] Editors must take all allegations and suspicions of misconduct seriously,[164] but they did not usually have either the legal legitimacy or the means to conduct investigations into serious cases.[165] Sanctions could be applied separately or combined. The following sanctions were ranked in approximate order of severity:[166]

1. A letter of explanation (and education) to the authors, where there appears to be a genuine misunderstanding of principles.

2. A letter of reprimand and warning as to future conduct.

3. A formal letter to the relevant head of institution or funding body.

4. Publication of a notice of redundant publication or plagiarism.

5. An editorial giving full details of the misconduct.

6. Refusal to accept future submissions from the individual, unit, or institution responsible for the misconduct, for a stated period.

7. Formal withdrawal or retraction of the paper from the scientific literature, informing other editors and the indexing authorities.

8. Reporting the case to the General Medical Council, or other such authority or organisation which can investigate and act with due process.

In the first 103 cases investigated by COPE there was evidence of misconduct in 80 cases. Several cases had been referred to employers and to regulatory bodies. Amongst the problems were undeclared redundant publication or submission (29),[167] disputes over authorship (18), falsification (15), failure to obtain informed consent (11), performing unethical research (11) and failure to gain approval from an ethics committee (10)

The conclusions reached by COPE were that research misconduct is a problem.[168] Most countries have not developed a coherent response to the problem and this was needed in order to avoid a collapse in public trust in medical research.[169]

Gøtzsche[170] and co-authors argued that ghostwriting was scientific misconduct and should be handled accordingly. Billions of dollars were being earned undeservedly by drug companies through flaws in research, research articles, reviews, and editorials; and many academic careers have been built on doubtful evidence. He listed suggestions that might help. Kassirer, after discussing the different degrees of ghostwriting, said that loss of trust may be the major victim. Neither the industry nor the profession could afford further damage to their reputations and both should "just say no" to ghostwriting.

Karen Woolley, Elizabeth Wager, Adam Jacobs, Art Gertel, and Cindy Hamilton argued for professional medical writers who must be distinguished from ghostwriters but agreed that the latter was dishonest and unacceptable. They supported disclosure rather than prohibition of medical writers. They felt that present guidelines were sufficient but suggested the mandatory use of a checklist that could help editors detect ghostwriting and help authors avoid ghostwriters. They requested that writing assistance was appropriate and adequately disclosed. Professional medical writers were trained to provide appropriate assistance and to insist on disclosure. In their opinion, professional medical writers could be valuable allies in the efforts to tackle ghostwriting.

Peer review

The integrity of the scientific record ultimately impacts on the health and well-being of society. Scientists are both entrusted and obliged to use the highest standards possible when proposing, performing, reviewing, and reporting research.

Peer review of articles is one way to find mistakes or problems in research but unfortunately, pressures on the peer review system compromise its effectiveness. Massively increasing numbers of articles require reviews.[171]

When mistakes escape detection and incorrect results are published, replication is supposed to safeguard the research record. If the research is important enough to attract the attention of other scientists replication will sometimes reveal problems. Hence, the value of the well-worn research adage, "Replication is the best statistic."

Koocher and others have recommended possible informal intervention to avert irresponsible scientific behaviour. Although not always the best course of action it is not as risky as people might fear.[172] For major cases of misconduct it is preferable, in their opinion, to take a formal route; "especially in people with combative or excessively arrogant personalities, those known to have a track record of scientific misbehaviour, extreme incompetence, mental or substance-abuse problems or those with much to lose." Others could be approached informally after careful consideration of the available options. It is crucial that a non-adversarial tone be used. The problem should be approached as an attempt at education and finding solutions, not as an attack, and the possibility that one's suspicions could be unfounded should be left open. They advise strongly against the sending of an anonymous note.

Preventing dissemination of fraudulent material

The scientific community has a duty to warn people to ignore an article containing faked data and must try to prevent inadvertent citation of it.[173]
The community accomplishes these tasks by publishing a retraction and linking it to the fraudulent article's citation in electronic indexes of the medical literature, such as *Pub Med*. but this mechanism is far from perfect. This was exemplified by the case of scientific fraud perpetrated by Eric Poehlman. His institution notified three journals that they had published tainted articles. Two journals failed to retract. The third journal retracted immediately, but other authors continued to cite the retracted article.

Governmental institutions should act if they have the authority to investigate and punish guilty scientists. Research institutions should investigate the alleged fraud and journal editors should issue a retraction. If even one fraudulent article has been published, research institutions must accept their responsibility and investigate every article published by the same author. Every article should be regarded as suspect until proven otherwise. All efforts must be made to prevent other authors from citing retracted articles and if this happens the appropriate correction must be made.

The United States is one of only a few countries with a Governmental system for evaluating allegations of scientific fraud. The U.S. Congress created the Office of Scientific Integrity in 1989. This was later renamed the Office of Research Integrity (ORI). It receives 30 to 40 new cases per year. Dishonesty in scientific research is a substantial ongoing problem. In March 2005, the ORI announced that Poehlman had published fabricated research in ten articles.[174] Furthermore, he had included fraudulent findings in National Institutes of Health grant applications, which is a federal criminal offence.

A three-year investigation into a University of Connecticut biology laboratory found its chief guilty of falsifying and fabricating data.[175] A 60,000-page report found Dipak Das,[176] director of the Cardiovascular Research Centre at the University of Connecticut Health Centre (UCHC) guilty of 145 counts of fabrication and falsification of data, involving at least 23 papers and 3 grant applications

Das studied the beneficial health effects of wine, including one component resveratrol, which has been linked to life extension and other health benefits. Fortunately, the alleged misconduct had nothing to do with wine. The misconduct involved manipulating experiments in other aspects of his research. The benefits of red wine live on! The report documented dozens of instances in published papers where protein bands from separate experiments were spliced and pasted together to suggest that they had been measured in the same experiment.

Members of Das's lab said that there was nothing wrong with digitally manipulating images.[177] The report cited e-mail exchanges between Das and lab members documenting data manipulation, and in one e-mail to Das, a student in the lab wrote: "I have changed the figures as you told me."[178] Das denied that he modified the images and he accused the University of racial discrimination.[179] He also complained that stress caused by the investigation had caused him to suffer a stroke.

The Office of Research Integrity (ORI) had notified the university, in November 2008, of a complaint involving a paper Das had published.[180] No papers have been retracted, but UCHC notified the journals in which Das's team published papers. UCHC also froze externally funded research in Das's lab,[181] and it turned away US$890,000 in federal grants while the investigation was underway. The university also began proceedings to fire Das. Fortunately for those of us who like the stuff, Nir Barzilai, a resveratrol researcher at the Albert Einstein College of Medicine in New York, said that the allegations of Das' research misconduct "will not have a significant impact on resveratrol research."

Few countries have anything like the ORI. When misconduct is alleged the responsible author's institution refuses to investigate and no national standard exists, Cox and co-authors ask, what does an editor do?[182,183,184,185]

As COPE have recognised, editors do not have the legal standing, expertise, time, or money to go into foreign institutions, secure evidence, and spend months or years uncovering misconduct, adjudicating, hearing appeals, and sanctioning offenders. Yet, if they refuse to publish work from institutions in countries lacking standard investigative procedures, which include, for example, the United Kingdom,[186] India and Japan, they would "limit the flow of good science, reduce the value of their journals, and be grossly unfair to honest authors."

Editors are encouraging their governments to set up systems like the ORI but, in the meantime, if local systems for investigating allegations of scientific misconduct fail, an editor can withdraw a journal's support for a suspected fraudulent article [187, 188] or publish an expression of concern.[189,190,191,192,193,194,195]

The United States Congress passed the Physician Payments Sunshine Act in 2010. This law compels all pharmaceutical companies and medical device manufacturers to reveal most of the money they give to physicians.

Plagiarism

Plagiarism poses a threat to the integrity of the scientific community.[196]

It is one of the most common offenses and often is the result of a lack of knowledge and understanding of the concepts. It is defined as "using someone else's words, ideas or results without attribution." It is unethical in scientific writing and qualifies as a form of scientific misconduct.[197] To be considered an infraction, the action must be a "serious deviation from accepted practices of the relevant research community" and "committed intentionally, knowingly or recklessly" and "proven by a preponderance of evidence."[198]

The ORI reported[199] that approximately 25 per cent of the total allegations of misconduct received concern plagiarism, and that these allegations typically represent misunderstandings of what exactly constitutes plagiarism and accurate citation procedures.[200]

Appropriate referencing is important in scientific writing.[201] Plagiarism can occur in various forms: plagiarism of ideas and plagiarism of text. Redundant or duplicate publication refers to the practice of substantial overlapping of text and/or data with another article(s) without full cross-referencing [202] in that they share the same hypothesis, data, discussion points, or conclusions.[203] It is a common issue in the scientific literature.

Bloemenkamp et al[204] reported that 20 per cent of articles published in a Dutch general medicine journal were also published elsewhere. Similarly, Schein and Paladugu[205] reported that one in six original articles published in three leading surgical journals represented a form of redundant publications. It is most certainly improper when done deceptively.

There are three major problems with this practice: deception and ethical issues, wasting of resources, and a negative impact on clinical decision making and future research.[206] Most importantly, duplicate publications can affect clinical decision making. It exaggerates the significance of the work in a qualitative manner and may skew the reader's perceived validity and reliability of the methods and results.[207]

Cicutto[208] suggested a list of 12 strategies for avoiding plagiarism. She concluded that "the responsibility for maintaining high standards of peer-reviewed published articles is a shared one, involving journal editors and reviewers, heads of university departments, professional societies, and individual scientists and authors."

References:

1. Research misconduct and biomedical journals Richard Smith
Editor, BMJ
www.bmj.com/talks Scientific Misconduct - The University of Tennessee Health ..,
http://www.uthsc.edu/research/research_administration/Seminar/doc/UTennMisconduct.pdf (accessed July 21, 2013).
2. Titus, Sandra L., Wells, James A., Rhoades, Lawrence J. Repairing research integrity. Nature 453, (19), 980-982 (19 June 2008) | doi:10.1038/453980a; Published online 18 June 2008
3. Scientific Misconduct - The University of Tennessee Health ..,
http://www.uthsc.edu/research/research_administration/Seminar/doc/UTennMisconduct.pdf (accessed July 21, 2013).
4. Office of Research Integrity. 20 Apr 2011 – Office of Science and Technology Policy. Executive Office of the President; Federal Policy on Research Misconduct. ori.hhs.gov/federal-research-misconduct-policy.
5. Integrity and misconduct in research: report of the ORI. US Committee on Research Integrity. ori.hhs.gov/images/ddblock/report_commission.pdf
Assurances, Representations, and Certifications - Sponsored ..,
http://www3.research.usf.edu/dsr/desk-manual/assurances.asp (accessed July 21, 2013).

6. Administration - Office of Sponsored Programs - Research ..,
http://www.wssu.edu/administration/sponsored-programs/research-compliance/miscon
duct-in-research.aspx (accessed July 21, 2013).
7. M Farthing. Research misconduct: Britain's failure to act. BMJ
v.321(7275); Dec 16, 2000 www.ncbi.nlm.nih.gov › ... ›
British science needs 'integrity overhaul' : Nature News ..,
http://nature.com/news/british-science-needs-integrity-overhaul-1.9803 (accessed July 21, 2013).
8. Jennifer Neuman,
Deborah Korenstein, Joseph S Ross and Salomeh Keyhani Prevalence of financial conflicts of interest among panel members producing clinical practice guidelines in Canada and United States: cross sectional study. BMJ 2011;343:d5621. doi: 10.1136/bmj.d5621 (Published 11 October 2011) Financial Conflicts 'Pervasive' On Key Medical Panels : Shots ..,
http://www.npr.org/blogs/health/2011/10/12/141264688/financial-conflicts-pervasive-on-key-medical-panels (accessed July 21, 2013).
9. Lock S, Wells F, Farthing M, eds. Fraud and misconduct in biomedical research. 3rd ed. London: BMJ Books, 2001.
10. A Tavare. Scientific misconduct is worryingly prevalent in the UK, shows BMJ survey. 12 January 2012. BMJ 2012;344:e377. Doi: 10.1136/bmj.e377
www.bmj.com/content/344/bmj.e377
11. Misconduct pervades UK research - FT.com - World business ..,
http://www.ft.com/cms/s/2/bc6f7204-3d1f-11e1-8129-00144feabdc0.html (accessed July 21, 2013).
12. Ibid.
13. A Tavare. J Med Ethics 2001;27:344-6
14. F Godlee and E Wager.BMJ 2012;344:d8357 doi:10.1136/bmj.d8357
15. Clive Cookson the Science Editor in the Financial Times of January 12th 2012 under the title "Misconduct pervades UK research" www.ft.com
Misconduct pervades UK research - FT.com - World business ..,
http://www.ft.com/cms/s/2/bc6f7204-3d1f-11e1-8129-00144feabdc0.html (accessed July 21, 2013).
16. Misconduct pervades UK research - FT.com - World business ..,
http://www.ft.com/cms/s/2/bc6f7204-3d1f-11e1-8129-00144feabdc0.html (accessed July 21, 2013).
17. Ibid.
18. British science needs 'integrity overhaul': Nature News ..,
http://nature.com/news/british-science-needs-integrity-overhaul-1.9803 (accessed July 21, 2013).
19. Misconduct pervades UK research - FT.com - World business ..,
http://www.ft.com/cms/s/2/bc6f7204-3d1f-11e1-8129-00144feabdc0.html (accessed July 21, 2013).
20. Daniel Cressey. British science needs "integrity overhaul": Nature News & Comment. 13 Jan 2012. www.nature.com/.../british-science-needs-integrity-overhaul-1.9803. doi:10.1038/nature.2012.9803. British science needs 'integrity overhaul': Nature News .., http://nature.com/news/british-science-needs-integrity-overhaul-1.9803 (accessed July 21, 2013).

21. British science needs 'integrity overhaul' : Nature News ..,
http://nature.com/news/british-science-needs-integrity-overhaul-1.9803 (accessed July 21, 2013).
22. Ibid.
23. Singh RB, Rastogi SS, Verma R, Laxmi B, Singh R, Ghosh S and Niaz MA. Randomised controlled trial of cardioprotective diet in patients with recent acute myocardial infarction: results of one year follow up. BMJ 1992; 304: 10159.
24. Al-Marzouki S, Evans S, Marshall T, Roberts I.
Are these data real? Statistical methods for the detection of data fabrication in clinical trials. BMJ 2005; 331: 267-70. Doi: 10.1136/bmj.331.7511.281
25. Jon Sudbø - Wikipedia, the free encyclopedia,
http://en.wikipedia.org/wiki/Jon_Sudbo (accessed July 21, 2013).
26. Sudbø, Jon. J Natl Cancer Inst 2006;98:374–6.
doi:10.1093/jnci/ ...Jon Sudbø - Wikipedia, the free encyclopedia,
http://en.wikipedia.org/wiki/Jon_Sudbo (accessed July 21, 2013).
27. K Travis Cancer Fraud Case Stuns Research Community, Prompts Reflection on Peer Review Process. J Natl Cancer Inst (15 March 2006) 98(6): 374-376
doi:10.1093/jnci/djj118
28. Kate Travis. Medscape. Recent Conference Addresses Research Integrity on Global Scale. J Natl Cancer Inst (2008) 100 (1): 7-10. Doi: 10.1093/jnci/djm300
29.Correcting the scientific record . Nature Chemical Biology 4, 381. 2008.
www.nature.com/nchembio/journal/v4/n7/.../nchembio0708-381.htm.
doi:10.1038/nchembio0708-381
30. Won J, Kim M, Kim N, Ahn JH, Lee WG, Kim SS, Chang KY, Yi YW, Kim TK Small molecule-based reversible reprogramming of cellular lifespan. 2006.
Nat. Chem. Biol. 2, 369–374, 2006
www.nature.com/uidfinder/10.1038/nchembio800. Published online: 11 June 2006 |Corrected online: 1 October 0613 | doi :10.1038/nchembio800.
www.ncbi.nlm.nih.gov/pubmed/16767085
31. De Angelis, Catherine D., Fontanarosa, Phil B. Editorial. Retraction:
Cheng B-Q, et al.
Chemoembolization combined with radiofrequency ablation for patients with hepatocellular carcinoma larger than 3 cm:
a randomized controlled trial.
JAMA, 301(18):1931, 2009. Published online April 20, 2009. Doi:
10.1001/jama.2009.640
32. Cheng B-Q, et al. Chemoembolization combined with radiofrequency ablation for patients with hepatocellular carcinoma larger than 3 cm: a randomized controlled trial. JAMA. 2008;299(14):1669-1677. Pmid:18398079.
33. Lock S, Wells F, Farthing M, eds. Fraud and misconduct in biomedical research. 3rd ed. London: BMJ Books, 2001.
34. Richard Smith. Research misconduct and biomedical journals. Editor, BMJ www.bmj.com/talks
35. Lock S, Wells F,Farthing M Rennie D,Gunsalus CK. . Regulations on scientific misconduct: lessons from the US experience. In: Lock S, Wells F, Farthing M, eds. Fraud and misconduct in biomedical research. 3rd edition. London: BMJ Books, 2001.
36. Ibid.
37. Martinson BC, Anderson MS, de Vries R. Scientists behaving badly. Nature 2005; 435: 7378.

38. Smith Richard. Investigating the previous studies of a fraudulent author. BMJ 2005, 331(7511):288-91.
39. Chandra, R. K . Effect of vitamin and trace-element supplementation on cognitive function in elderly subjects. Nutrition 2001; 17: 70912.
40. Meguid, M. Retraction of: Chandra RK. Nutrition 2001; 17: 70912.
41. Lock S, Wells F, Farthing M. Research misconduct 1974–1990: an imperfect history. In: Lock S, Wells F, Farthing M, eds. Fraud and misconduct in biomedical research. 3rd ed. London: BMJ Books, 2001.
42. Payne D. Nutrition retracts 2001 paper. Scientist 2005 Mar 3. http://www.the-scientist.com/news/20050303/02.
43. McCall Smith A. What is the legal position? J R Coll. Physicians Edinb. 2000; 30(suppl 7):22.
44. Alexander McCall Smith - ABC Perth - Australian Broadcasting .., http://www.abc.net.au/local/audio/2009/02/12/2489919.htm (accessed July 21, 2013).
45. David Cyranoski. Research ethics: Zero tolerance. Nature News & Comment. A university cracks down on misconduct in China. 11 January 2012. www.nature.com/news/research-ethics-zero-tolerance-1.9756
46. Research ethics: Zero tolerance: Nature News & Comment, http://www.nature.com/news/research-ethics-zero-tolerance-1.9756?WT.ec_id=NEWS-20120117 (accessed July 21, 2013).
47. Ibid.
48. David Cyranoski. Named and shamed. Nature2006. 441, 392–393. www.nature.com/nature/journal/v441/n7092/. doi:10.1038/441392a
Research ethics: Zero tolerance: Nature News & Comment, http://www.nature.com/news/research-ethics-zero-tolerance-1.9756?WT.ec_id=NEWS-2
0120117 (accessed July 21, 2013).
49. David Cyranoski. Policing the plagiarists.
Nature. 12 January 2012. Volume 481, Pages: 134–136. Doi:10.1038/481134a
50. Research ethics: Zero tolerance: Nature News & Comment, http://www.nature.com/news/research-ethics-zero-tolerance-1.9756?WT.ec_id=NEWS-2
0120117 (accessed July 21, 2013).
51. Y. Zhang Nature 467, 153; 2010. Research ethics: Zero tolerance: Nature News & Comment, http://nature.com/news/research-ethics-zero-tolerance-1.9756 (accessed July 21, 2013).
52. Research ethics: Zero tolerance: Nature News & Comment, http://www.nature.com/news/research-ethics-zero-tolerance-1.9756?WT.ec_id=NEWS-2
0120117 (accessed July 21, 2013).
53. Ibid.
54. Ibid.
55. Ibid.
56. Ibid.
57. Ibid.
58. Ibid.
59. Ibid.
60. Ibid.
61. David Cyranoski. Policing the plagiarists.

Nature. 12 January 2012. Volume 481, Pages: 134–136. Doi:10.1038/481134a
Research ethics: Zero tolerance : Nature News & Comment, http://www.nature.com/news/research-ethics-zero-tolerance-1.9756?WT.ec_id=NEWS-20120117 (accessed July 21, 2013).
62. Research ethics: Zero tolerance: Nature News & Comment, http://www.nature.com/news/research-ethics-zero-tolerance-1.9756?WT.ec_id=NEWS-2 0120117 (accessed July 21, 2013).
63. Ibid.
64. Ibid.
65. Ibid.
66. Scientific American. January 2012. Vol 306. No. 1 p 75. Research ethics: Zero tolerance: Nature News & Comment, http://www.nature.com/news/research-ethics-zero-tolerance-1.9756?WT.ec_id=NEWS-2 0120117 (accessed July 21, 2013).
67. Jobs at Macmillan, http://jobs.macmillan.com/VacancyDetail.aspx?VacancyUID=000000002353 (accessed July 21, 2013).
68. Ibid.
69. Ibid.
70. Ibid.
71. Richard Smith.
Editor, Fraud in medical research - BMJ resources. GMC & Committee on Publication Ethics. BMJ
www.bmj.com/talks resources.bmj.com/files/talks/fraudcardiff.ppt
72. Ibid.
73. Barnes,
D. E., Bero, L. A. Why review articles on the health effects of passive smoking reach different conclusions. JAMA 1998; 279: 1566-1570
74. Stelfox HT, Chua G, O'Rourke K, Detsky AS. Conflict of interest in the debate over calcium channel antagonists. N Engl J Med 1998; 338: 101-105
75. Vandenbroucke JP, Helmerhorst FM, Frits R Rosendaal FR. Competing interests and controversy about third generation oral contraceptives. BMJ 2000; 320: 381
76. Richard Smith.
Editor, Fraud in medical research - BMJ resources. GMC & Committee on Publication Ethics.
BMJ
www.bmj.com/talks resources.bmj.com/files/talks/fraudcardiff.ppt
77. Richard Smith
Editor, BMJ
Research misconduct and biomedical journals. www.bmj.com/talks
PLOS ONE: How Many Scientists Fabricate and Falsify Research .., http://www.plosone.org/article/info:doi/10.1371/journal.pone.0005738 (accessed July 21, 2013).
78. Fanelli D. How Many Scientists Fabricate and Falsify Research?
A Systematic Review and Meta-Analysis of Survey Data. (2009) Science 299: 31–31. PLoS ONE 4(5): e5738.
www.plosone.org/.../info%3Adoi%2F10.1371%2Fjournal.po...
doi:10.1371/journal.pone.0005738

79. Saunders R, Savulescu J (2008) Research ethics and lessons from Hwanggate: what can we learn from the Korean cloning fraud? Journal of Medical Ethics 34: 214–221.
PLOS ONE: How Many Scientists Fabricate and Falsify Research .., http://www.plosone.org/article/info:doi/10.1371/journal.pone.0005738 (accessed July 21, 2013).
80. Service RF (31st Jan 2003) Scientific misconduct - More of Bell Labs physicist's papers retracted. Science 299: 31–31.
www.sciencemag.org/content/299/5603/31.2.short. DOI: 10.1126/science.299.5603.31b ...
81. Marshall E (2000) Scientific misconduct - How prevalent is fraud? That's a million-dollar question. Science 290: 1662–1663.
82. Sovacool BK (2008) Exploring scientific misconduct: isolated individuals, impure institutions, or an inevitable idiom of modern science? Journal of Bioethical Inquiry 5: 271–282. PLOS ONE: How Many Scientists Fabricate and Falsify Research .., http://www.plosone.org/article/info:doi/10.1371/journal.pone.0005738 (accessed July 21, 2013).
83. Bogner A, Menz W (2006) Science crime: the Korean cloning scandal and the role of ethics. Science & Public Policy 33: 601–612.
84. Koshland DE (1987) Fraud in Science. Science 235: 141.
85. La Follette MC (2000) The evolution of the "scientific misconduct" issues: an historical overview. Procedings of the Society for Experimental Biology and Medicine 224: 211–215. 86. PLOS ONE: How Many Scientists Fabricate and Falsify Research .., http://www.plosone.org/article/info:doi/10.1371/journal.pone.0005738 (accessed July 21, 2013).
87. Smith R (2000) What is research misconduct? The COPE Report 2000: the Committee on Publication Ethics.
88. Kalichman MW, Friedman PJ (1992) A pilot study of biomedical trainees' perceptions concerning research ethics. Academic Medicine 67: 769–775.
89. COPE (2000) The COPE report 2000. Committee on Publication Ethics. PLOS ONE: How Many Scientists Fabricate and Falsify Research .., http://www.plosone.org/article/info:doi/10.1371/journal.pone.0005738 (accessed July 21, 2013).
90. Berk RA, Korenman SG, Wenger NS (2000) Measuring consensus about scientific research norms. Science and Engineering Ethics. Springer 6: 315–340.
91. Eastwood S, Derish P, Leash E, Ordway S (1996) Ethical issues in biomedical research: Perceptions and practices of postdoctoral research fellows responding to a survey. Science and Engineering Ethics 2: 89–114.
92. PLOS ONE: How Many Scientists Fabricate and Falsify Research .., http://www.plosone.org/article/info:doi/10.1371/journal.pone.0005738 (accessed July 21, 2013).
93. Kalichman MW, Friedman PJ (1992) A pilot study of biomedical trainees' perceptions concerning research ethics. Academic Medicine 67: 769–775. PLOS ONE: How Many Scientists Fabricate and Falsify Research .., http://www.plosone.org/article/info:doi/10.1371/journal.pone.0005738 (accessed July 21, 2013).
94. PLOS ONE: How Many Scientists Fabricate and Falsify Research .., http://www.plosone.org/article/info:doi/10.1371/journal.pone.0005738 (accessed July 21, 2013).

95. Angell M (2000) Is academic medicine for sale? New England Journal of Medicine 342: 1516–1518.
96. Bekelman JE, Li Y, Gross CP (2003) Scope and impact of financial conflicts of interest in biomedical research - A systematic review. Jama-Journal of the American Medical Association 289: 454–465.
97. Sismondo S (2008) Pharmaceutical company funding and its consequences: a qualitative systematic review. Contemporary Clinical Trials 29: 109–113.
98. Angell M. Is academic medicine for sale? 2000. New England Journal of Medicine 342: 1516–1518. Is Academic Medicine for Sale? MARCIA ANGELL, MD / Editorial .., http://www.mindfully.org/Health/Academic-Medicine-Sale18may00.htm (accessed July 21, 2013).
99. Skeptical Investigations - Scientific Objectivity - Flawed .., http://www.skepticalinvestigations.org/Flawedevidence/index.html (accessed July 21, 2013). 100. Rescuing Science from Politics Edited by Wendy Wagner Cambridge University Press (2006) 274 pages ISBN: 0521855209, 9780521855204
101. Center for Progressive Reform :: CPR Perspective: Clean Science, http://www.progressivereform.org/perspScience.cfm (accessed July 21, 2013).
102. Ibid.
103. Ibid.
104. Is Academic Medicine for Sale? MARCIA ANGELL, MD / Editorial .., http://www.mindfully.org/Health/Academic-Medicine-Sale18may00.htm (accessed July 21, 2013).
105. Ibid.
106. Ibid.
107. Ibid.
108. Ibid.
109. Ibid.
110. Schwartz, L., Woloshin, S. and Moynihan, R. Who's watching the watchdogs? : BMJ 2008;337:a2535 ; 337 doi: 10.1136/bmj.a2535 (Published 19 November 2008. Who's watching the watchdogs? | BMJ, http://www.bmj.com/content/337/bmj.a2535 (accessed July 21, 2013).
111. Who's watching the watchdogs? | BMJ, http://www.bmj.com/content/337/bmj.a2535 (accessed July 21, 2013).
112. Hoskins Z. UNC-CH chooses professor to head new medical journalism program. University of North Carolina at Chapel Hill News Services. www.unc.edu/news/archives/jun97/linden.html. Who's watching the watchdogs? | BMJ, http://www.bmj.com/content/337/bmj.a2535 (accessed July 21, 2013).
113. University of North Carolina School of Journalism and Mass Communication. Pfizer minority medical journalism scholarship. www.jomc.unc.edu/medicaljournalism/scholarship.html. Who's watching the watchdogs? | BMJ, http://www.bmj.com/content/337/bmj.a2535 (accessed July 21, 2013).
114. American Medical Writers Association. The resource for medical communicators. www.amwa.org/default.asp?Mode=DirectoryDisplay&id=1. Who's watching the watchdogs? | BMJ, http://www.bmj.com/content/337/bmj.a2535 (accessed July 21, 2013).
115. Schwitzer health news blog: Search Results, http://blog.lib.umn.edu/cgi-bin/mt-search.cgi?IncludeBlogs=704&search=sanjay%20gupta (accessed July 21, 2013).

116. Boehringer Ingelheim. Winners of the second Embrace journalism award for reporting on urinary incontinence are announced. www.boehringer-ingelheim.com/corporate/news/press_releases/detail.asp?ID=4274.
117. Boehringer Ingelheim. Eloquium COPD communication award. www.boehringer-ingelheim.com/corporate/news/awards.asp. Schwitzer health news blog: Search Results, http://blog.lib.umn.edu/cgi-bin/mt-search.cgi?IncludeBlogs=704&search=sanjay%20g upta (accessed July 21, 2013).
118. Mental Health America. About us. www.mentalhealthamerica.net/go/about-us. Schwitzer health news blog: Search Results, http://blog.lib.umn.edu/cgi-bin/mt-search.cgi?IncludeBlogs=704&search=sanjay%20g upta (accessed July 21, 2013).
119. Wazana A. Physicians and the pharmaceutical industry: is a gift ever just a gift? JAMA2000;283:373-80.
120. Schwartz, L., Woloshin, S. and Moynihan, R. Who's watching the watchdogs? : BMJ 2008;337:a2535 ; 337 doi: 10.1136/bmj.a2535 (Published 19 November 2008)
121. Patient View. Fundraising and the growth of industry involvement. HSC News International2004:4;7-62.
122. Moynihan R, Bero L, Ross-Degnan D, Henry D, Lee K, Watkins J, et al. Coverage by the news media of the benefits and risks of medications. N Engl J Med 2000;342:1645-50. 123. Wager E (2007) Authors, Ghosts, Damned Lies, and Statisticians. PLoS Med 4(1): e34. doi:10.1371/journal.pmed.0040034. Published: January 16, 2007. PLOS Medicine: Authors, Ghosts, Damned Lies, and Statisticians, http://www.plosmedicine.org/article/info%3Adoi%2F10.1371%2Fjournal.pmed.0040034 (accessed July 22, 2013).
124. PLOS Medicine: Authors, Ghosts, Damned Lies, and Statisticians, http://www.plosmedicine.org/article/info%3Adoi%2F10.1371%2Fjournal.pmed.0040034 (accessed July 22, 2013).
125. Woolley KL, Ely JA, Woolley MJ, Findlay L, Lynch FA, et al. (2006) Declaration of medical writing assistance in international peer-reviewed publications. JAMA 296: 932–934.
126. Healy DT (2004) Transparency and trust: Figure for ghost written articles was misquoted. BMJ 329: 1345. doi:10.1136/bmj.329.7478.134
127. Ross JS, Hill KP, Egilman DS, Krumholz HM. Guest authorship and ghostwriting in publications related to rofecoxib: a case study of industry documents from rofecoxib litigation. JAMA 2008;299(15):1800–12.
128. Rennie D, Flanagin A. Authorship! authorship! guests, ghosts, grafters, and the two-sided coin. JAMA 1994;271(6):469–71.
129. Rennie D, Yank V, Emanuel L. When authorship fails: a proposal to make contributors accountable. JAMA 1997;278 (7):579–85.
130. Gøtzsche PC, Hróbjartsson A, Johansen HK, Haahr MT, Altman DG (2007) Ghost authorship in industry-initiated randomised trials. PLoS Med 4: e535. doi:10.1371/journal.pmed.0040019.
131. Jef Feeley and Sophia Pearson, Wyeth used ghostwritten Prempro articles, files show (Update3), Bloomberg.com, Aug. 5, 2009, available at www.bloomberg.com/apps/news?pid=newsarchive&sid= abGoyhK2PAes
132. Marvin A. Konstam, Matthew R. Weir, Alise Reicin, Deborah Shapiro, Rhoda S Sperling, Eliav Barr, and Barry J Gertz, Cardiovascular thrombotic events in controlled, clinical trials of rofecoxib, 104 CIRCULATION 2280, 2287 (2001).

133. Joseph S. Ross, Kevin P. Hill, David S. Egilman, and Harlan M. Krumholtz, Guest authorship and ghostwriting in publications related to rofecoxib: A case study of industry documents from rofecoxib litigation, 299(15) JAMA 1800 (2008).
134. Harris Gardiner and Berenson Alex. 10 Voters on panel backing pain pills had industry ties. New York Times2005 Feb 25.
www.nytimes.com/2005/02/25/politics/25fda.html. Sources by F.D.A.; Center for Science in the Public Interest)(pg. A20)
November 23, 2011, 5:00 pm
135. Ross JS, Hill KP, Egilman DS, Krumholz HM. Guest authorship and ghostwriting in publications related to rofecoxib: a case study of industry documents from rofecoxib litigation. JAMA 2008;299(15):1800–12.
136. Flanagin A, Carey LA, Fontanarosa PB, et al. Prevalence of articles with honorary authors and ghost authors in peer reviewed medical journals. JAMA 1998;280(3):222–4.
137. Mowatt G, Shirran L, Grimshaw JM, et al. Prevalence of honorary and ghost authorship in Cochrane reviews. JAMA 2002;287(21):2769–71.
138. Shapiro DW, Wenger NS, Shapiro MF. The contributions of authors to multiauthored biomedical research papers. JAMA 1994;271(6):438–42.
139. Scheife, Richard T. A Ghost in the Machine. Pharmacotherapy 2009;29(4):363-364.
140. Larry D. Claxton. Scientific authorship: Part 1. A window into scientific fraud? Mutation Research/Reviews in Mutation Research, January 2005, Volume 589, Issue 1, Pages 17-30.
141. Larry D. Claxton
Scientific authorship: Part 2. History, recurring issues, practices, and guidelines Mutation Research/Reviews in Mutation Research, January 2005, Volume 589, Issue 1, Pages 31-45. ScienceDirect.com - Mutation Research/Reviews in Mutation .., http://www.sciencedirect.com/science/article/pii/S1383574204000559 (accessed July 22, 2013).
142. ScienceDirect.com - Mutation Research/Reviews in Mutation .., http://www.sciencedirect.com/science/article/pii/S1383574204000559 (accessed July 22, 2013).
143. Ibid.
144. Ibid.
145. Al-Marzouki S, Evans S, Marshall T, Roberts I. Are these data real? Statistical methods for the detection of data fabrication in clinical trials. BMJ. 2005 July 30; 331(7511): 267–270. doi:
10.1136/bmj.331.7511.267
146. Buyse M, George SL, Evans S, Geller NL, Ranstam J, Scherrer B, Lesaffre E, Murray G, Edler L, Hutton J, Colton T, Lachenbruch P, Verma BL. The role of biostatistics in the prevention, detection and treatment of fraud in clinical trials. Stat Med. 1999 Dec 30;18(24):3435-51.
147. Wager E (2007) Authors, Ghosts, Damned Lies, and Statisticians. PLoS Med 4(1): e34. doi:10.1371/journal.pmed.0040034. January 16, 2007. PLOS Medicine: Authors, Ghosts, Damned Lies, and Statisticians, http://www.plosmedicine.org/article/info%3Adoi%2F10.1371%2Fjournal.pmed.0040034 (accessed July 22, 2013).
148. Biagioli M (1998) The instability of authorship: Credit and responsibility in contemporary medicine. FASEB J 12: 3–16. PLOS Medicine: Authors, Ghosts, Damned Lies, and Statisticians,

http://www.plosmedicine.org/article/info%3Adoi%2F10.1371%2Fjournal.pmed.0040034 (accessed July 22, 2013).
149. PLOS Medicine: Authors, Ghosts, Damned Lies, and Statisticians, http://www.plosmedicine.org/article/info%3Adoi%2F10.1371%2Fjournal.pmed.0040034 (accessed July 22, 2013).
150. Abbasi K (2004) Transparency and trust. BMJ. 329. doi:10.1136/bmj.329.7472.0-g.
151. International Committee of Medical Journal Editors (2006) Uniform requirements for manuscripts submitted to biomedical journals: Writing and editing for biomedical publication. Available: http://www.icmje.org.
152. Huth E, Case K (2004) The URM: Twenty-five years old. Science Editor 27: 17–21.
PLOS Medicine: Authors, Ghosts, Damned Lies, and Statisticians, http://www.plosmedicine.org/article/info%3Adoi%2F10.1371%2Fjournal.pmed.0040034 (accessed July 22, 2013).
153. Gøtzsche PC, Hróbjartsson A, Johansen HK, Haahr MT, Altman DG (2007) Ghost authorship in industry-initiated randomised trials. Ibid.
154. International Committee of Medical Journal Editors (2006) Uniform requirements for manuscripts submitted to biomedical journals: Writing and editing for biomedical publication. Available: http://www.icmje.org.
155. PLOS Medicine: Authors, Ghosts, Damned Lies, and Statisticians, http://www.plosmedicine.org/article/info%3Adoi%2F10.1371%2Fjournal.pmed.0040034 (accessed July 22, 2013).
156. Wikipedia (2006) Lies, damned lies, and statistics. Available: http://en.wikipedia.org/wiki/Lies,_damned_lies,_and_statistics. Accessed 11 December 2006.
PLOS Medicine: Authors, Ghosts, Damned Lies, and Statisticians, http://www.plosmedicine.org/article/info%3Adoi%2F10.1371%2Fjournal.pmed.0040034 (accessed July 22, 2013).
157. Richard Smith
Editor, BMJ
www.bmj.com/talks
Fraud in medical research - Upload & Share PowerPoint .., http://www.slideshare.net/Medresearch/fraud-in-medical-research-5870848 (accessed July 22, 2013).
158. Fraud in medical research - Upload & Share PowerPoint .., http://www.slideshare.net/Medresearch/fraud-in-medical-research-5870848 (accessed July 22, 2013).
159. McMillan A. Committee on Publication Ethics: the COPE report. Sex Transm Infect 2000;76:68-72 doi:10.1136/sti.76.2.68
160. United Kingdom Code: Committee on Publication Ethics .., http://www.rjionline.org/MAS-Codes-UK-COPE (accessed July 22, 2013).
161. Ibid.
162. Ibid.
163. Ibid.
164. Ibid.
165. Ibid.
166. Ibid.

167. Fraud in medical research - Upload & Share PowerPoint ..,
http://www.slideshare.net/Medresearch/fraud-in-medical-research-5870848 (accessed July 22, 2013).
168. Ibid.
169. Ibid.
170. Gøtzsche PC, Kassirer JP, Woolley KL, Wagner E, Jacobs A, et al. (2009) What Should Be Done To Tackle Ghostwriting in the Medical Literature? PLoS Med 6(2): e1000023. doi:10.1371/journal.pmed.1000023
171. Anderson, Melissa S.
Scientific Integrity:
Maintaining the Legitimacy of the Research Enterprise.
Proceedings of the 4th International Barcelona Conference on High Education, 1, 2008.
172. Koocher, Gerald and Keith-Spiegel, Patricia.
Peers nip misconduct in the bud.
Nature, Vol. 466, July 22, 2010.
173. Harold C. Sox, MD, and Drummond Rennie, MD. Research Misconduct, Retraction, and Cleansing the Medical Literature: Lessons from the Poehlman Case. Ann Intern Med. 2006;144:609-613. www.annals.org
174. Office of Research Integrity, U.S. Department of Health and Human Services. Papers affected by Dr. Poehlman's misconduct.2005.Accessedathttp://ori.dhhs.gov/documents/pubmed_list.pdfon24March2005.
175. Ewen Callaway.In vino non veritas? Red wine researcher implicated in misconduct case. Nature News & Comment. 12 Jan 2012. Red-Wine Researcher Implicated in Data Misconduct Case ..,
https://www.scientificamerican.com/article.cfm?id=red-wine-researcher-implicated-misconduct (accessed July 22, 2013).
176. Red-Wine Researcher Implicated in Data Misconduct Case ..,
https://www.scientificamerican.com/article.cfm?id=red-wine-researcher-implicated-misconduct (accessed July 22, 2013).
177. Ibid.
178. Ibid.
179. Ibid.
180. Ibid.
181. Ibid.
182. Smith J, Godlee F. Investigating allegations of scientific misconduct [Editorial]. BMJ.2005;331:245-6.[PMID:16051990]
183. White C. Suspected research fraud: difficulties of getting at the truth.BMJ.2005;331:281-8.[PMID:16052022]
184. Smith R. Investigating the previous studies of a fraudulent author. BMJ.2005; 331:288-91. [PMID:16052023]
185. Horton R. Expression of concern: Indo-Mediterranean Diet Heart Study. Lancet. 2005; 366:354-6.[PMID:16054927]
186. Smith J, Godlee F. Investigating allegations of scientific misconduct [Editorial]. BMJ.2005;331:245-6.[PMID:16051990]
187. Hammerschmidt DE, Gross AG. Allegations of impropriety in manuscripts by AwsS.Salim: examination and withdrawal of journal aegis. The Executive Editorial Committee of the Journal of Laboratory and Clinical Medicine [Editorial]. JLabClinMed. 1994;123:795-9.[PMID:8201253]

188. Hammerschmidt DE, Gross AG. Withdrawal of aegis? So what's that?[Editorial] JLabClinMed. 1994;123:792-4.[PMID:8201252]
189. International Committee of Medical Journal Editors. Uniform requirements For manuscripts submitted to biomedical journals: writing and editing for bio-medical publication. Accessedatwww.icmje.org/index.html#topon16January 2006.
190. Smith J, Godlee F. Investigating allegations of scientific misconduct [Editorial]. BMJ.2005;331:245-6.[PMID:16051990]
191. Horton R. Expression of concern: Indo-Mediterranean Diet Heart Study. Lancet. 2005; 366:354-6.[PMID:16054927]
192. Kennedy D. Editorial expression of concern [Letter].Science.2006;311:36. [PMID: 16373531]
193. Curfman GD, Morrissey S, Drazen JM. Expression of concern: Bombardier,et al. Comparison of upper gastrointestinal toxicity of rofecoxib and naproxenin patients with rheumatoid arthritis. NEnglJMed.2000;343:1520-8.NEnglJMed.2005;353:2813-4. [PMID:16339408]
194. Curfman GD, Morrissey S, Drazen JM. Expression of concern: Sudbø J,et al.DNA content as a prognostic marker in patients with oral leukoplakia. NEnglJMed.2001;344: 1270-8andSudbøJ,etal.The influence of resection and aneuploidy on mortality in oral leukoplakia.NEnglJMed.2004;350:1405-13. NEnglJMed.2006;354:638.[PMID:16428677]
195. Horton R. Expression of concern: non-steroidal anti-inflammatory drugs and the risk of oral cancer. Lancet.2006;367:196.[PMID:16427477]
196. Cicutto, Lisa.
Plagiarism. Avoiding the Peril in Scientific Writing.
CHEST, 133:579-581, 2008. CHEST Journal | Article, http://journal.publications.chestnet.org/article.aspx?articleid=1085699 (accessed July 22, 2013).
197. CHEST Journal | Article, http://journal.publications.chestnet.org/article.aspx?articleid=1085699 (accessed July 22, 2013).
198. Steneck N. H. Introduction to the responsible conduct of research. Washington, DC: US Government Printing Office. Available at:
http://ori.hhs.gov/documents/rcrinto.pdf. Accessed January 10,
199. CHEST Journal | Article, http://journal.publications.chestnet.org/article.aspx?articleid=1085699 (accessed July 22, 2013).
200. Office of Research Integrity. Annual report 2006. Department of Health and Human Services, May 2007. Available at:
http://ori.hhs.gov/documents/annual_reports/ori_annual_report_2006.pdf. Accessed January 10, 2008
201. Foote, MA Why references: giving credit and growing the field. Chest 2007;132,344-346
202. CHEST Journal | Article, http://journal.publications.chestnet.org/article.aspx?articleid=1085699 (accessed July 22, 2013).
203. Committee on Publication Ethics (COPE). Guidelines on good publication practice. J Postgrad Med 2000;46,217-221
204. Bloemenkamp, DG, Walvroot, HC, Hart, W, et al Duplicate publication of articles in the Dutch Journal of Medicine in 1996. Ned Tidchr Geneeskd 1999;23,2150-2153

205. Schein, M, Paladugu, R Redundant surgical publications: tip of the iceberg. Surgery 2001;129,655-661
206. CHEST Journal | Article, http://journal.publications.chestnet.org/article.aspx?articleid=1085699 (accessed July 22, 2013).
207. Tramer, MR, Reynolds, DJ, Moore, RA, et al Impact of covert duplicate publication on meta-analysis: a case study. BMJ 1997;315,635-640
208. Cicutto, Lisa.
Plagiarism. Avoiding the Peril in Scientific Writing.
CHEST, 133:579-581, 2008. CHEST Journal | Article, http://journal.publications.chestnet.org/article.aspx?articleid=1085699 (accessed July 22, 2013).

Chapter nine - Quackery - Food Supplements and Vitamins

Supplements; food or drugs?

Buy two and receive a third "absolutely free"! How often do we see or hear this? Something is free or it is not free. There are not different degrees of free. If something is received as a condition that one purchases or receives something else how can that item be "absolutely" free? We buy "special offers" not for $300 or $400 but for $299.99 or $399.99. What is one cent in three or four hundred dollars? How gullible can we be? This is all so obvious everybody knows it but we still purchase the goods believing that we are getting a bargain. The average man in the street is conned by advertising but no more than he is when purchasing pharmaceutical products or supplements.

Professor Arnold Bender the Professor of Nutrition and Dietetics and Head of Department at Queen Elizabeth died in 1999. He was the author of some 150 research publications and major academic reviews, and 14 books, many of which have become major reference works and standard textbooks at school and university level. Professor Bender was also an editor of professional journals, and a committee member of the Nutrition Society, The Institute of Food Science and Technology, The Royal Society of Health and Hygiene and many others. In the first sentence in his book titled *Health or Hoax: The Truth about Health Foods and Diets*[1] he said: "There is no such thing as a health food. The term is both false and misleading, misleading because it suggests that other foods are unhealthy."

Dietary supplements, their ingredients, safety, and claims are a continual source of controversy.[2] Are they necessary? Vitamins are generally recommended for very young children until they are eating solid foods that contain enough vitamins. After that it is seldom necessary to continue supplements. In 1980, the Committee on Nutrition of the American Academy of Pediatrics stated that supplements might be appropriate in certain circumstances. These included fluoride supplements in children not drinking fluoridated water, multivitamin tablets for children with poor eating habits and those using weight-reduction diets or those on strict vegetarian diets.[3]

The U.S. Preventive Services Task Force has recommended that all women planning or capable of pregnancy should take a daily supplement of folic acid in order to reduce the risk of birth defects in their offspring.[4] Pregnant women may also need to take iron. Elderly individuals of both sexes who may not be receiving sufficient nutrients may also benefit from multivitamin-mineral supplementation. Older women need an adequate intake of calcium to help to prevent osteoporosis and if they do not have adequate exposure to sunlight they may benefit from a vitamin D supplement. Vegetarians and vegans may need dietary supplements. Antioxidants have been mentioned in an earlier chapter. They have received a lot of favourable publicity but swallowing antioxidant supplements does not make sense.[5]

As the late John H. Renner, president of the National Council against Health Fraud, aptly pointed out: "Nutrition is awfully important in a variety of illnesses as prevention and, in a few, as treatment. But you don't put out a fire with the same things you use to keep it from starting".[6] For by far the greater number of people, supplements are not necessary in any way whatsoever other than to fill the pockets of the supplement manufacturing companies.

In December 1995 the BBC's Food and Drink Program exposed the dubious quality of some so-called "nutrition consultants." As part of a survey carried out with the help of the British Dietetic and Diabetic Associations, five such consultants were randomly selected from the classified advertisement section of consumer health magazines.[7] A woman with non-insulin dependent diabetes made appointments with each, explained the common symptoms of diabetes as her presenting complaint and waited for their diagnosis and prescription. Only one suggested diabetes as a possible diagnosis, all gave inappropriate advice and most actively discouraged contact with the woman's doctor.

How does one become a qualified nutritionist or, even better, a nutrition consultant? The British Dietetic Association's Public Relations Advisor, Lyndel Costain went undercover to check out the training offered by a correspondence course for would-be "nutrition consultants."[8] It cost her £215 to enroll as a student of a ten-week correspondence nutrition course from the British School of Yoga.[9] The course consisted of reading often haphazardly put together lesson notes, then answering ten questions. As the exact answers were found in the text, it was hard to get them wrong.[10]

According to *HealthWatch,* no application of knowledge was required, and much of the nutritional science was flawed.[11] The lessons covered included the Natural Therapists' Approach to Health;[12] The Digestive System; Iron Deficiency; Vitamins and Minerals; What to do About Stress and The Healing Crisis; Self Diagnostic Procedures; The Sugar Menace; Allergies; Disease States and Food Combining.

Lyndel Costain likened the course to a word-search puzzle rather than anything resembling a course that would "qualify" her to diagnose and treat disease.[13] Diagnostic tools included kinesiology (which relies upon changes in muscular resistance in the presence of a possible allergen) and swinging pendulums. A pendulum was held over a food or drug, the question is asked, "Is this good for me?" and the pendulum will, it is said, swing to indicate "yes or no".[14] Treatments, she was "taught" ranged from fasting and cleansing diets, through food combining, to mega-doses of vitamins and minerals.[15]

Her "undisputed favourite" was "The Gall Bladder Flush."[16] It was claimed that gallstones could be broken down, flushed out and "passed" as greenish shale. Where this shale was supposed to be passed out was not mentioned. The method was described as follows: "take a cleansing diet (fruit, vegetables, brown rice) for five days with daily lecithin, apple juice and water; on the fifth afternoon (after skipping lunch) take a teaspoon of Epsom salts in warm water at 4pm and 6pm; then from 8pm take 50 ml olive oil shaken with 15 ml. lemon juice every 15 minutes until eight doses are taken: go to bed and lie on the right side with right knee pulled up; try not to move, and go to sleep."

After following these instructions one presumably also found that the tooth fairy had visited!

Assuming that the diagnosis of gallstones was correct in the first place, and not a misdiagnosis of gastric cancer, pancreatitis, heart disease or indigestion, large volumes of olive oil as described could well cause vomiting. Similarly odd treatments were detailed for an extensive range of other health problems such as colds, cancer, heart disease, food intolerance, diabetes, yeast infections and gastro-intestinal disorders, to name a few.[17]

Potentially harmful doses of vitamins and minerals were sometimes advised for treatment of infections such as "heavy colds, pneumonia or AIDS." For example supplementation with vitamin C was recommended in quantities from 10 g/day and rising to 180 g/day (equivalent to more than 2,000 oranges!).[18] The United Kingdom recommended daily allowance of vitamin C is 40 mg/day and doses of 10 g/day can cause problems in patients with kidney disease.[19] The dangers of nutrient supplementation were entertained in cavalier fashion. Probably the greatest safeguard against the potentially harmful effects of these high dose supplement practices was said to be that "many people get bored or lose confidence in the programs" and stop taking the supplements.[20] The advice about drinking water, according to Costain, was "positively alarming".[21] "Tap water is not suitable for human consumption - it is heavily laden with inorganic salts, additives and toxic chemicals and is a slow poison."

She stated that "On the basis of the information given in this course, I fear that anyone who consults a British School of Yoga trained "nutrition consultant" could be at risk "of misdiagnosis, inappropriate treatment of medically diagnosed diseases, unnecessarily restrictive and unbalanced dietary advice, potentially harmful doses of some vitamins and minerals and bombardment with anecdotal information."[22]

It is worth remembering that, while anyone can call themselves a "nutrition consultant", state registered dietitians are the only profession with a recognised and regulated graduate qualification in nutrition and dietetics.[23]

Patrick Holford is a self-styled "nutritionist," and, according to Ben Goldacre, "probably the second most famous of the bunch".[24] He writes "plausible, reference-laden, sciencey-looking books," and is used as an "authority" but his only academic qualification is an undergraduate degree in psychology from York in 1976. In 1995 he did receive a "diploma in nutritional therapy" from the Institute of Optimum Nutrition, an institute which he founded himself but this remains his only qualification in nutrition, since he failed to complete a master's degree in nutrition from Surrey 20 years ago. In the United Kingdom, "nutritionist" is not a title covered by any registered professional body, so Patrick Holford's qualifications and expertise have been questioned. For example he has been criticised for the preposterous claim that AZT, the first prescribable anti-HIV drug, is "potentially harmful, and proving less effective than vitamin C."[25]

It is estimated that 40 per cent of people in Britain take supplements, spending between £340 and £360 million a year, and the market is growing.[26] Healthy adults use supplements to promote "optimum health."

Katherine Harmon[27] in an article titled "Worts and All" claimed that Americans spent $14.8 billion on herbal supplements and other natural health products in 2007, "even though numerous recent studies have shown that ginkgo, echinacea, St. John's wort, saw palmetto and others are relatively ineffective against many of the ills they have claimed to help". Saw palmetto is used by over two million men in the United States for the treatment of benign prostatic hyperplasia and is commonly recommended as an alternative to drugs approved by the Food and Drug Administration.[28]

In a double-blind trial,[29] 225 men over the age of 49 years who had moderate-to-severe symptoms of benign prostatic hyperplasia were randomly assigned to one year of treatment with saw Palmetto extract or placebo. The authors concluded that saw palmetto "did not improve symptoms or objective measures of benign prostatic hyperplasia."

Ginkgo biloba is sometimes claimed to help in cases of Alzheimer's disease. It has also been widely credited with improving memory and concentration. Beth Snitz and others writing in the *Journal of the American Medical Association*[30] stated that ginkgo biloba "has no effect on memory". Their study investigated 3,069 people, aged between 72 and 96 and showed that elderly people who took the supplement every day for six years had as many difficulties with recall as those who took a fake supplement. They said: "Ginkgo biloba is marketed widely and used with the hope of improving, preventing, or delaying cognitive impairment associated with aging and neurodegenerative disorders such as Alzheimer's disease. We found no evidence that ginkgo biloba slows the rate of cognitive decline in older adults." According to the article thousands of people who take this herbal supplement to ward off memory problems in old age are wasting their time. They are also wasting their money. In Britain, at least 100,000 people are thought regularly to take ginkgo biloba.

According to Paul G. Shekelle, an internist and director of the Southern California Evidence-Based Practice Centre.[31] Under the 1994 Dietary Supplement Health and Education Act the United States Food and Drug Administration regulates all dietary supplements as food products. Not as drugs. The Act says that the manufacturers are only responsible for making sure a supplement is safe and meets efficacy claims. The supplement makers are not required to present any information about how they arrived at these conclusions. Although they cannot claim a product will cure, treat or prevent a specific condition (the act prohibits unauthorised claims about disease) the labels on their products can boast of improvement of general body function such as "aids digestion," "improves heart health" or "boosts brain function" or, my favourite, "enhances the immune system."

The herb ephedra has been purported to enhance athletic performance and increase weight loss. In recent years some athletes and other individuals who apparently had ingested the herb have collapsed and, in some cases, died.[32] The Baltimore Orioles pitcher Steve Bechler apparently died in this way. Since then government officials and the public at large have become increasingly louder in demanding proof of the safety and efficacy of the herb. Unfortunately, this proof has become exceedingly difficult to obtain. As a result of the 1994 Act, ephedra is classified as a "dietary supplement" and is not considered to be a "drug". No evidence of the efficacy or safety of the product needs to be provided prior to marketing. Therefore, the usual regulatory controls do not exist.

The same Katherine Harmon mentioned earlier quoted an investigation by the Government Accountability Office in the United States, part of which employed undercover staff members and senior citizens, which revealed how loose regulations and questionable sales tactics were more persuasive than science, potentially putting consumers' health at risk.[33] They used undercover consumers over the age of 65 because most of them take prescription medication with which a supplement could interact. They asked common questions of supplement retailers such as: Is ginkgo biloba safe to take with aspirin? Can ginseng fend off cancer? What about replacing prescribed blood pressure medication with garlic supplements?

Although the United States National Institutes of Health warns against all three of these statements, the queries received resounding affirmative answers from sales staff. A combination of Ginkgo and aspirin can increase the risk of internal bleeding. Ginseng has not been scientifically proven to cure any diseases and, according to the National Institutes of Health, should be avoided for those with breast and uterine cancers. Garlic has not been shown to significantly lower high blood pressure and supplements are not intended to replace prescribed drugs.[34]

The statements by supplement sales staff amounted to "unequivocal deception" according to Marcus M. Reidenberg, Chief of the Division of Clinical Pharmacology at New York Presbyterian Hospital/Weill Cornell Medical Centre. The Government Accountability Office report, which was delivered as testimony to the United States Congress stated that both the Food and Drug Administration and the Federal Trade Commission found the practices "improper and likely in violation of statutes and regulations."

Answering this accusation, Steve Mister, President and chief executive officer of the Council for Responsible Nutrition, one of several supplement trade groups, noted in the US Congress that "making false or misleading statements about a dietary supplement in a consumer transaction violates many states' consumer protection, antifraud and unfair competition statutes." He added that he was not sure "whether the retailers in the Government Accountability Office's investigations are aware that they are breaking the law." What price honesty? Which of the two parties is legally allowed to lie?

Of the 40 herbal supplements tested for the Government Accountability Office investigation, 37 contained trace levels of at least one hazardous compound. Other analyses found contaminants that included steroids and even active pharmaceuticals. Dietary supplements are not necessarily safe.

Sensitivity to certain foods is said to be detectable using a Vega machine. This machine, it is claimed, measures the body's energy levels.[35] These levels are meant to decrease when the body comes into contact with certain foods. Holland and Barrett in the U.K. are one such company offering these tests. Hundreds of thousands of people take a food sensitivity test every year to discover if their ill health is a direct result of their diets.[36] Most walk away with a list of foods to avoid. How accurate are these food sensitivity tests? In 2003, the BBC did its own investigation to determine their accuracy.[37]

They sent an investigator from *Inside Out*, Chris Packham to three Holland and Barrett stores across the South of England.[38] He took a Vega test in Newbury, Chichester and Farnborough, only to discover that the allergy results from this test differed from store to store. In total, he was found to be sensitive to over 33 different foods, including staples like wheat, potatoes, milk, tomatoes, tea and coffee.[39] But out of the 33 products, there were only two that all three testers agreed on - cheese and chocolate! Poor Chris Packham, what allergies to have! He was also advised by Holland and Barrett staff to take a total of 20 different vitamins and minerals.[40] But again, the testers could not agree as all three testers advised different supplements. It seems that one's allergies may not be determined by food alone, but also by location.[41]

This test was repeated by sending another member of the *Inside Out* team to stores in Southampton, Brighton and Dorchester. Once again the Vega machine showed different results in different stores and this time the testers could only agree on one food product.[42] *Inside Out* put these findings to Holland and Barrett, who informed them that the tests carried out in the stores were actually conducted by another company called Health Screening UK Ltd. (HSL). Holland and Barrett also responded by saying: "In light of the issues raised, we are already carrying out a full review of the services that HSL provide."[43]

The chairman of HSL, Roy Harris admitted that the food sensitivity tests were only about 70 per cent accurate! "We have an imperfect system that works in the end because people eliminate certain things from their diet," he said.[44] "It may just be the discipline of sitting down with somebody and agreeing to cut out the nasty things in their diet."[45]

If this is the case, what use is the Vega machine?

Quality of supplements

The production of modern pharmaceuticals is strictly regulated to ensure that medicines contain a standardised quantity of active ingredients and are free from contamination.[46] Alternative medicine products are not subject to the same governmental quality control. Standards and consistency between doses can vary. This lack of oversight means that alternative health products are vulnerable to adulteration and contamination.[47]

"Nutritional supplements" are among the most profitable of all scams. An editorial on Food makers and Supplements in *Scientific American*[48] stated that food makers should have to prove the validity of their claims. Sales of so-called "functional foods", those that manufacturers have modified to provide supposed health benefits, generated $31 billion in the USA in 2008, a 14 per cent increase over 2006; according to a market research firm, Packaged Facts.

Science does not support the health claims made by the manufacturers of many of these products and the US government, for example, does not endorse them. Many of the products are nutritionally bereft and they may also give consumers a false sense of security that discourages them from taking more effective measures to maintain health. Forty per cent of people think that herbal remedies are safe because they are said to be "natural"[49] but herbal remedies may be medicines and, as with any other medicine, if they are used, they should be used with care. Herbal remedies or herbal medicines are made up of plants, trees and fungi which, in certain circumstances may be poisonous to humans.

The Traditional Herbal Registration (THR) certification mark is a type of trade mark indicating that a herbal medicine has been registered with the MHRA under the Traditional Herbal Registration (THR) Scheme and meets the required standards relating to its quality, safety, evidence of traditional use and other criteria.[50, 51]

With the increase in information on the internet, people are increasingly going online to check their symptoms and research possible treatments.[52] There is a higher risk of buying a poor-quality herbal remedy when buying over the internet especially if the remedy does not have a THR certification mark.[53] It may be a fake and it may be dangerous. Drugs and herbal remedies sold online may contain active ingredients, banned ingredients and toxic substances.[54] They may be copies of licensed drugs but made in unlicensed factories with no quality control. Some websites may appear to be legitimate but are fronted by bogus doctors or pharmacists.

Since 2005, the MHRA in Britain has tested 138 unlicensed "herbal" remedies sold as treatments for erectile dysfunction.[55] Of the products tested, 65 per cent[56] were found to contain prescription only medicines, such as sildenafil, tadalafil, vardenafil, or their analogues, or lignocaine. Quantities varied widely and in some cases amounted to what would be regarded as toxic overdose levels of prescription medicines.

The MHRA warned that traditional Chinese medicine (TCM) shops had been found to have in stock a "herbal" product containing undeclared pharmaceuticals at four times the level found in legally prescribed medicine.[57]

The product, called Jia Yi Jian and manufactured by HU NAN AIMIN Pharmaceutical Ltd, claimed to contain only herbal ingredients but on laboratory analysis was revealed to contain dangerously high levels of Tadalafil and Sibutramine. In one particular case, the product was seized by an MHRA Enforcement investigator during an inspection of a TCM shop where it was being advertised as "Herbal Viagra". The undeclared ingredients in this product, particularly to the dangerously high dosage levels identified, could cause many side effects including serious effects on the heart and blood pressure and also may interact with other prescription drugs (such as those for high blood pressure or heart disease and certain antidepressants). When purchased and taken in an uncontrolled way, as is the case with TCM shops selling Jia Yi Jian, this presents a significant risk to the health of the unsuspecting patient/consumer. The MHRA advised anyone using this product to stop taking it and to consult their healthcare professional immediately with the details contained in this notification.[58]

One man collapsed after consuming a herbal product called Tian Li, which claimed to provide sexual enhancement.[59] He was also taking Viagra on prescription. Whilst no permanent ill health was suffered the product when analysed showed both hydroxyhomosildenafil and tadalafil to be present. These are both prescription only ingredients. They can interfere with heart medication and can be fatal for some people.[60] Many of these "medicines" originate in the Far East. In 2010, the MHRA made 378 interceptions of unlicensed erectile dysfunction drugs and seized 2,173,442 tablets! Of the products tested "many include unlicensed products that are not authorised for sale such as herbs, or that include prescription only ingredients" said Mick Deats, head of enforcement at The Medicine and Healthcare products Regulators Agency (MHRA).

The websites often feature doctors in white coats with stethoscopes around their necks but in reality the compounds are often manufactured and packaged in garages, lock ups and, often accompanied by appalling hygiene practices.[61] "In one place a man was replacing his clutch on one side of the garage and packing medicine on the other" said Mick Deats. The MHRA is responsible for tracking down and prosecuting the people behind the impressive websites and emails promising to cure all ailments.[62] At any one time they have under surveillance about 100 websites which sell into the United Kingdom. Test purchases are made and then tested in the laboratory.[63] In one investigation, from 100 test purchases, 15 never arrived, 10 resulted in identity theft or credit card details being stolen and in 15 the orders were received but with a different product to the one ordered.[64]

Sales of chondroitin and glucosamine as treatment for osteoarthritis are worth billions of dollars, but the evidence that they work has never been good. Clegg[65] and others concluded that "Glucosamine and chondroitin sulfate alone or in combination did not reduce pain effectively in the overall group of patients with osteoarthritis of the knee" but they did suggest that the combination might be effective in a subgroup of patients with moderate-to-severe knee pain. A later meta-analysis of clinical trials showed that effects of chondroitin on the symptoms of osteoarthritis is "minimal or nonexistent".[66] A Cochrane review[67] did not entirely rule out some benefit, but again the effects seemed to get smaller as the trials improved.

ConsumerLab.com[68] has reported that eight out of 20 products said to contain chondroitin failed its quality tests, with four containing between zero and eight per cent of amount stated on the label. Glucosamine shows a similar trend. It is a synthetic chemical, but it is not a licensed medicine in the United Kingdom. It is marketed as a "food supplement" and not as a drug. It is not approved for prescription on the National Health Service. Glucosamine and chondroitin have been widely sold and have increasingly been prescribed by family practitioners and rheumatologists in the last decade but have been shown to be no better than placebo at reducing joint pain.[69]

This systematic review and network meta-analysis carried out by researchers from the University of Bern, Switzerland and published in the peer-reviewed *British Medical Journal* looked at whether glucosamine and chondroitin could help with joint pain associated with osteoarthritis of the hip or knee. They included randomised controlled trials with at least 200 patients with hip or knee osteoarthritis which was treated with either glucosamine, chondroitin or both. They excluded studies that used sub-therapeutic doses (less than 800mg a day of chondroitin and less than 1,500 mg a day of glucosamine) and only included trials in which the patients did not know whether they were receiving the treatment or the placebo. The review contained 12 reports describing ten trials that met the inclusion criteria.

The researchers concluded that chondroitin, glucosamine or a combination of both, do not have a useful clinical effect in the treatment of osteoarthritis but the supplements were also not found to be harmful. The conclusions reached were in keeping with guidance from the National Institute for Health and Clinical Excellence (NICE), which does not recommend treating osteoarthritis with these supplements.

The study findings were widely reported in the British television and press. On September 16th 2010, *BBC News* announced that "Supplements for osteoarthritis do not work". "Arthritis supplements have no clinical impact" said *The Daily Telegraph* on September 17th, 2010. "Supplements to ease pain of arthritis do not work' ran *The Independent* on the same day. Nevertheless these products are still extensively prescribed and used. Despite large-scale, methodologically sound trials indicating that the symptomatic benefit of chondroitin and glucosamine are minimal or non-existent they are still used. Their use in routine clinical practice should be discouraged unless the patient is paying for the placebo effect.

On *Sky News* on the 27th January 2012 there was an item concerning the deaths of nearly 100 patients in Pakistan.[70] The illness and deaths were "due to a reaction to heart drugs" said Shahbaz Sharif, the head of the government in central Punjab province. This was not a reaction to the drugs. The locally made drugs themselves were faulty. The victims were mostly poor patients who had received free drugs from the state run Punjab Institute of Cardiology (PIC), he said. The government said another 287 people had been admitted to hospitals in Lahore, Pakistan's second largest city, after taking the drugs. Police arrested owners of three pharmaceutical companies suspected of supplying the medicine. Initial investigations showed that the drugs were sub-standard. The problem was first detected in December 2011 when contaminated drugs in at least one batch of medicine caused 23 deaths. 46,000 patients receive drugs from PIC every month and, on that basis, it was thought that the number of patients affected by sub-standard drugs may rise. Drugs made in various countries are sold all over the world. This type of incident could occur anywhere.

Counterfeit herbal or pharmaceutical medicines can be reported to the MHRA on a dedicated 24-hour hotline on 0203 080 6701 or email counterfeit@mhra.gsi,gov.uk with the reference "Stay Safe".

In March 2010 the United States Food and Drug Administration issued warning letters to 17 food and beverage manufacturers[71] concerning false or misleading health and nutrition claims on their products. The labeling for 22 of their food products violated the Federal Food, Drug, and Cosmetic Act. This was an unusually expansive crackdown for the agency. Their regulatory power over food companies had declined over the past decades due to support for the latter by Congress and the courts. The Food and Drug Administration's move, accompanied by an open letter from Commissioner Margaret Hamburg about the importance of accurate nutrition labelling, was "a significant step toward halting the exploitation of science by food marketers, but it does not go far enough in protecting consumers from deceptive marketing".

In 2006 Europe began holding food makers to rigorous scientific standards. Since then, the European Food Safety Authority has rejected, on the basis of insufficient evidence, a whopping 80 per cent of the more than 900 claims they have assessed. Among the rejects were claims about probiotic ingredients and, the extremely popular fish oil, Omega 3.

Fish Oil

Quoting *The Times* David Colquhoun[72] reported: "Fat pupils on fish oils make a mental leap", with a subtitle "Fatty acids can help children in exams and improve their behaviour in class and at home, a study suggests.". But the "study" was on only four very atypically heavy children, it had no control group, and it did not measure behaviour or examination performance, but rather a chemical in the brain.[73]

Professor Basant Puri, who led the study is head of the Lipid Neuroscience Group at Imperial College London, and MRC Clinical Sciences Centre, Hammersmith Hospital.[74] Dr Alex Richardson (Oxford), who had worked with Professor Puri, dissociated herself from this study.

Ben Goldacre wrote in *The Guardian*[75] that the entire British news media had been claiming for several years that there were trials showing that Omega 3 improved school performance and behaviour in mainstream children, despite the fact that no such trial had ever been published. He describes the story as "possibly the greatest example of scientific incompetence ever documented from a local authority."

The pill company Equazen together with Durham Council had said that they were doing a trial on children doing their GCSE year but this was not a proper trial. There was no control group and, when asked, Durham Council refused to release the detailed information one would expect from a proper piece of research. There still has never been a single controlled trial of omega 3 fish oil supplements in normal children but what were the GCSE results in Durham, for the 3,000 children signed up for their trial?

Goldacre points out that this was an area of failing schools, receiving a huge amount of input of all forms. The preceding year, with no fish oil, the number of kids getting five GCSE grades A to C had improved by 5.5 per cent. After the fish oil intervention there was only a 3.5 per cent improvement. And this is against a backdrop of a two per cent increase nationally. One could argue that this "trial" had a negative result.

Goldacre suggests that the fish oils may even have retarded the progress of the children. It's a possibility he considers we must always be alive to. He has recently pointed out that positive results of even more trials of fish oils have started appearing all over the media. Toft Hill school in, of course, Durham, had a nice write up "in the *Daily Mail*, with a picture of the smiling headmaster holding a nice big box of Equazen brand fish oil. Even the *Mirror* gave it a nice page. This stuff costs 50p a child a day (and Durham only spends 70p on school meals)."

At the time, Goldacre suggested this so-called trial in GCSE candidates was meaningless, as "there was no control group taking placebo tablets. Getting the cameras in, raising expectations, and showering lots of extra attention is bound to elicit a massive placebo benefit." It was argued by Equazen and the Durham Council that a placebo control group would be "unethical", since that would deprive some children of the benefit. This, according to Goldacre, was "absurd: we do not know if there is a benefit, that's why we needed a proper trial."

Goldacre was very concerned as there "is a genuine ethical issue at stake now: nonsense research undermines the credibility of trial research. It propagates cynicism and encourages people to believe trials are only a sham marketing exercise. People consent to take part in a trial on the grounds they will be contributing to human knowledge, not a marketing exercise. If the results of this "trial" of fish oil pills are not published in full, it will be a betrayal of the faith put in the researchers by Durham's parents and children."

A survey conducted by *Which?* showed that 45 per cent of shoppers[76] were more likely to buy a product that was claimed to be high in Omega 3 than the same food without this claim but, in fact, there are different types of Omega 3 fatty acids. Only the longer-chain ones, EPA (Eicosapentaenoic acid) and DHA (Docosahexaenoic acid) found in fish and seafood have clear health benefits. Vegetarian sources of DHA come from seaweed. Increased consumption of EPA and DHA from fish and seafood is associated with a healthier heart and circulation,[77,78] better vision, reduced inflammation (and better joint mobility) and improved brain function (most notably in the areas of mood and memory).[79]

ALA is a shorter-chain Omega 3 derived from plant sources (usually flax or canola oil). It does not have the same health benefits as EPA and DHA, but it is much cheaper.[80] Unscrupulous companies can therefore add ALA to their products and then boast "Omega 3" on the label and some do! The *Which?* survey showed that many consumers were being misled by claims about Omega 3 on food labels.[81]

Which? examined a range of foods that are promoted as containing, or being high in, Omega 3 and found that labeling on Asda's Healthy wholegrain bread made statements relating to Omega 3 that were incorrect. Asda agreed the label may be confusing to customers and said they would withdraw the bread from sale while the packaging was redesigned.[82] The difference between plant-based and oily fish-based sources of Omega 3 is all too rarely made clear on food labels. So Good Soya Essential Omega 3 drink, for example, does not make it clear that the nutrient in its product is not the type that is proven to help keep one's heart healthy.[83]

Even products with added fish oil often fail to make it clear how much you would have to consume to obtain a useful amount of Omega 3.[84] One would need to drink one and a half litres every day of Tesco's Healthy Living pomegranate juice to have a beneficial measure of Omega 3.[85] Neil Fowler, editor of *Which?* magazine, said: "Our research shows that many shoppers will snap up products that claim to be high in Omega 3.[86]

Many food manufacturers are adding Omega 3 to all sorts of foods but they do not mention that it may not be the right sort of omega 3, or enough of it, to be as beneficial as simply eating oily fish."[87] Asda claimed that four slices of their special bread provided 31.3g of Omega 3 but *Which?* tests revealed that this bread had just 0.009g of DHA/EPA per 100g, so one would have to eat just over 11 loaves a day to get a required daily amount of EPA/DHA from this product.[88]

Asda admitted a typing error with the claimed amount of Omega 3 in four slices.[89] It acknowledged that the Omega 3 in its product was from plant-based sources. New European Union (EU) laws will in the future prevent food companies from making misleading health and nutrition claims on labels, but these will not be fully implemented for several years and they do not yet contain anything specific to Omega 3.[90]

European Union (EU) Food supplements directive

The European Court decided in 2002, by means of the Food Supplements Directive, approved by EU governments, to tighten rules on the sale of natural remedies, vitamin supplements and mineral plant extracts. Only vitamins and minerals on an approved list could now be used in supplements. Restrictions on the upper limits of vitamin dose would also be imposed. This was done in an attempt to reduce the fraud perpetrated on a gullible public by the "supplements" industry but even with this ruling it remained legal to sell medicines dishonestly labeled as "supplements" without producing any evidence at all that they worked. It is illegal to sell washing machines or television sets that do not work but ineffective supplements are considered differently. One need only ensure that they do no harm.

The European directive to limit the fraud perpetrated by the nutritional supplement industry was opposed by the British Health Food Manufacturers Association (HFMA), National Association of Health Stores (NAHS) and Alliance for Natural Health (ANH).[91]

Retailers, consumer groups and celebrities such as Sir Elton John and Sir Paul McCartney joined in the opposition. The Directive aimed to standardise regulations across Europe but the group, Consumers for Health Choice (CHC) believed that the legislation would effectively ban any herbal medicinal product that had not been on the market for 30 years and would mean long established remedies being taken out of health food shops, until they had been subjected to a long, expensive testing process. The damage to the United Kingdom's £70 million a year herbal medicine industry was also a consideration!

Professor John Garrow, in his capacity as Honorary Secretary of HealthWatch, in a response letter to Lord Hunt at the Department of Health said, among other topics, that; "Concerning herbal products that have not been used in EU countries for the required 30 years we do not think that the requirements under the proposed Directive are unreasonable. The evidence of purity, safety and efficacy are certainly less stringent than those required for new prescription drugs."

David Colquhoun has said that to create a market in nutrition all that is needed is a plausible idea and a little bit of evidence. Such is "the megaphone of marketing and the influence of countless 'healthy eating' articles that these ideas, even the half-baked ones, can lodge very firmly in the national psyche."[92]

He quotes from *Natural Causes,* a book by Dan Hurley, which sets out dramatically the harm, sometimes serious harm that untested "supplements" have done to some individuals. The book, according to Colquhoun, also reveals the political lobbying in the US by the $20 billion supplement industry; "with the aim (largely successful) of undermining the Food and Drug Administration and escaping from any effective regulation of its absurd, but exceedingly profitable, claims. The supplements industry puts the Prince of Wales in the shade when it comes to subverting common sense and good science."

Colquhoun also describes how he was instrumental in the Hertfordshire Trading Standards Department shutting down a local Noni juice marketing organisation on the basis of quite extraordinarily dishonest claims the manufacturers were making, including alleged benefits in cancer. He compiled a dossier on the dishonest literature which they were distributing.[93] As a result the promotional web site they used was closed down although he said that it had reappeared, operating from the same address, but this time marketing "miracle shampoo!"

He became aware that the noni-juice was still being marketed door-to-door in his area because they had tried to recruit his son as a salesman. A booklet his son was given to aid the sales purported to give medical advice about the use of noni-juice. The booklet was written by a Dr Neil Solomon MD, PhD. Colquhoun's investigations[94] revealed that Neil Solomon gave up his United States Medical Licence in 1993, after admitting to sexual malpractices with his patients.

Morinda citrifolia[95] or Noni as it is called in Hawaii is also found by different names in Tamil Nadu, India, Barbados, Indonesia, Malaysia, Philippines, Bali, Java, Honolulu and Australasia. The green fruit, leaves, and root/rhizome were traditionally used in Polynesian cultures to treat menstrual cramps, bowel irregularities, diabetes, liver diseases, and urinary tract infections.

M. citrifolia fruit contains a number of phytochemicals,[96] but although these substances have been studied for bioactivity, current research is insufficient to conclude anything about their effects on human health.[97, 98, 99, 100, 101] These phytochemicals also exist in various other plants.

Slimming tablets

The supply of fraudulent claims for "health foods" is endless.[102] Another "plausible idea and a little bit of evidence" has lead to "slimming" medications. Thyroid hormones, with concomitant dangers, are sometimes given for this purpose. Although possibly dangerous and harmful when used in this way, the use of thyroid hormones does not even approach the extent to which fraudsters went to in relieving a Mrs Jarvis and many other clients of their money in a case brought by the North Yorkshire Country Council. John Garrow, the Emeritus Professor of Human Nutrition at the University of London described the case in a *HealthWatch* newsletter.[103]

In May 1999,[104] Mrs Jarvis in North Yorkshire received a telephone call inviting her to buy slimming tablets from the Regional Health and Diet Centre (RHDC), 12 Harley Street, London W1N 1AA. She was told that the tablets were natural and 100 per cent safe and that she would lose 15 pounds in a fortnight even though she continued to eat all her favourite high calorie foods. She was assured that when she stopped the tablets she would not put the weight back on.

She sent £93 for a six month supply (180 tablets). She received a package with only 90 tablets but with 14 pages of dietary advice. She took the tablets for six weeks but gained weight, and did not receive the remainder of the tablets she had paid for. On the 6th July 1999 she contacted the North Yorkshire Trading Standards Department, who started a prosecution of the management of the RHDC for conspiracy to defraud. On 12th July 2002 (three years after the initial complaint) in Teesside Crown Court the chief defendant was given a 12-month prison sentence after pleading guilty, and his assistant, who was given legal aid, also pleaded guilty and was given a six-month jail sentence. The slimming formula was initially hydroxy-citric acid and chromium, but later repackaged capsules containing vitamins, zinc and iron were substituted. The advertising claims had no scientific or experimental basis and the Harley Street address served merely as a post box.

There was a three-year interval between the complaint and sentencing. What had at first appeared to be a simple complaint was in fact the tip of an iceberg of a complex fraud which took time to unravel. Regional Health and Diet Centre was in fact an amalgamation of four separate companies. Three of these were set up for the primary purpose of selling bogus diet pills to members of the public with the fourth company being an associated debt collecting company. The fraud took in some 6,000 consumers and netted at least £300,000. The selling operation by Regional Health had been undertaken across the country. The main perpetrator who established the fraud, Madjide Khalik, had been a disqualified director of a previous fraudulent operation. He entered guilty pleas to the substantive charges of fraud against him and his co-accused Marcella Hynes, although initially pleading not guilty later changed this to a guilty plea on the very first day of the trial.

Professor John Garrow reported on another case this time resulting in a successful outcome for Shropshire Trading Standards officers.[105] A mail-order company which used amazing claims to market food supplements with names such as Speedslim CP-2000 and The Australian Anti-fat Miracle was prosecuted in the Shropshire Crown Court. The task of prosecuting companies which use misleading advertisements to promote their healthcare products is, according to Garrow, rather like that confronting Hercules in his attempt to slay the many-headed hydra: when one head was cut off two grew in its place.

Mail-order companies can easily be wound up if found guilty of Trading Standards offences, but another company springs up in its place to sell similar goods by similar advertisements. The Shropshire Trading Standards officers discovered various organisations trading from two premises in London under the names of Tobyward Ltd, City Trading Ltd and Quietlynn Ltd. They were using the trading names Natural Herbal Research, A.A.F. and Dialbuy.

The Australian Antifat Miracle and Speedslim were said to enable a person to lose as much weight as he or she liked within three weeks without cutting out the foods that person liked, going on a starvation diet or taking strenuous exercise.[106] An advertising leaflet explained, "its unique formula contains a special anti-fat starch blocking ingredient that works by inhibiting enzymes in your digestion thus decreasing your calorific absorption-this blocking action does not cause you unwanted health problems because the valuable vitamins, essential minerals and proteins are still freely absorbed". Speedslim was described as a "pure natural protein legume concentrate." Tobyward were applying a false trade description to several types of goods, contrary to section 1(1)(a) of the Trade descriptions Act 1968.[107]

In addition, the company, when trading as Natural Herbal Research, was making medicinal claims for foods contrary to the Food Labelling Regulations 1984. For example, Evening Primrose Oil was said, "to have far-reaching benefits for those who use it for the relief of headaches, tension, insomnia and depression." Radical Defence was promoted with the comment, "So why gamble with your health when help is at hand from a new supplement called RADICAL DEFENCE which contains the required Beta Carotene, vitamins and minerals to neutralise harmful free radicals.[108] Just one capsule per day will help safeguard your body from the potentially lethal action of free radicals and the cancer or heart disease which can follow. It is a convenient, cost-effective method of promoting for you, and your family, a long and healthy life."

In the United Kingdom it is illegal to claim that a food is capable of "preventing, treating or curing human disease" unless that food has a product licence issued under the provisions of the Medicines Act 1968.[109] After nearly two years of legal wrangling the defendants indicated that they would be pleading guilty to the charges.[110] The Judge, Michael Mander, imposed fines totalling £85,000 and ordered the defendants to pay prosecution costs of £12,245.[111] In the magistrates court Tobyward were fined a further £3,000. Passing sentence, the Judge said the false claims about the slimming tablets were "a disgraceful and cynical attempt to play on the weakness and vanity of a gullible public."[112] It remains to be seen if these fines will have any effect on the promotion of health products by misleading advertising claims. It is very doubtful.

Perhaps the worst piece of advertising I have ever seen was that of the uniquely South African sausage, the boerewors. This word is Afrikaans for "farmer's sausage" but I saw a picture of one draped in a Union Jack and advertised as "The British sausage. Uniquely Australian" and with the selling price of Australian $5.89!

The Royal Pharmaceutical Society's (RPS) Statutory Committee, in 1997, warned registered pharmacists that they would be struck off the Royal Pharmaceutical Society's roll if they associated themselves "in any way" with a remedy called Spagyrik therapy. This was after a disciplinary hearing in which the widely sold alternative medicine system by this name was described as unscientific "quackery." An account of a couple who practised this "quackery" from a registered pharmacy in rural England was reported in the British Medical Journal.[113]

Spagyrik therapy was sold by Signalysis Ltd, of Stroud, Gloucestershire. The therapy involved taking blood and urine samples. These were used for diagnosis and in the manufacture of liquid remedies. The company operated through a large national network of "practitioners", some of whom were registered medical doctors, who took samples and then administered the remedies to patients.

At a series of disciplinary hearings the company claimed that their sale of spagyrik liquids as medicinal products was lawful without a product licence because they were produced at a registered pharmacy and under the supervision of a superintending pharmacist, Mrs Jacqueline Wells. This was done "as though this meant that they were scientifically based and worked." Mrs Wells told the committee that she did not attend during the process and only worked in the pharmacy for about two hours a week. The committee found her guilty of serious professional misconduct. The spagyrik "pharmacy" did not produce or sell any other type of medicine.

The directors of Signalysis Ltd, Kenneth Spellman, a retired town planner, and Rosemary Spellman, who ran the service, were told that they were guilty of "misconduct" under [Section 80(1)(b) of] the Medicines Act. Their premises would no longer be registered as a pharmacy. Had they been pharmacists they would have been struck off the roll, the committee ruled.[114]

They had been "practising quackery from the premises of a licensed pharmacy." The company's claim to be exempt from licensing requirements under Section 10 of the Medicines Act was, said the RPS, "a mere device [because] the product being dispensed and made is quackery." The committee concluded that the "spagyrik treatment and therapy has no pharmacological basis at all. It is not supported by any clinical trials. It is not scientific. It has no credible or respectable place in scientific literature."[115]

Spagyrik therapy had been claimed to diagnose and treat all types of illness using boiled extracts of blood and urine. Described as a "system of diagnosis and treatment in one", the process involved distilling then evaporating the blood and urine sample by heating to 400 degrees Celsius. The resulting ash is moistened and studied under a powerful microscope. Mrs Spellman had been "trained to read" patterns to produce "an individualised patient-oriented diagnosis". Subsequently, the distillate ash and evaporated fraction were combined, mixed with herbs, diluted and posted back for oral administration to the patient.

Signalysis Ltd had also claimed exemption under the Medicines Act because the company employed and used medical doctors. Dr Alec Forbes, a registered medical practitioner and formerly the Medical Director of the Bristol Cancer Help Centre, was listed on stationery as the Medical Consultant of Signalysis Ltd. Mrs Spelman told the committee that she had worked at the Bristol Centre for three years before setting up her business. Advertisments for spagyrik were later published by the Centre. The committee did not further consider the position of registered doctors who prescribed spagyrik therapy or who acted as advisers to the company.

The committee conceded that Mr and Mrs Spellman had responded to criticism and altered their presentation of the therapy over the years and, although their references suggested that they were well-intentioned and compassionate people, what they had done was "reprehensible." They had also "connived" at their misconduct. They had originally claimed that "in all chronic illnesses regarded as incurable, Spagyrik is able to offer help and the alleviation of pain", and that it had a "high success rate ... in practically all illnesses of humans."

These and similar claims were dismissed as "exceptionally dangerous nonsense" by Dr Charles Shepherd, a Gloucestershire general practitioner who had provided most of the evidence which the committee considered. "If they could do any of that, they would be in line for the Nobel prize. I am very glad that the RPS shares my view on this quackery. I hope that the General Medical Council will now look at the role of registered medical practitioners in this affair." He then added the obvious that "Spagyrik was clearly being aimed at very vulnerable patients, many of whom may not have had a precise diagnosis. They were being relieved of their savings rather than their suffering."

Vitamins

Ben Goldacre states that the vitamin industry was legendary in the world of economics as the setting of the most outrageous price-fixing cartel ever documented.[116] During the 1990s the main offenders were forced to pay the largest criminal fines ever levied in legal history - $1.5 billion in total, after entering guilty pleas with the US Department of Justice and regulators in Canada, Australia and the European Union.

In the Unites States a high potency Vitamin E intravenous injection named E-Ferol, was associated with adverse reactions in about 100 premature infants, 40 of whom died., In response to this in November of 1984, a congressional oversight committee issued a report to the Food and Drug Administration expressing the committee's concern regarding the thousands of unapproved drug products in the marketplace.

A spokesman for the Health Supplements Information Service reportedly said: "People should get all the vitamins and minerals they need from their diet, but for the millions who are not able to do that, vitamins can be a useful supplement and they should not stop taking them."[117]

However, Catherine Collins, of the British Dietetic Association, said: "This study is deeply worrying and shows that there should be more regulation for vitamins and minerals. The public can buy vitamins as easily as sweets. They should be treated in the same way as Paracetamol with maximum limits on the dosage." High doses of vitamins should be regarded as drugs rather than supplements and should only be given under medical supervision. Most high-dose recommendations by the health-food industry are not valid.[118]

Arnold Bender's son, David Bender[119] followed in his father's footsteps as a nutritional biochemist at University College London. It is fitting that this chapter started with Arnold Bender and will now be followed with comments by his son. David Bender wrote a position paper on multivitamin supplements. He discussed the use of vitamin supplements in addition to a normal diet and not the pharmacological use of vitamins to treat disease.

Recommended or reference intakes of vitamins are calculated to ensure that no-one suffers from deficiency; reference intakes are derived on the basis of average requirement plus twice the standard deviation around that requirement, so are higher than the requirements of almost everyone in the population[120,121, 122,123,124,125,126]

There are difficulties with the definition of the word requirement. The United States usage differs from that used by the World Health Organisation but the important questions are whether levels of intake higher than current reference intakes may provide health benefits, and whether higher intakes are safe.[127]

Vitamins A, D, B6 and niacin are all known to be toxic in excess.[128,129]

The UK report on Dietary Reference Intakes[130] gave "guidance on higher intakes" while the US/Canadian reports[131,132,133,134] give "tolerable upper levels of intake" derived from the highest level of intake at which there is no adverse recommended level, and there is no established benefit for healthy individuals consuming more than the recommended daily allowance.[135]

In the UK, the Foods Standards Agency set up an Expert Group on Vitamins and Minerals[136] "to establish principles on which controls for ensuring the safety of vitamin and mineral supplements sold under food law can be based; to review the levels of individual vitamins and minerals associated with adverse effects; and to recommend maximum levels of intakes of vitamins and minerals from supplements if appropriate". This "Expert Group" published a series of working documents evaluating the evidence of safety or hazard.[137]

In similar vein the European Federation of Health Food Manufacturers published upper limits of vitamins and minerals for use in over-the-counter supplement[138] and, although these are voluntary, responsible manufacturers are likely to abide by them.

Are there benefits to be derived from higher levels of intake of vitamins? A review in 2002 found little convincing evidence in favour of supplements.[139]

Vitamin E and beta-carotene

David Bender states that there is clear epidemiological evidence that people with a high plasma concentration of vitamin E are less at risk from cardiovascular disease.[140]

The Cambridge Heart Antioxidant Study[141] found a reduction in non-fatal, but not in fatal, myocardial infarctions but this is hardly convincing evidence of the benefits of vitamin E supplements. Other large intervention trials have found no beneficial effect of vitamin E in coronary heart disease.[142,143,144] In the alpha-tocopherol beta-carotene study,[145] there was a lower incidence of, and mortality from, prostate cancer in those people taking a vitamin E supplement[146] but there is no clear evidence from other intervention trials that vitamin E reduces cancer risk.

There is evidence that high intakes of beta-carotene are associated with a lower incidence of lung, prostate and other cancers, but beta-carotene may simply be a marker of fruit and vegetable consumption. Supplements of beta-carotene, vitamin E and selenium to a marginally malnourished population in China,[147] however, led to a reduction in mortality from a variety of cancers, especially gastric cancer.

On the other hand, the results of two major intervention studies with beta-carotene, one in Finland among smokers[148] and the other in the USA among people who had been exposed to asbestos,[149] both yielded unexpected, and unwelcome, results. More people receiving supposedly protective beta-carotene supplements died from lung cancer than those receiving placebo in a major intervention trial of smokers in Finland. The US Physicians' Health Study[150] was a 12-year trial of beta-carotene supplements which found no effect on the incidence of cardiovascular disease or cancer. The results of both these trials were unexpected. Both vitamin E and carotene are antioxidants and might be expected to reduce the damage caused by the action of free radicals.[151] It is this damage that leads to the development of both cancer and cardiovascular disease.

Vitamin C

Vitamin C is an antioxidant, and it might therefore be expected to give some protection against the development of cancer and cardiovascular disease. The epidemiological evidence of a protective effect of vitamin C against cancer may be a result of the fact that fruits and vegetables that are sources of vitamin C are also rich in a variety of other compounds that may be protective.[152]

Vitamin C deficiency is associated with an increased risk of atherosclerosis,[153] but there is little evidence of protective effects on the incidence of strokes or coronary heart disease at intakes greater than needed to meet daily requirements[154, 155] High doses of vitamin C are popularly recommended for the prevention and treatment of the common cold.[156]

This originated from the work of Linus Pauling, the only person awarded two unshared Nobel prizes and one of only four persons to win more than one Nobel prize. He won the Nobel prize in chemistry in 1954 for 'his research into the nature of the chemical bond and its application to the elucidation of the structure of complex substances." His second prize was the Nobel peace prize in 1962. He must have known something as he lived to the age of 93. He is, however, more widely and unfortunately, known more for his work on Vitamin C. The "great grandfather of modern nutritionism," as Pauling became known, "cherry-picked" the literature for his work on vitamin C and the common cold[157] quoting only the studies that agreed with his thinking. Paul Knipschild, Professor of Epidemiology at the University of Maastricht, published a chapter in *Systematic Reviews* in 1993.[158]

He investigated the literature as it was when Pauling did his work and Knipschild subjected this literature to rigorous systematic review as is now current practice.[159] He found that while some trials did suggest that vitamin C had some benefits, Pauling had selectively quoted from the literature to prove his point.[160] He had "cherry picked"! In Pauling's defence, he worked at a time when people knew no better, and he was probably quite unaware of what he was doing.[161] Cherry-picking is one of the most common dubious practices in alternative therapies, and particularly in nutritionism.[162]

The evidence from controlled trials that vitamin C is of benefit in the prevention or treatment of colds is unconvincing [163,164] and Hemila in 1992[165] concluded that there was no evidence that Vitamin C lowered the incidence of colds. He did, however, find consistent evidence of a beneficial effect in reducing the severity and duration of symptoms. A systematic review[166] similarly concluded that there was no beneficial effect in terms of preventing infection, but a modest benefit in terms of reducing the duration of symptoms.

Vitamin D

Vitamin D and calcium delay the loss of bone with increasing age. Supplements may be advisable to prevent osteoporosis and osteomalacia.[167] For most people increased sunlight exposure is probably more effective than supplements.

Folic acid

The benefits of folic acid supplements taken periconceptually in preventing neural tube defects in the fetus have been demonstrated convincingly.[168] In the USA and elsewhere cereal products are fortified with folic acid.

David Bender concluded that daily supplements apart from folic acid taken periconceptually and possibly vitamin D for the elderly are probably of no use for adults.[169] For children, supplements of vitamins A and D are desirable. It worried him that multivitamin tablets are promoted as an aid to "optimum nutrition" or to make good a diet that is inadequate.[170]
He considered that it was not possible to show that supplements promoted optimum nutrition if the diet is already adequate by WHO standards. If the diet was not adequate or if health risks were increased by other factors (e.g. smoking or obesity) then taking a multivitamin tablet was unlikely to help. It was even more hazardous to take a cocktail containing many nutritional supplements "to be on the safe side".[171]
Overloading with one nutrient (e.g. a particular amino acid, vitamin or mineral) might cause disorders of metabolism of other amino acids vitamins or minerals. Human beings evolved on a diet of mixed animal and plant foods in which the balance of nutrients is about right; to alter that balance markedly is, according to Bender, not "to be on the safe side".[172]
Physicians, pharmacists and the news media should not fall victim to the fad for vitamin supplements. Doctors were not immune to being swayed by fashion. Pharmacists tended to depend on vitamin supplements for a considerable proportion of their profit. Newspapers and magazines tended to abandon journalistic scepticism when it came to articles on health. It was incumbent, he said, on all these groups to recognise that their actions in respect of vitamin supplements can be tantamount to the promotion of quackery.

Vitamins and Mortality

Although most vitamin supplements are not associated with a higher risk of death, multivitamins, vitamin B_6, and folic acid, as well as minerals such as iron, magnesium, zinc, and copper are.[173] Vitamin B_6, folic acid, iron, magnesium, and zinc were associated with about a three to six per cent increased risk for death, whereas copper was associated with an 18 per cent increased risk for total mortality when compared with corresponding non-use. In contrast, the use of calcium was inversely related to risk for death.
Known as the Iowa Women's Health Study, the authors found that 66 per cent of women investigated used at least one dietary supplement at baseline in 1986. More than 38,000 women who were, on average, age 62, were followed for up to 22 years. There were more than 15,000 deaths during the follow-up period. The study showed very few benefits of any of these vitamin or mineral

supplements. Most of the supplements studied were not associated with a reduced total mortality rate in older women.[174]

In contrast, they found that several commonly used dietary vitamin and mineral supplements, including multivitamins, vitamins B_6, and folic acid, as well as minerals iron, magnesium, zinc, and copper, were associated with a higher risk of total mortality.

The study also showed that older women who used dietary supplements were more likely to be active, non-smokers, have a lower body mass index (BMI), and were less likely to have diabetes or high blood pressure. In addition, they had higher education, and were more likely to use estrogen replacement therapy!

Why are we so gullible?

"Doubt is our product," a cigarette executive once observed,[175] "since it is the best means of competing with the 'body of fact' that exists in the minds of the general public. It is also the means of establishing a controversy." In the book of the same title, David Michaels reveals how the tobacco industry's duplicitous tactics have spawned a multimillion dollar industry. He shows how consultants in various industries, and this would include the pharmaceutical companies, have increasingly "skewed the scientific literature, manufactured and magnified scientific uncertainty and influenced policy decisions to the industry's advantage."[176]

To keep the public confused about the hazards posed by global warming, second-hand smoke, asbestos, lead, plastics, and many other toxic materials, industry executives have hired unscrupulous scientists and lobbyists to dispute scientific evidence about health risks.[177] By these actions these scientists and lobbyists have delayed action on specific hazards and they have also constructed barriers making it more difficult for lawmakers, government agencies, and courts to respond to future threats. All in the interests of profit.

These underhand methods aim to create confusion about the nature of scientific inquiry and undermine the public's confidence in science's ability and the truth. Michaels considers the regulatory system in the USA to be broken but he offers concrete, workable suggestions for how it can be restored by taking the politics out of science and ensuring that concern for public safety, rather than private profits, becomes the guiding policy.[178]

A fool and his money are easily parted but some of these victims are not fools. Some are extremely intelligent. Others are desperate ...

References:

1. A. Bender. Health or Hoax: The Truth About Health Foods and Diets." Elvendon Press, 1985.
2. "Nutritionist calls for tighter regulation of supplements". CNN. http://www.cnn.com/HEALTH/alternative/9909/17/supplement.drug.journal/index.html. Retrieved 2010-04-23.
3. American Academy of Pediatrics Committee on Nutrition. Vitamin and mineral supplement needs of normal children in the United States. Pediatrics 66:1015-1020, 1980.

4. U.S Preventive Services Task Force. Folic acid to prevent neural tube defects. USPSTF Web site, May 2009. FPM Documents with MESH term: Medical History Taking - Family .., http://www.aafp.org/fpm/viewRelatedDocumentsByMesh.htm?meshId=D008487&page=9 (accessed July 22, 2013).

5. Barrett S. Antioxidants and other phytochemicals: Current scientific perspective. Quackwatch. Jan 22, 2010.

6. Renner JH. Interview in Jenkin D. Dietary supplements: Cure or curse. The Oakland Press, Jan 10, 1999. HealthWatch Newsletter no 21, http://www.healthwatch-uk.org/newsletters/nlett21.html (accessed July 22, 2013).

7. HealthWatch Newsletter no 21, http://www.healthwatch-uk.org/newsletters/nlett21.html (accessed July22, 2013).

8. HealthWatch. You too can be a nutritionist ... for £215. Newsletter no 21: April 1996.
HealthWatch Newsletter no 21, http://www.healthwatch-uk.org/newsletters/nlett21.html (accessed July 22, 2013).

9. HealthWatch Newsletter no 21, http://www.healthwatch-uk.org/newsletters/nlett21.html (accessed July 22, 2013).

10. Ibid.
11. Ibid.
12. Ibid.
13. Ibid.
14. Ibid.
15. Ibid.
16. Ibid.
17. Ibid.
18. Ibid.
19. Ibid.
20. Ibid.
21. Ibid.
22. Ibid.
23. Ibid.

24. Ben Goldacre. Doctored information on celebrity nutritionist | Science | The Guardian. www.guardian.co.uk/science/2007/jan/.../badscience.wikipedi...

25. Ben Goldacre. "Bad Science". Fourth Estate. London. 2009. p 163.

26. Ransley J, Donnelly J et al. Food and Nutritional Supplements: their Role in Health and Disease. Berlin: Heidelberg; New York: Springer-Verlag, 2001.

27. Katherine Harmon. Worts and All.
False claims still pervade the supplements industry. Medicine & Health. www.ScientificAmerlcan.com or editors@SciAm.com. August 2010.

28. Saw palmetto for benign prostatic hyperplasia, http://www.ncbi.nlm.nih.gov/pubmed/16467543 (accessed July 22, 2013).

29. Stephen Bent, M.D., Christopher Kane, M.D., Katsuto Shinohara, M.D., John Neuhaus, Ph.D., Esther S. Hudes, Ph.D., M.P.H., Harley Goldberg, D.O., and Andrew L. Avins, M.D., M.P.H. "Saw Palmetto for Benign Prostatic Hyperplasia". New England Journal of Medicine. February 9th 2006. 354, p 557 – 566. Saw palmetto for benign prostatic hyperplasia, http://www.ncbi.nlm.nih.gov/pubmed/16467543 (accessed July 22, 2013).

30. Beth E. Snitz, Ellen S. O'Meara, Michelle C. Carlson, Alice M. Arnold, Diane G. Ives, Stephen R. Rapp, Judith Saxton, Oscar L. Lopez, Leslie O. Dunn, Kaycee M.

Sink, Steven T. DeKosky. Ginkgo biloba for Preventing Cognitive Decline in Older Adults JAMA. 2009;302(24):2663-2670.
31. Paul G. Shekelle, Margaret Maglione, and Sally C. Morton. RAND Review: Spring 2003: Preponderance of Evidence: Judging What to Do About Ephedra
32. Ibid.
33. Katherine Harmon. worts and all.False claims still pervade the supplements industry. Medicine & health. www.ScientificAmerlcan.com or editors@SciAm.com. August 2010.
34. High blood pressure | Define High blood pressure at .., http://dictionary.reference.com/browse/high+blood+pressure?s=t (accessed July 22, 2013).
35. BBC Inside Out - Food Sensitivity, http://www.bbc.co.uk/insideout/south/series2/food_sensitivity_allergy_vega_tests.shtml (accessed July 22, 2013).
36. Ibid.
37. BBC 1 page. Inside Out - South: Monday 17th February, 2003.
38. BBC Inside Out - Food Sensitivity, http://www.bbc.co.uk/insideout/south/series2/food_sensitivity_allergy_vega_tests.shtml (accessed July 22, 2013).
39. Ibid.
40. Ibid.
41. Ibid.
42. Ibid.
43. Ibid.
44. Ibid.
45. Ibid.
46. Regulation of alternative medicine - Wikipedia, the free .., http://en.wikipedia.org/wiki/Regulation_of_alternative_medicine (accessed July 22, 2013).
47. Agin, Dan (2006-10-03). Junk Science: how politicians, corporations, and other hucksters betray us. Thomas Dunne Books. pp. Ch. 8. ISBN 978-0-312-35241-7. Regulation of alternative medicine - Wikipedia, the free .., http://en.wikipedia.org/wiki/Regulation_of_alternative_medicine (accessed July 22, 2013).
48. Snake Oil in the Supermarket. Perspectives. Editorial comment. editors@SciAm.com. September 2010.
49. MHRA. Herbal medicines. Advice for consumers. Ipsos MORI / MHRA, 2008.
50. Search results: MHRA - Medicines and Healthcare products .., http://www.mhra.gov.uk/SearchHelp/Search/Searchresults/index.htm?within=Yes&Query (accessed July 22, 2013).
51. How to register your product under the Traditional Herbal .., http://www.mhra.gov.uk/Howweregulate/Medicines/Herbalmedicinesregulation/RegisteredTraditionalHerbalMedicines/HowtoregisteryourproductundertheTraditionalHerbalMedicinesRegistrationScheme/Traditionaluse/index.htm (accessed July 22, 2013).
52. Risks of buying herbal remedies online: MHRA, http://www.mhra.gov.uk/Safetyinformation/Generalsafetyinformationandadvice/Herbalmedicines/Staysafeusingnaturalremedies/Risksofbuyingherbalremediesonline/index.htm (accessed July 22, 2013).
53. Ibid.
54. Ibid.

55. Ibid.
56. MHRA. Advice to consumers - safe use of herbal medicines. Herbal sexual dysfunction products warnings and alerts. Unlicensed Traditional Chinese Medicine (TCM) product found with dangerously high levels of undeclared prescription pharmaceuticals. Risks of buying herbal remedies online: MHRA, http://www.mhra.gov.uk/Safetyinformation/Generalsafetyinformationandadvice/Herbalmedicines/Staysafeusingnaturalremedies/Risksofbuyingherbalremediesonline/index.htm (accessed July 22, 2013).
57. Herbal sexual dysfunction products warnings and alerts: MHRA, http://www.mhra.gov.uk/Safetyinformation/Generalsafetyinformationandadvice/Herbalmedicines/Herbalsafetyupdates/Herbalerectilesexualdysfunctionproductswarningsandalerts/index.htm (accessed July 22, 2013).
58. MHRA. Herbal sexual dysfunction products warnings and alerts: www.mhra.gov.uk/.../...
59. Risks of buying herbal remedies online: MHRA, http://www.mhra.gov.uk/Safetyinformation/Generalsafetyinformationandadvice/Herbalmedicines/Staysafeusingnaturalremedies/Risksofbuyingherbalremediesonline/index.htm (accessed July 22, 2013).
60. Ibid.
61. Ibid.
62. Ibid.
63. Ibid.
64. Ibid.
65. Clegg DO, Reda DJ, Harris CL, Klein MA, O'Dell JR, Hooper MM, Bradley JD, Bingham CO 3rd, Weisman MH, Jackson CG, Lane NE, Cush JJ, Moreland LW, Schumacher HR Jr, Oddis CV, Wolfe F, Molitor JA, Yocum DE, Schnitzer TJ, Furst DE, Sawitzke AD, Shi H, Brandt KD, Moskowitz RW, Williams HJ. Glucosamine, chondroitin sulfate, and the two in combination for painful knee osteoarthritis. N Engl J Med. 2006 Feb 23;354(8):795-808. (ClinicalTrials.gov number, NCT00032890.)
66. Reichenbach S and others. Meta-analysis: Chondroitin for osteoarthritis of the knee or hip. Annals of Internal Medicine 146:580-590, 2007.
67. Towheed T, Maxwell L, Anastassiades TP, Shea B, Houpt J, Welch V, Hochberg MC, Wells GA. summaries.cochrane.org/CD002946 . Published Online: 7 Oct 2009.
68. ConsumerLab.comProduct Review: Joint Health Supplements with Glucosamine, Chondroitin, and/or MSM. Contamination and Mislabeling Discovered in Over 20% of Arthritis Supplements Selected for Review. Initial Posting: 7/6/09, Updated: 9/22/11.
69. Wandel S, Jüni P, Tendal B et al. Effects of glucosamine, chondroitin, or placebo in patients with osteoarthritis of hip or knee: network meta-analysis. BMJ 2010; 341:c46.
70. Sky News: Faulty drug toll nears 100 in Pakistan. www.skynews.co.nz/world/article .aspx?id=711793&vId= - Cached .
71. FDA Press release. FDA Calls on Food Companies to Correct Labeling Violations; FDA Commissioner Issues an Open Letter to the Industry. www.fda.gov/newsevents/newsroom/.../ucm202814.htm. 3 Mar 2010
72. David Colquhoun's Improbable Science page.dcscience.net/improbable.html - 12th Sep 2007.
The quack page - UCL - London's Global University, http://www.ucl.ac.uk/pharmacology/dc-bits-old/quack-01-06-07.html (accessed July 22, 2013).

73. Ibid.
74. Ibid.
75. Ben Goldacre. Omega-3 and the GCSE year trial? It still smells fishy ...The Guardian Saturday September 22nd 2007. www.guardian.co.uk/science/2007/sep/22/1
76. Which? magazine. "Omega 3 claims confusing shoppers."25 Oct 2007.
77. Fatty fish consumption and ischemic heart disease mortality in older adults: The cardiovascular heart study. Presented at the American Heart Association's 41st annual conference on cardiovascular disease epidemiology and prevention. AHA. 2001.
78. Harper CR, Jacobson TA. The fats of life: the role of omega-3 fatty acids in the prevention of coronary heart disease. Arch Intern Med. 2001;161(18):2185-2192.Food and Behaviour Research: 25 Oct 2007 - Which magazine .., http://www.fabresearch.org/1389 (accessed July 22, 2013).
79. Food and Behaviour Research: 25 Oct 2007 - Which magazine .., http://www.fabresearch.org/1389 (accessed July 22, 2013).
80. Ibid.
81. Ibid.
82. Ibid.
83. Ibid.
84. Ibid.
85. Ibid.
86. Ibid.
87. Ibid.
88. Ibid.
89. Ibid.
90. Ibid.
91. HealthWatch for treatment that works.
Registered charity. Newsletter no 47: October 2002. The quack page - UCL - London's Global University, http://www.ucl.ac.uk/pharmacology/dc-bits-old/quack-01-06-07.html (accessed July 22, 2013).
92. David Colquhoun. DC's Improbable Science page. http://dcscience.net/.
93. The quack page - UCL - London's Global University, http://www.ucl.ac.uk/pharmacology/dc-bits-old/quack-01-06-07.html (accessed July 22, 2013).
94. DC's IMPROBABLE SCIENCE page. http://dcscience.net/.
95. ^ Wang MY, West BJ, Jensen CJ, Nowicki D, Su C, Palu AK, Anderson G (2002). "Morinda citrifolia (Noni): a literature review and recent advances in Noni research". Pharmacol Sin 23 (12): 1127–41. PMID 12466051. Morinda citrifolia - Wikipedia, the free encyclopedia, http://en.wikipedia.org/wiki/Vomit_fruit (accessed July 22, 2013).
96. Morinda citrifolia - Wikipedia, the free encyclopedia, http://en.wikipedia.org/wiki/Vomit_fruit (accessed July 22, 2013).
97. ^ Saleem, Muhammad; Kim, Hyoung Ja; Ali, Muhammad Shaiq; Lee, Yong Sup (2005). "An update on bioactive plant lignans". Natural Product Reports 22 (6): 696. doi:10.1039/b514045p. PMID 16311631.
98. ^ Deng, Shixin; Palu, 'Afa K.; West, Brett J.; Su, Chen X.; Zhou, Bing-Nan; Jensen, Jarakae C. (2007). "Lipoxygenase Inhibitory Constituents of the Fruits of Noni (Morindacitrifolia) Collected in Tahiti". Journal of Natural Products 70 (5): 859–62. doi:10.1021/np0605539. PMID 17378609.
99. ^ Lin, Chwan Fwu; Ni, Ching Li; Huang, Yu Ling; Sheu, Shuenn Jyi; Chen, Chien Chih (2007). "Lignans and anthraquinones from the fruits ofMorinda

citrifolia". Natural Product Research 21 (13): 1199–204. doi:10.1080/14786410601132451. PMID 17987501.
100. ^ Levand, Oscar; Larson, Harold (2009). "Some Chemical Constituents of Morinda citrifolia". Planta Medica 36 (06): 186–7. doi:10.1055/s-0028-1097264. Morinda citrifolia - Wikipedia, the free encyclopedia, http://en.wikipedia.org/wiki/Vomit_fruit (accessed July 22, 2013).
101. ^ Mohd Zin, Z.; Abdul Hamid, A.; Osman, A.; Saari, N.; Misran, A. (2007). "Isolation and Identification of Antioxidative Compound from Fruit of Mengkudu (Morinda citrifoliaL.)". International Journal of Food Properties 10 (2): 363–73. doi:10.1080/10942910601052723.
102. The quack page - UCL - London's Global University, http://www.ucl.ac.uk/pharmacology/dc-bits-old/quack-01-06-07.html (accessed July 22, 2013).
103. HealthWatch Newsletter no 21, http://www.healthwatch-uk.org/newsletters/nlett21.html (accessed July 22, 2013).
104. John Garrow. Trading Standards. Food fraud, and the law's delay. HealthWatch. Registered charity. Newsletter no 47: October 2002.
105. John Garrow "Miracle" slimming pill company prosecuted. HealthWatch. Newsletter no 21: HealthWatch Newsletter no 21, http://www.healthwatch-uk.org/newsletters/nlett21.html (accessed July 22, 2013).
106. HealthWatch Newsletter no 21, http://www.healthwatch-uk.org/newsletters/nlett21.html (accessed July 22, 2013).
107. Ibid.
108. Ibid.
109. Ibid.
110. Ibid.
111. Ibid.
112. Ibid.
113. Reported by Duncan Campbell from the BMJ 13th Sept. 1997. 315 7 109.
114. HealthWatch Newsletter no 27, http://www.healthwatch-uk.org/newsletters/nlett27.html (accessed July 22, 2013).
115. Ibid.
116. Global Pricefixing: Our Customers Are the Enemy. Springer (2001). John M Connor. The Nonsense du Jour for [Ben Goldacre] Bad Science, http://www.scribd.com/doc/145552156/6/The-Nonsense-du-Jour (accessed July 22, 2013). 117. T h e L i b e r t a r i a n: Vitamins Will Kill You, Have .., http://2164th.blogspot.com/2008/04/vitamins-will-kill-you-have-apple.html (accessed July 22, 2013).
118. Barrett S, Herbert V. The Vitamin Pushers: How the "Health Food" Industry Is Selling Americans a Bill of Goods. Amherst, NY: Prometheus Books, 1994.
119. David Bender. Position paper on multi-vitamin supplements. HealthWatch. Newsletter no. 47: October 2002. This review is an expanded version of David Bender's editorial published in the British Medical Journal in July 2002
120. Department of Health Dietary Reference Values for Food Energy and Nutrients for the United Kingdom. London: Her Majesty's Stationery Office, 1991.
121. Scientific Committee for Food Nutrient and Energy Intakes for the European Community. Luxemburg: Commission of the European Communities, 1993.
122. Institute of Medicine Dietary Reference Intakes for Calcium, Phosphorus, Magnesium, Vitamin D and Fluoride. Washington DC: National Academy Press, 1997.

123. Institute of Medicine Dietary Reference Values for Thiamin, Riboflavin, Niacin, Vitamin B6, Folate, Vitamin B12, Pantothenic Acid, Biotin and Choline. Washington DC: National Academy Press, 1998.
124. Institute of Medicine. Dietary Reference Values for Vitamin C, Vitamin E, Selenium and Carotenoids. Washington DC: National Academy Press, 2000. HealthWatch Newsletter no 21, http://www.healthwatch-uk.org/newsletters/nlett21.html (accessed July 22, 2013).
125. Institute of Medicine. Dietary Reference Intakes for Vitamin A, Vitamin K, Arsenic, Boron, Chromium, Copper, Iodine, Iron, Manganese, Molybdenum, Nickel, Silicon, Vanadium and Zinc. Washington DC: National Academy Press, 2001. FAO/WHO. Human Vitamin and Mineral Requirements: Report of a joint FAO/WHO expert consultation, Bankok, Thailand. Rome: Food and Nutrition Division of the United Nations Food and Agriculture Organization, 2001.
126. FAO/WHO. Human Vitamin and Mineral Requirements: Report of a joint FAO/WHO expert consultation, Bangkok, Thailand. Rome: Food and Nutrition Division of the United Nations Food and Agriculture Organization, 2001. Position paper: Multi-vitamin supplements, http://www.healthwatch-uk.org/Vitamin%20supplements.pdf (accessed July 22, 2013).
127. Position paper: Multi-vitamin supplements, http://www.healthwatch-uk.org/Vitamin%20supplements.pdf (accessed July 22, 2013).
128. Chesney RW. Requirements and upper limits of vitamin D intake in the term neonate, infant, and older child. Journal of Pediatrics 1990; 116: 159–66.
129. Holick MF. The use and interpretation of assays for vitamin D and its metabolites. Journal of Nutrition 1990; 120 (Suppl 11): 1464–9. Position paper: Multi-vitamin supplements, http://www.healthwatch-uk.org/Vitamin%20supplements.pdf (accessed July 22, 2013).
130. Department of Health Dietary Reference Values for Food Energy and Nutrients for the United Kingdom. London: Her Majesty's Stationery Office, 1991.
131. Institute of Medicine Dietary Reference Intakes for Calcium, Phosphorus, Magnesium, Vitamin D and Fluoride. Washington DC: National Academy Press, 1997.
132. Institute of Medicine Dietary Reference Values for Thiamin, Riboflavin, Niacin, Vitamin B6, Folate, Vitamin B12, Pantothenic Acid, Biotin and Choline. Washington DC: National Academy Press, 1998.
133. Institute of Medicine. Dietary Reference Values for Vitamin C, Vitamin E, Selenium and Carotenoids. Washington DC: National Academy Press, 2000.
134. Institute of Medicine. Dietary Reference Intakes for Vitamin A, Vitamin K, Arsenic, Boron, Chromium, Copper, Iodine, Iron, Manganese, Molybdenum, Nickel, Silicon, Vanadium and Zinc. Washington DC: National Academy Press, 2001 Position paper: Multi-vitamin supplements, http://www.healthwatch-uk.org/Vitamin%20supplements.pdf (accessed July 22, 2013).
135. Institute of Medicine Dietary Reference Intakes for Calcium, Phosphorus, Magnesium, Vitamin D and Fluoride. Washington DC: National Academy Press, 1997.
136. EXPERT GROUP ON VITAMINS AND MINERALS PAPER FOR DISCUSSION .., http://archive.food.gov.uk/dept_health/pdf/evmpdf/evm11fin.pdf (accessed July 22, 2013).
137. Expert Group on Vitamins and Minerals. http://www.foodstandards.gov.uk/science/ouradvisors/vitandmin/
138. Shrimpton D. Vitamins and Minerals: A Scientific Evaluation of the Range of Safe Intakes. Thames Ditton Surrey, Brussels: European Federation of Health Product

Manufacturers Associations, 1997. Position paper: Multi-vitamin supplements, http://www.healthwatch-uk.org/Vitamin%20supplements.pdf (accessed July 22, 2013). Position paper: Multi-vitamin supplements, http://www.healthwatch-uk.org/Vitamin%20supplements.pdf (accessed July 22, 2013).

139. Fairfield KM & Fletcher RH. Vitamins for chronic disease prevention in adults: scientific review. Journal of the American Medical Association 2002; 287: 3116–26.

140. Gey KF. Cardiovascular disease and vitamins. Concurrent correction of 'suboptimal' plasma antioxidant levels may, as important part of 'optimal' nutrition, help to prevent early stages of cardiovascular disease and cancer, respectively. Biblio Nutritio et Dieta 1995; 52: 75–91. Position paper: Multi-vitamin supplements, http://www.healthwatch-uk.org/Vitamin%20supplements.pdf (accessed July 22, 2013).

141. Stephens NG, Parsons A et al. Randomised controlled trial of vitamin E in patients with coronary disease: Cambridge Heart Antioxidant Study (CHAOS). Lancet 1996; 347: 781–6.

142. Meydani M. Vitamin E and prevention of heart disease in high-risk patients. Nutrition Reviews 2000; 58: 278–81.

143. Kaul N, Devaraj S et al. Alpha-tocopherol and atherosclerosis. Experimental Biology and Medicine (Maywood) 2001; 226: 5–12.

144. Pruthi S, Allison TG et al. Vitamin E supplementation in the prevention of coronary heart disease. Mayo Clinic Proceedings 2001; 76: 1131–6.

145. Alpha-Tocopherol Beta-Carotene Cancer Prevention Study Group. The effect of vitamin E and beta carotene on the incidence of lung and other cancers in male smokers. New England Journal of Medicine 1994; 330: 1029–35.

146. Heinonen OP, Albanes D et al. Prostate cancer and supplementation with alpha-tocopherol and beta-carotene: incidence and mortality in a controlled trial. Journal of the National Cancer Institute 1998; 90: 440–6. Position paper: Multi-vitamin supplements, http://www.healthwatch-uk.org/Vitamin%20supplements.pdf (accessed July 22, 2013).

147. Blot WJ, Li JY et al. Nutrition intervention trials in Linxian, China: supplementation with specific vitamin/mineral combinations, cancer incidence, and disease-specific mortality in the general population. Journal of the National Cancer Institute 1993; 85: 1483–92.

148. Alpha-Tocopherol Beta-Carotene Cancer Prevention Study Group. The effect of vitamin E and beta carotene on the incidence of lung and other cancers in male smokers. New England Journal of Medicine 1994; 330: 1029–35.

149. Omenn GS, Goodman BE, et al. Effects of a combination of beta carotene and vitamin A on lung cancer and cardiovascular disease. New England Journal of Medicine 1996; 334: 1150–5.

150. Hennekens CH, Buring JE, et al. Lack of effect of long-term supplementation with beta carotene on the incidence of malignant neoplasms and cardiovascular disease. New England Journal of Medicine 1996; 334: 1145–9. Position paper: Multi-vitamin supplements, http://www.healthwatch-uk.org/Vitamin%20supplements.pdf (accessed July 22, 2013).

151. Position paper: Multi-vitamin supplements, http://www.healthwatch-uk.org/Vitamin%20supplements.pdf (accessed July 22, 2013).

152. Ibid.

153. Ibid.

154. Jacob RA. Vitamin C nutriture and risk of atherosclerotic heart disease. Nutrition Reviews 1998; 56: 334–7.

155. Ness AR, Powles JW, et al. Vitamin C and cardiovascular disease: a systematic review. Journal of Cardiovascular Risk 1996; 3: 513–21.
156. Position paper: Multi-vitamin supplements, http://www.healthwatch-uk.org/Vitamin%20supplements.pdf (accessed July 22, 2013).
157. Pauling L. How to live longer and feel better. New York: Freeman, 1986.
158. Chalmers I, Altman DG, eds. Systematic reviews. London: BMJ Publishing Group. 1995. The Nonsense du Jour for [Ben Goldacre] Bad Science, http://www.scribd.com/doc/145552156/6/The-Nonsense-du-Jour (accessed July 22, 2013).
160. The Nonsense du Jour for [Ben Goldacre] Bad Science, http://www.scribd.com/doc/145552156/6/The-Nonsense-du-Jour (accessed July 22, 2013).
161. Ibid.
162. Ibid.
163. Scientific Committee for Food Nutrient and Energy Intakes for the European Community. Luxemburg: Commission of the European Communities, 1993.
164. Institute of Medicine Dietary Reference Intakes for Calcium, Phosphorus, Magnesium, Vitamin D and Fluoride. Washington DC: National Academy Press, 1997.
165. Hemila H. Vitamin C and the common cold. British Journal of Nutrition 1992; 67: 3–16.
166. Institute of Medicine Dietary Reference Values for Thiamin, Riboflavin, Niacin, Vitamin B6, Folate, Vitamin B12, Pantothenic Acid, Biotin and Choline. Washington DC: National Academy Press, 1998. Position paper: Multi-vitamin supplements, http://www.healthwatch-uk.org/Vitamin%20supplements.pdf (accessed July 22, 2013).
167. Institute of Medicine. Dietary Reference Values for Vitamin C, Vitamin E, Selenium and Carotenoids. Washington DC: National Academy Press, 2000.
168. FAO/WHO. Human Vitamin and Mineral Requirements: Report of a joint FAO/WHO expert consultation, Bankok, Thailand. Rome: Food and Nutrition Division of the United Nations Food and Agriculture Organization, 2001. Position paper: Multi-vitamin supplements, http://www.healthwatch-uk.org/Vitamin%20supplements.pdf (accessed July 22, 2013).
169. Position paper: Multi-vitamin supplements, http://www.healthwatch-uk.org/Vitamin%20supplements.pdf (accessed July 22, 2013).
170. Ibid.
171. Ibid.
172. Ibid.
173. Mursu et al. Vitamin, Mineral Supplements Linked With Increased Mortality Risk. Arch Intern Med. 2011;171:1625-1633,1633-1634
174. Dietary Supplements and .., http://michaelscally.blogspot.com/2011/10/dietary-supplements-and-mortality-rate. (accessed July 22, 2013).
175. David Michaels. Doubt is their product. Oxford University Press, 23 Apr,2008 Doubt is Their Product | Defending Science, http://defendingscience.org/writing-and-speeches/doubt-their-product (accessed July 22, 2013).
176. Doubt is Their Product | Defending Science, http://defendingscience.org/writing-and-speeches/doubt-their-product (accessed July 22, 2013).
177. Ibid.
178. Ibid.

CHAPTER TEN - QUACKERY - PHARMACEUTICAL COMPANIES

Pharmaceutical companies

Criticism of the big drug companies is common and well earned. This criticism comes, not only from people without adequate knowledge of the industry but also from very knowledgeable people. Some severe critics, until recently, were editors of very well known medical journals. In 2004 Marcia Angell lambasted the industry for becoming "primarily a marketing machine" and co-opting "every institution that might stand in its way."[1] She was formerly Editor in chief of the *New England Journal of Medicine*. Richard Smith felt that "Journals have devolved into information laundering operations for the pharmaceutical industry."[2] He was until 2004, editor of the *British Medical Journal*. Richard Horton[3] was editor of *The Lancet*.

Advertisements certainly influence physicians but a favourable drug trial is worth thousands of pages of advertising. This has to be worrying when one considers that the majority of drug trials published in major medical journals are funded by the pharmaceutical industry. In December 2005, the financial journal, Bloomberg Markets[4] published a lengthy investigative report which contended that "the clinical trial drug industry is poorly regulated, riddled with conflicts of interest, and sometimes deadly."

In 1991, 80 percent of industry-sponsored drug trials were conducted by universities, with protection for participants provided by the university's ethics committee or "oversight boards".[5] Now, according to CenterWatch, a Boston-based compiler of clinical trial data, more than 75 percent of all clinical trials paid for by pharmaceutical companies are done in private test centers or doctors' offices.[6] The U.S. Food and Drug Administration has farmed out much of the responsibility of policing the safety of human drug testing to a network of private companies and groups called institutional review boards or IRBs.[7,8] The IRBs that oversee drug company trials operate in such secrecy that the names of their members are often not disclosed to the public.[9]

These IRBs are paid by "Big Pharma" just like the testing centers they are regulating.[10] Pharmaceutical companies sponsored 36,839 new clinical trials from 2001 to 2004 and every year, trial participants are injured or killed. Few doctors dispute that testing drugs on people is necessary.[11]

Animal testing is not adequate. Human testing has resulted in the development of huge numbers of highly effective treatments but every year trial participants are injured or killed. Every year, Big Pharma spends $14 billion to test experimental drugs on humans. In the U.S., 3.7 million people have been human guinea pigs.[12]

The oldest and largest review company in the USA is Western Institutional Review Board (WIRB), founded in 1977 by Angela Bowen, an endocrinologist. WIRB is responsible for protecting people in 17,000 clinical trials in the United States.[13] The company oversaw tests in California and Georgia in the 1990s for which doctors were criminally charged and jailed for lying to the FDA and endangering the lives of trial participants. No action was taken against WIRB.

In 1978, the National Commission for the Protection of Human Research Subjects, an advisory committee appointed by President Richard Nixon, recommended, in what became known as the Belmont Report, that clinical trial participants be fully informed of risks and sign a consent form.[14] So-called informed consent was not required by the Food and Drug Administration until 1981. Interviews with people in clinical trials and relatives of participants who died in medical experiments across the U.S. suggest that researchers often do not fully explain risks and potential side effects. Laura Dunn, a professor of psychiatry at the University of California, San Diego, who wrote an article on informed consent that appeared in the *Journal of the American Medical Association* said "Decades of research show that poor understanding of informed consent documents is widespread."[15, 16] Money is the main reason people sign up for these clinical trials. Some even enroll in two or more trials being run concurrently. They may even be taking drugs with conflicting aims thus endangering their health.

Professor Martin Keller. Head of Psychiatry at Brown University in the USA was implicated in a dramatic scandal involving the drug Seroxat. Starting in 2002, BBC's *Panorama* made four programs about this anti-depressant drug: "The Secrets of Seroxat" (2002)[17] "Seroxat: Emails from the Edge" (2003);[18] "Taken on Trust" (2004)[19] and "Secrets of the Drug Trials" (2007).[20] "The Secrets of Seroxat" elicited a record response from the public as 65,000 people called the BBC helpline and 1,300 people e-mailed Panorama directly. The leading mental health charity, "Mind" collaborated with Panorama in a survey of those who e-mailed the program.

Anonymous findings from the 239 responses were sent to the Medicines and Healthcare Products Regulatory Agency (MHRA) and the second *Panorama* program on Seroxat, "E-mails from the Edge", included a report of the survey.[21] It showed widespread experiences of suicidal feelings and other severe reactions, very bad withdrawal symptoms and lack of warnings from doctors.[22] Following the broadcast users of the drug and members of "Mind" protested outside the offices of the MHRA. This scandal had been unearthed by television journalists and lawyers whereas the Medicine and Healthcare products Regulators Agency (MHRA) had been working on the case for three years and had still not produced its report.

On 29th January 2007, the fourth documentary in the series about Seroxat (Paroxetine) was broadcast. Presented by Jeremy Vine this exposed the huge drug scandal.[23] The program showed the suppression of evidence of the side effects of Seroxat by GlaxoSmithKline (GSK).

Seroxat was originally hailed as a wonder drug to treat depression and anxiety in the 1990's.

GSK promoted it as a cure for everything from stress to shyness. By the new millennium 100 million Seroxat prescriptions had been written worldwide bringing in two billion dollars a year but this treatment was confined to adults. If GlaxoSmithKline tested Seroxat for children they could get a six month extension on their patent which meant enormous profits. It would become the antidepressant being used worldwide for children with depression.

For the first 10 years of Seroxat's availability, GlaxoSmithKline's marketing of the drug stated falsely that it was "not habit forming"[24] but in 2001, the BBC reported the World Health Organisation had found it to have the hardest withdrawal problems of any anti-depressant.[25] A series of legal challenges by lawyers had forced many of these "secret" e-mails into the open. They contained details about clinical trials that GlaxoSmithKline (GSK) had begun over a decade previously for its antidepressant, Seroxat. GSK had organised three large scale paediatric clinical trials of this drug on children and adolescents with depression. The e-mails showed how results of drug trials were glossed over to cover up a link with suicide in teenagers.[26] Data from the trials showed that Seroxat could not be proven to work for teenagers. In addition, one clinical trial indicated that they were six times more likely to become suicidal after taking it.[27]

Panorama revealed the secret trail of internal e-mails which showed how GlaxoSmithKline manipulated the results of the trials for its own commercial gain. The documents revealed how hundreds of children with depression were recruited from around the world to take part in three large scale clinical trials of Seroxat.[28]

The biggest of these was in the USA and came to be known as "Study 329". The company had tested the drug on depressed children six years previously and Seroxat had proved to be no better than placebo. In one study seven of the 93 children who took Seroxat had to be taken to hospital. Some had self-harmed.[29]

In an internal memo to senior executives as far back as 1998, the product director for Seroxat in the UK admitted there was a problem. He had said "The results of the studies were disappointing. The possibility of obtaining a safety statement from this data was considered but rejected. The best which could have been achieved was a statement that although safety data was reassuring, efficacy had not been demonstrated."[30]

The BBC reporter, Shelley Jofre, commented that inside GSK the discussion was all about what a failure the study had been. Another of GSK's public relations people wrote in an e-mail dated 5th March 2001: "Originally we had planned to do extensive media relations surrounding this study until we actually viewed the results. Essentially the study did not really show it was effective in treating adolescent depression which is not something we want to publicise."[31]

Publishing the data in full would put profits for the company at risk.[32] Instead they preferred to state that Seroxat was safe and worked for teenagers. The inconvenient facts would be buried and the marketing people would spread the good news around the world. They would downplay the risks, exaggerate the supposed benefits and really minimise the negative findings. This is bad as any quackery and the collusion of an academic amplifies this many times over. GSK used a supposedly independent medical academic, Professor Martin Keller. Head of Psychiatry at Brown University.

His name was worth a lot to companies like GSK. They knew if they used respected academics to sell their product, doctors would be far more influenced than by regular sales representatives. Professor Keller himself said: "You're respected for being a... um... how to put this, an honourable person, and therefore when you give an opinion about something, people tend to listen and say oh, this individual gave their opinion, it's worth considering."[33]

But how independent was Professor Keller? In a single year he had earned half a million dollars from drug companies including GSK.[34] His name is at the head of GSK's study 329 but how much input he had is questionable. In a memo he thanked a ghost writer for the initial preparation of the manuscript; a ghost writer who worked for a public relations company hired by GSK. He said: "You did a superb job with this. Thank you very much. It is excellent. Enclosed are some rather minor changes from me ..."[35] Another letter from the ghost writer to Professor Keller said that all the necessary materials were enclosed so that Professor Keller could submit study 329 for publication. A covering letter stated: "please re-type on your letterhead. Revise if you wish."[36]

Ghost-written medical research like this is becoming a real problem. Professor Keller later excused himself by claiming that: "I've reviewed data analytic tables; I don't recall how raw it was. The huge printouts that list items by item number... you know, item numbers, invariable numbers and don't even have words on 'em. I tend not to look at those. I do better with words than I do with symbols."[37] It seems that Professor Keller did not really scrutinise the data in his own study as well as he could have. It is apparent that the public relations expert made crucial decisions about how to present the data. In one of the e-mails one of the GSK executives actually protested: "She's going too far in burying bad news."[38] In another e-mail dated 19th July 1999 it was stated that "It seems incongruous that we state it as safe yet report so many serious adverse events."[39]

There were actually 11 side-effects including self-harm, aggression and suicidal thoughts. GSK suggested to the public relations person that she make it clear Seroxat may have caused these side effects but the final article merely says: "Of the 11 patients, only headache (one patient) was considered to be related to the treatment."[40] The article never mentioned how many children became suicidal nor did it explore whether the drug was to blame. Instead it concluded that Seroxat is "generally well tolerated and effective."

The next step was to have the study published. Doctors rely on medical journals to give them advice they can trust.[41] Fiona Godlee, editor of the *British Medical Journal*, spoke on the *Panorama* program. She had declined to publish the paper. She commented: "Another journal had peer reviewers who also spotted a number of the problems but the paper was published nonetheless relatively unchanged, and I think the journal must take some responsibility for that."[42] The "other journal" was the *Journal of the Academy of Child and Adolescent Psychiatry*. Dr Mina Dulcan Editor of this journal accepted the article for publication. According to her the journal ranked "number one in child mental health and number two in paediatrics worldwide".[43] The journal's reviewers wrote on 3rd November 2000: "Overall results do not clearly indicate efficacy.

Authors need to clearly note this. A relatively high rate of serious adverse effects was not addressed in the discussion."[44] Despite these reviews the article was published in this world ranked journal! The same month the journal article was published, the third of the company's clinical trials in depressed children reported back.[45]

It actually showed the children on Seroxat did worse than the ones on placebos.[46]

Yet doctors at this time asking GSK for advice on treating children were told that study 329 involving Seroxat showed that the drug... "was superior to placebo by several assessment methods."[47] No mention of the serious side-effects or of the two failed studies. Meanwhile GSK was telling its American sales representatives who were promoting their drugs direct to doctors that Seroxat: "demonstrates remarkable efficacy and safety in the treatment of adolescent depression."

In June 2003 the USA Government's drug safety advisers warned that Seroxat should not be given to anyone under 18 years of age.[48] The medicines regulator had discovered this from examination of the secret clinical trial data that GSK had finally handed over, two years after the last depression study had ended. Seroxat had been found to treble the risk of suicidal thoughts and behaviour in depressed children. In 2004, when forced by the US medicines regulator to go back through its own trial results, the company discovered a further four children on Seroxat who had become suicidal during study 329.They discovered that there was actually a six fold increase in events relating to suicide.[49]

Dr Alastair Benbow,[50] medical director for GSK Europe, said: "The safe use of our medicines is paramount to everyone who works for GSK and the company is committed to ensuring that all appropriate information is made available to regulators, doctors and patients. We firmly believe we acted properly and responsibly in first carrying out this important clinical trials programme and then informing the regulatory agencies when we identified a potential increased risk of suicidal thinking and behaviour in patients under 18." He added: "Whilst there are substantive and rigorous requirements in place regarding disclosure of clinical trial data, it is clear that there is a need and benefit to strengthen the confidence of decision-makers and the general public that all pharmaceutical industry clinical trial data are disclosed promptly and transparently."

On 1st February, 2007, Charles Medawar wrote to the General Medical Council (GMC),[51] under the letterhead of the organisation (Social Audit Ltd) which employed him, enquiring what action could be taken against Alistair Benbow for offering inappropriately reassuring advice about the safety profile of Seroxat, in programmes broadcast on television (*Panorama*: BBC-TV), distributed worldwide. Medawar complained that Benbow's statements were (by omission and/or commission) inaccurate, misleading and possibly reckless; that the statements he made did not reflect the evidence to which he had unique access[52] and that substantial harm very probably resulted from his failure either to critically assess the evidence available to him,[53] and/or to his presumption that there was no cause for concern.

Medawar felt that Benbow's statements left the impression that "he conceived his primary duty of care to be to his employers, rather than to the many people (including health professionals) likely to have trusted his judgment as a doctor, and to have been influenced by the reassurances he gave."[54] Anna Neill, the Investigation Manager replied on behalf of the GMC stating that the GMCs main statutory objective was "to protect, promote and maintain the health and safety of the public" but they felt that there was nothing in the complaint "in its current form" suggesting that Dr Benbow's medical abilities were affected, as a result of the comments he made, to warrant action against him.[55] They requested further details.

Charles Medawar wrote again on 28th February 2007 emphasising that Dr Benbow had "publicly and emphatically denied the existence of risks with Seroxat when his employers were in possession of evidence that those risks were substantial and real."[56] He said that "With apparent sincerity, but also quite deviously,"[57] Dr Benbow had denied their significance. Dr. Benbow also denied the available evidence of the risk of Seroxat-induced violence and self harm including suicidal behaviour, especially in children and adolescents[58] though a few weeks after the second *Panorama* program, the UK regulators required Seroxat to be contraindicated for use by under 18-year olds.[59]

Medawar[60] felt that there would be no grounds for complaint had Dr Benbow complied with the terms of the pharmaceutical industry's codes of practice for drug sales representatives – e.g. "Information, claims and comparisons must be accurate, balanced, fair, objective and unambiguous and must be based on an up-to-date evaluation of all evidence and reflect that evidence clearly. They must not mislead either directly or by implication." Medawar questioned to what extent the public should trust a doctor's "professional commitment to procuring health and doing no harm" when substantial conflicts of interest are involved? Tim Cox-Brown, an investigation officer at the GMC replied on the 11th May stating that the GMC could not "identify any issues that would enable us to conduct an investigation into Dr Benbow's practice.[61] In the absence of any clear criminal or other regulatory proceedings relating to the research into, and/or production or marketing of, Seroxat, to which Dr Benbow can be directly linked, there is no information available to us which could amount to an allegation of misconduct capable of calling into question Dr Benbow's fitness to practise."

In a fiercely worded reply Charles Medawar replied to Mr Cox-Brown on May 24th. He stated that his view was that the response of the General Medical Council cast doubt on their fitness for purpose. He was "struck by the emptiness" of Cox-Brown's letter and considered that the letter "to date signals to me lack of competence, capacity, imagination, independence and commitment to health." He said that everything in the letter "emphasised that the GMC believes nothing can or should be done.[62]

The available evidence was sufficient to persuade *Panorama* to complain that Dr Benbow, representing himself as expert, had broadcast false and misleading statements about the safety of Seroxat. Yet the GMC seems unconcerned." He questioned whether this was really "in the public interest, and in line with public expectations of the GMC."[63] He also stated that it seemed absurd that the GMC should be satisfied with the conduct of a registered medical practitioner, even when he falls short of pharmaceutical industry standards for drug sales representatives that: "Information, claims and comparisons must be accurate, balanced, fair, objective and unambiguous and must be based on an up-to-date evaluation of all evidence and reflect that evidence clearly.[64] They must not mislead either directly or by implication."

Medawar expressed extreme concern that any doctor should so uncritically "toe the company line," when evidence of drug risk and harm is so strong.[65] He asked "are doctors who speak for drug companies under too much pressure or otherwise professionally compromised?[66] Are they simply to be regarded as company spokespeople, owing correspondingly less to the public by way of duty of care?" before adding that "It seems really feeble that the GMC should conclude so blandly, authoritatively and emphatically that there is nothing to be said, case closed."[67]

The Medicines and Healthcare Products Regulatory Agency launched an investigation into GSK in May 2003 alleging that it had known of the drug's dangers for several years but failed to pass the information on. Professor Kent Woods, chief executive of the MHRA, said: 'I remain concerned that GSK could and should have reported this information earlier than they did." No prosecution followed. In Parliament it was stated that "immediate steps" would be taken to strengthen the law making it clear that drugs firms must disclose any information they had which could have a bearing on the protection of health. GlaxoSmithKline responded by saying that "it noted" the conclusions of the MHRA. This scandal shows just how tightly the drug companies control medical research.[68]

In the US, bereaved families joined together to sue GSK claiming it acted fraudulently. If the case succeeds the company could be forced to pay out millions of dollars to the families.[69] On 22 December 2006, a US court decided in *Hoorman, et al. v. SmithKline Beecham Corp* that individuals who purchased Paxil or Paxil CR (paroxetine) for a minor child may be eligible for benefits under a $63.8 million Proposed Settlement.[70]

On Friday, January 27, 2012 it was announced by Glaxo that multi-millionaire media mogul James Murdoch who in 2011 was at the centre of a phone hacking scandal, had decided not to stand for re-election to GlaxoSmithKline's board at the annual general meeting of the company in 2012.

Marianne Barriaux[71] reported in *The Guardian* that GlaxoSmithKline, the UK's biggest pharmaceutical firm, had labelled allegations in the *Panorama* program as "defamatory." The company had looked into taking legal action an official said, "but there wouldn't be much to gain from taking action against the BBC." The company said: "GSK utterly rejects any suggestion that it has improperly withheld drug trial information."

David Healy, a professor of psychiatry at Cardiff University, said: "During the course of the last five years, the pharmaceuticals industry has gone from being very highly regarded to looking little better than the tobacco industry."[72]

In 2003 GSK signed a corporate integrity agreement and paid $88 million in a civil fine for overcharging Medicaid for Paxil, and nasal-allergy spray Flonase.[73] Later that year GSK also ran afoul of the Internal Revenue Service (IRS) and was facing a demand for $7.8 billion in backdated taxes and interest, the highest in IRS history. The company has settled some suicide claims, though terms of the settlements have not been released. In 2004, it agreed to pay the state of New York $2.5 million to resolve claims that officials suppressed research showing Paxil may increase suicide risk in young people. The settlement also required Glaxo to publicly disclose the studies.

The company's provision for legal and other non-tax disputes as of June 30 was £1.7 billion ($2.8 billion), the company said in a July 22 regulatory filing that did not mention the Paxil litigation. It is being sued for as much as £15.7 million ($31 million) by several hundred U.K. patients.[74] The claims were brought by people who alleged withdrawal symptoms and found it difficult to stop taking Seroxat. The U.K. lawsuit sought between £15,000 and £50,000 each on behalf of 314 people who alleged personal injury from Seroxat. GlaxoSmithKline is also the target of more than 4,000 lawsuits in the U.S., combined in a federal court in Los Angeles, that allege Paxil (Seroxat) users suffered withdrawal symptoms. GlaxoSmithKline said in a statement "We believe there is no merit in this litigation. Seroxat has benefited millions of people worldwide who have suffered from depression."[75]

On 26 August 2004, New York State Attorney General Eliot Spitzer's office announced it had settled legal action against GlaxoSmithKline.[76] The settlement required GSK to post a registry which would include much more information about pretrial and clinical drug study results than which the U.S. Food and Drug Administration and other pharmaceutical companies had thus far been willing to make public.[77] Attorney General Spitzer hailed the settlement as "transformational in that it will provide doctors and patients access to the clinical testing data necessary to make informed judgments." As for the monetary compensation, both sides finally agreed to $2.5 million.[78] On 12 September 2006 GSK settled the largest tax dispute in IRS history agreeing to pay $3.1 billion.[79]

The U.S. Department of Justice announced in October 2010 that GlaxoSmithKline would pay $150 million in criminal fines and $600 million in civil penalties.[80] GlaxoSmithKline agreed to pay the $750 million settlement in response to criminal and civil complaints against the company stemming from production of improperly made and adulterated drugs at their subsidiary SB Pharmco Puerto Rico Inc in Cidra, Puerto Rico.[81] On January 3, 2012, Argentinian justice fined GSK with 400,000 AR$ (US$92,000) for irregularities in documentation of a clinical trial for the Synflorix vaccine.[82]

Not all is bad. In February 2009, the GlaxoSmithKline head, Andrew Witty, announced that the company "would cut drug prices by 25 percent in 50 of the poorest nations,[83] release intellectual property rights for substances and processes relevant to neglected disease into a patent pool to encourage new drug development, and invest 20 per cent of profits from the least developed countries in medical infrastructure for those countries."[84] The decision has received mixed reactions from medical charities.[85, 86] Médecins Sans Frontières welcomed the decision, encouraging other companies to follow suit, but criticised GSK for failing to include HIV patents in their patent pool, and for not including middle-income countries in the initiative.[87] In addition GlaxoSmithKline has been short-listed for awards such as the Worldaware Business Award for its work to eliminate malaria in Kenya.[88]

They also recently donated money to the British flood appeal, and were ranked first on the 2006 UK Corporate Citizenship Index for donations.[89]

GSK was formed in 2000 by the merger of GlaxoWellcome and SmithKline Beecham plc.[90] The company is the world's third-largest pharmaceutical company measured by revenues (after Johnson & Johnson and Pfizer).[91] It has a revenue of £28.392 billion (2010),[92] an operating income of £5,128 billion (2010) and a net income of £1.853 billion (2010) It has 99,000 employees (2009)[93] including over 40,000 in sales and marketing. The company has a presence in almost 70 countries. As of December 2011, it had a market capitalisation of £73.8 billion, the fifth-largest of any company listed on the London Stock Exchange.[94]

Originally Glaxo, founded in Bunnythorpe, New Zealand in 1904,[95] was a baby food manufacturer processing local milk into a baby food by the same name: the product was sold in the 1930s under the slogan "Glaxo builds bonny babies."

Even Ribena

On 27 March 2007, GSK pleaded guilty in an Auckland District Court to 15 charges relating to misleading conduct brought against them under the Fair Trading Act by New Zealand's Commerce Commission.[96] The charges related to the popular blackcurrant fruit drink Ribena which the company had led consumers to believe contained high levels of vitamin C.[97] As part of a school science project, two 14-year-old school girls, Anna Devathasan and Jenny Suo, from Pakuranga College in Auckland discovered that ready-to-drink juice sold in 100ml containers contained very little vitamin C.[98]

Approaches by the two teens to the company failed to resolve the issue but after the matter was publicised on a national consumer affairs television show (*Fair Go*) the matter came to the attention of the Commerce Commission (a government funded "consumer watch-dog"). The commission's testing found that ready-to-drink Ribena contained no detectable vitamin C.[99] The company was fined $217,000. GSK was also ordered to run an advertising campaign to provide the facts after it admitted misleading the public.[100]

A Journal of the American Medical Association article that reviewed 102 clinical trials found that 50 percent of efficacy outcomes and 65 percent of harm outcomes were incompletely reported. The article concluded that trial outcomes are frequently incomplete, biased and inconsistent with protocols.

Pharmaceutical company gifts

About 90 percent of the pharmaceutical industry's $21 billion marketing budget is directed at physicians.[101] As part of a reaction against corporate influence on medicine, at a time of growing concern over the safety and rising cost of drugs and medical devices, radical changes took place in 2006.[102] Stanford University Medical Centre, Yale and the University of Pennsylvania prohibited its physicians from accepting even small gifts like pens and mugs from pharmaceutical sales representatives under a new policy intended to limit industry influence on patient care and doctor education.[103] Many faculty members and departments had become dependent on sponsored meals from industry in order to run seminars.[104]

Doctors were also prohibited from accepting free drug samples and from publishing articles in medical journals that were ghost-written by industry contractors. The policy would also apply not just to pharmaceutical company's sales representatives but makers of medical devices and other companies as well. Doctors buying medical equipment would have to report any financial relationships with equipment suppliers and could be excluded from the decision-making, the university said.[105]

In 2002 the Bush administration planned to restrict gifts and other rewards that pharmaceutical manufacturers gave doctors and insurers to encourage the prescribing of particular drugs. The USA Department of Health and Human Services said many gifts and gratuities were suspect because they looked like illegal kickbacks.[106]

Some consumer groups supported the move for the proposed restrictions but they were outnumbered by the drug makers, doctors and health maintenance organisations that criticised the proposal.[107] Marketing practices that had long been shrouded in secrecy became discussed openly. Pharmaceutical companies acknowledged that "they routinely made payments to insurance plans to increase the use of their products,[108] to expand their market share, to be added to lists of recommended drugs or to reward doctors and pharmacists for switching patients from one brand of drug to another." This was sometimes in the form of financial rewards. Insurers, doctors and drug makers said that such payments were so embedded in the structure of the health care industry that the Bush Administration plan would be profoundly disruptive.[109]

Some doctors argued that the drug manufacturing companies contributed markedly financially towards their professional education programs, and that the administration proposal could drastically reduce such subsidies. Dr. Michael D. Maves, executive vice president of the American Medical Association said[110] that "Without financial support from industry, medical societies would most likely be forced to curtail or stop offering these important educational activities." Doctors of all types echoed that concern.[111]

The United States government warned drug makers not to offer financial incentives to doctors, pharmacists or other health care professionals to prescribe or recommend particular drugs.[112] The government said the industry's aggressive marketing practices could improperly drive up costs for Medicare and Medicaid, the federal health programs for 75 million people who were elderly, disabled or poor.[113] But a coalition of 19 pharmaceutical companies, including Pfizer, Eli Lilly and Schering-Plough, said the Bush administration proposal was "not grounded in an understanding of industry practices." They said that the payments and incentives are standard in the drug industry. Merck & Company were even more explicit. They said that they routinely gave discounts and payments to health plans to reward "shifts in market share" favoring its products.[114]

Merck complained that the administration proposal would "criminalize a wide range of commercial conduct" that the industry regards as normal and entirely proper. The Pharmaceutical Research and Manufacturers of America, the chief lobby for brand-name drug companies, acknowledged that these payments created a strong incentive to prescribe certain drugs, or to shift patients from one drug to another. But, it said, that did not make the payments "illegal kickbacks." Solvay Pharmaceuticals of Marietta, Ga., told the government: "We understand that bribes and other hidden remuneration should be prohibited. However, a policy statement that declares well-established commercial practices potentially criminal creates a chilling effect on commerce and ultimately harms all consumers."

Drug manufacturers said they often encouraged the use of their products by making payments or giving discounts to pharmacy benefit managers and others.[115] They could exert immense influence over what drugs were prescribed and dispensed. The manufacturer might agree to a higher payment if the drug achieved a larger share of the market. This appeared to be standard practice. Alissa Fox, policy director for the Blue Cross and Blue Shield Association, whose members insure more than 84 million people, said the proposal would impede what it described as legitimate cost-control measures; "Pharmaceutical companies may be less willing to offer large discounts if those discounts cannot be tied to movements in market share."[116]

LaVarne A. Burton,[117] President of the Pharmaceutical Care Management Association, which represents pharmacy benefit managers like Express Scripts and AdvancePCS, said that "manufacturers may cease offering discounts," rather than run the risk of liability under the proposed guidelines. But the Food Marketing Institute, whose members operate 12,000 supermarket pharmacies, applauded the proposal. "Pharmacy benefit managers routinely refuse to disclose their financial arrangements with drug companies," said Tim Hammonds, president of the institute, "and they do not wish to be subjected to any kind of accountability, such as an annual audit." As a result, Mr. Hammonds said, "it is not possible to know with any certainty whether Pharmacy benefit managers are helping to control drug costs for the federal government or if these middlemen are contributing to skyrocketing drug costs."[118]

The administration proposal said that when drug executives discovered evidence of illegal conduct, they should report it to federal authorities within 60 days.[119] It also said that drug manufacturers should consider offering rewards to whistle-blowers and should prominently display the phone number for reporting Medicare fraud to the government. The coalition of drug makers objected to these recommendations, saying they would undercut the companies' efforts to police themselves.[120]

Other pharmacy benefit managers sometimes sent letters to doctors recommending that they shift patients from generic drugs to brand-name medicines. For each letter sent to a doctor the pharmacy benefit manager received an administrative fee, and additional remuneration might be given for converting patients from one drug to another. Pharmacy benefit managers said they typically received money from the manufacturer of a drug if sales of that drug reached a certain level, say 40 percent of all the prescriptions for cholesterol-lowering agents.[121] The manufacturer may agree to a higher payment if the drug achieves a larger share of the market. AdvancePCS, a pharmacy benefit manager based in Irving, Texas, confirmed that it received payments from drug companies for letters sent to doctors and patients urging them to use particular drugs but it said the payments, typically a flat fee for each letter, were for educational services that could help control drug spending.[122]

Kaiser Permanente, a nonprofit H.M.O. based in Oakland, Calif., said the administration plan would impair its ability to negotiate lower drug prices for its 8.5 million members because it suggested that discounts and rebate payments create "a prosecutorial risk" under the kickback law. The American Medical Association said drug companies should not be forbidden to give doctors pens, notepads and other items of nominal value that have "no correlation to any service provided by the physician to the pharmaceutical company." Such "giveaway items" are harmless, it said but the Massachusetts Medical Society suggested that "these items would not be so readily produced if they were not an effective form of advertising."[123]

The society asked: "Is the physician who writes a prescription with a company's logo on the pen more likely to write a prescription for that advertiser? Are patients more likely to request a certain drug because they see the notepad on the doctor's desk?"

For many years the drug industry spent billions of dollars annually, far more than it spends on research, trying to persuade doctors to prescribe its pills.[124] While it is illegal for drug makers to pay physicians directly for prescriptions, they once routinely offered "free dinners, gasoline and even Christmas trees" to doctors. Doctors were often given tickets to Broadway shows and professional sporting events. In 2002 the industry publicly forswore many of these practices with a voluntary code of conduct that discouraged expensive gifts but even though the American Medical Association instructs doctors not to take such gifts, marketing "abuses" continued.

Gardiner Harris reported that three years after the drug industry said it would stop giving expensive gifts to doctors a top federal drug official told a Senate panel that such marketing efforts continued.[125] Dr. Janet Woodcock, acting deputy commissioner for operations of the Food and Drug Administration, said that drug companies still invited doctors on cruises and to resorts in exotic places, all free.[126]

In early 2011, the Academy of Medical Royal Colleges (AoMRC) and many member Colleges signed a statement supporting the changes to the Association of the British Pharmaceutical Industry (ABPI) code on the provision of branded promotional aids and greater transparency.[127] The statement highlighted all parties' commitment to driving this agenda forward,[128] including collecting and declaring information about payments to healthcare professionals for services such as speaker fees, consultancy and sponsorship as well as declaring the number of health professionals a company works with. The first annual declaration of payments was to be made in 2013 for payments made in 2012. The AoMRC intends to continue its discussions with ABP1 over the evolution of the code and the requirements for greater transparency. The Academy has also recently advised that Her Majesty's Revenue and Customs (HMRC) in the United Kingdom have asked them to provide information on all payments made to individual clinicians over the last two tax years.

References:

1. The Truth About the Drug Companies. Marcia Angell M.D., Random House, 2004 (ISBN 0-375-50845-3). Alliance for Human Research Protection - Big Pharma's .., http://www.ahrp.org/cms/content/view/335/9/ (accessed July 22, 2013).
2. Smith R (2005) Medical journals are an extension of the marketing arm of pharmaceutical companies. PLoS Med 2(5): e138.
3. Horton R (2004) The dawn of McScience. NewYork Review of Books 51(4): 7-9.
4. David Evans, Michael Smith and Liz Willen. Big Pharma's Shameful Secret. Special Report Cover story. Bloomberg Markets. December 2005.
5. Alliance for Human Research Protection - Big Pharma's .., http://www.ahrp.org/cms/content/view/335/9/ (accessed July 22, 2013).
6. Ibid.
7. Ibid.
8. In the U.S., 37 million people have been human guinea pigs .., http://www.laleva.org/eng/2006/01/in_the_us_37_million_people_have_been_human_guinea_pigs.html (accessed July 22, 2013).
9. Alliance for Human Research Protection - Big Pharma's .., http://www.ahrp.org/cms/content/view/335/9/ (accessed July 22, 2013).
10. In the U.S., 37 million people have been human guinea pigs .., http://www.laleva.org/eng/2006/01/in_the_us_37_million_people_have_been_human_guinea_pigs.html (accessed July 22, 2013).
11. Alliance for Human Research Protection - Big Pharma's .., http://www.ahrp.org/cms/content/view/335/9/ (accessed July 22, 2013).
12. In the U.S., 37 million people have been human guinea pigs .., http://www.laleva.org/eng/2006/01/in_the_us_37_million_people_have_been_human_guinea_pigs.html (accessed July 22, 2013).
13. Ibid.
14. Alliance for Human Research Protection - Big Pharma's .., http://www.ahrp.org/cms/content/view/335/9/ (accessed July 22, 2013).
15. Ibid.
16. In the U.S., 37 million people have been human guinea pigs .., http://www.laleva.org/eng/2006/01/in_the_us_37_million_people_have_been_human_guinea_pigs.html (accessed July 22, 2013).
17. "The secrets of seroxat". BBC News. 10 October 2002. http://news.bbc.co.uk/1/hi/programmes/panorama/2310197.stm. Panorama (TV series) - Wikipedia, the free encyclopedia, http://en.wikipedia.org/wiki/North_Korea_Undercover (accessed July 22, 2013).
18. "Seroxat: Emails from the edge". BBC News. 28 April 2003. http://news.bbc.co.uk/1/hi/programmes/panorama/2982797.stm.
19. "Taken on trust". BBC News. 21 September 2004. http://news.bbc.co.uk/1/hi/programmes/panorama/3677792.stm.
20. "Secrets of the drug trials". BBC News. 29 January 2007. http://news.bbc.co.uk/1/hi/programmes/panorama/6291773.stm.
21. Panorama (TV series) - Wikipedia, the free encyclopedia, http://en.wikipedia.org/wiki/North_Korea_Undercover (accessed July 22, 2013).
22. Ibid.
23. "Secrets of the drug trials". BBC News. 29 January 2007. http://news.bbc.co.uk/1/hi/programmes/panorama/6291773.stm

SSRI DISCUSSION FORUM: REPOSTING: WATCH ONLINE VIDEO OF BBC ..,
http://www.network54.com/Forum/281849/thread/1170159897/REPOSTING-++WATCH+ONLINE+VIDEO+OF+BBC+PANORAMA+SECRET+OF+THE+DRUG+TRIALS+%28Seroxat+Paxil%29 (accessed July 22, 2013).

24. ^ "Judge: Paxil ads can't say it isn't habit-forming". USA Today. 20 August 2002. http://www.usatoday.com/news/health/2002-08-20-paxil-ads_x.htm. Retrieved 3 May 2010.

GlaxoSmithKline : definition of GlaxoSmithKline and synonyms .., http://dictionary.sensagent.com/GlaxoSmithKline/en-en/ (accessed July 22, 2013).

25. ^ Anti-depressant addiction warning, BBC News, 11 June 2001.

26. SSRI DISCUSSION FORUM: REPOSTING: WATCH ONLINE VIDEO OF BBC .., http://www.network54.com/Forum/281849/thread/1170159897/REPOSTING-++WATCH+ONLINE+VIDEO+OF+BBC+PANORAMA+SECRET+OF+THE+DRUG+TRIALS+%28Seroxat+Paxil%29 (accessed July 22, 2013).

27. Panorama (TV series) - Wikipedia, the free encyclopedia, http://en.wikipedia.org/wiki/North_Korea_Undercover (accessed July 22, 2013).

28. SSRI DISCUSSION FORUM: REPOSTING: WATCH ONLINE VIDEO OF BBC .., http://www.network54.com/Forum/281849/thread/1170159897/REPOSTING-++WATCH+ONLINE+VIDEO+OF+BBC+PANORAMA+SECRET+OF+THE+DRUG+TRIALS+%28Seroxat+Paxil%29 (accessed July 22, 2013).

29. Ibid.
30. Ibid.
31. Ibid.
32. Ibid.
33. Ibid.
34. Ibid.
35. Ibid.
36. Ibid.
37. Ibid.
38. Ibid.
39. Ibid.
40. Ibid.
41. Ibid.
42. Ibid.
43. Ibid.
44. Ibid.
45. Ibid.
46. Ibid.
47. Ibid.

48. Not Suicide, just plain Murder (depression dialogues .., http://www.paxilprogress.org/forums/showthread.php?p=320876 (accessed July 22, 2013).

49. SSRI DISCUSSION FORUM: REPOSTING: WATCH ONLINE VIDEO OF BBC .., http://www.network54.com/Forum/281849/thread/1170159897/REPOSTING-++WATCH+ONLINE+VIDEO+OF+BBC+PANORAMA+SECRET+OF+THE+DRUG+TRIALS+%28Seroxat+Paxil%29 (accessed July 22, 2013).

50. The Press Association.http://www.which.co.uk/news/2008/03/anti-depressant-drug-firm-criticised-134081/#ixzz1eHKwU2O4
51. Correspondence between Charles Medawar [Director of Social Audit Ltd] and the GMC. www.socialaudit.org.uk/6070201.htm. Alastair Benbow « seroxat secrets…, http://seroxatsecrets.wordpress.com/category/alastair-benbow/ (accessed July 22, 2013).
52. Alastair Benbow « seroxat secrets…, http://seroxatsecrets.wordpress.com/category/alastair-benbow/ (accessed July 22, 2013).
53. Ibid.
54. Ibid.
55. Ibid.
56. Ibid.
57. Ibid.
58. Ibid.
59. Ibid.
60. Ibid.
61. Ibid.
62. Ibid.
63. Ibid.
64. Ibid.
65. Ibid.
66. Ibid.
67. Ibid.
68. SSRI DISCUSSION FORUM: REPOSTING: WATCH ONLINE VIDEO OF BBC .., http://www.network54.com/Forum/281849/thread/1170159897/REPOSTING-++WATCH+ONLINE+VIDEO+OF+BBC+PANORAMA+SECRET+OF+THE+DRUG+TRIALS+%28Seroxat+Paxil%29 (accessed July 22, 2013).
69. Ibid.
70. ^ Paxil Pediatric Settlement website
71. Marianne Barriaux. GSK rebuts Panorama claims it distorted Seroxat trial results.The Guardian, Tuesday 30 January 2007. www.guardian.co.uk/business/2007/.../ broadcasting.socialcare. Not Suicide, just plain Murder (depression dialogues .., http://www.paxilprogress.org/forums/showthread.php?p=320876 (accessed July 22, 2013).
72. paxil timeline…we all need to be aware of this .., http://www.paxilprogress.org/forums/showthread.php?t=57649 (accessed July 22, 2013).
73. GlaxoSmithKline: definition of GlaxoSmithKline and synonyms .., http://dictionary.sensagent.com/GlaxoSmithKline/en-en/ (accessed July 22, 2013).
74. Caroline Byrne. GlaxoSmithKline Is Sued in U.K. Over Antidepressant Seroxat ... 8 Jan 2008. www.bloomberg.com/apps/news?pid=newsarchive&sid...
75. GlaxoSmithKline - Wikipedia, the free encyclopedia. en.wikipedia.org/wiki/GlaxoSmithKline
76. GlaxoSmithKline: definition of GlaxoSmithKline and synonyms .., http://dictionary.sensagent.com/GlaxoSmithKline/en-en/ (accessed July 22, 2013).
77. Ibid.

78. GlaxoSmithKline: Map (The Full Wiki) - Google Maps meets .., http://maps.thefullwiki.org/GlaxoSmithKline (accessed July 22, 2013).
79. ^ GSK settles largest tax dispute in history for $3.1bn. The Times (UK). 12 Sept 2006. GlaxoSmithKline - SourceWatch, http://www.sourcewatch.org/index.php/GlaxoSmithKline (accessed July 22, 2013).
80. GlaxoSmithKline: definition of GlaxoSmithKline and synonyms .., http://dictionary.sensagent.com/GlaxoSmithKline/en-en/ (accessed July 22, 2013).
81. ^ "Drugwatch. Paxil and Other Popular Drugs Subject of $750 Million Settlement". Drugwatch.com. http://www.drugwatch.com/news/2010/10/27/paxil-and-other-popular-drugs-subject-750-million-settlement/. Retrieved 18 April 2011. GlaxoSmithKline: definition of GlaxoSmithKline and synonyms .., http://dictionary.sensagent.com/GlaxoSmithKline/en-en/ (accessed July 22, 2013).
82. ^ "Argentina fines drug company over vaccine trial". CNN. January 3, 2012. http://www.cnn.com/2012/01/03/world/americas/argentina-drug-company-fined/index.htmlLawsuits - past/pending - Topix - Topix: Your town. Your news .., http://www.topix.com/forum/drug/effexor/TRT0NBBQO1RD5V9LE (accessed July 22, 2013). GlaxoSmithKline: definition of GlaxoSmithKline and synonyms .., http://dictionary.sensagent.com/GlaxoSmithKline/en-en/ (accessed July 22, 2013).
83. GlaxoSmithKline: definition of GlaxoSmithKline and synonyms .., http://dictionary.sensagent.com/GlaxoSmithKline/en-en/ (accessed July 22, 2013).
84. ^ Drug giant GlaxoSmithKline pledges cheap medicine for world's poor, The Guardian, 13 February 2009
85. ^ UNITAID Statement on GSK Patent Pool For Neglected Diseases, 16 Feb 2009
86. ^ GSK Access to Medicines: The Good, the Bad, and the Illusory Prof. Brook K. Baker, Health GAP, 2009-2-15
GlaxoSmithKline - Wikipedia, the free encyclopedia, http://en.wikipedia.org/wiki/Gsk.com (accessed July 22, 2013).
87. ^ MSF response to GSK patent pool proposal, Médecins Sans Frontières, 2009-2-16.
88. ^ The Shell Technology for Development Award Worldware Business Award. GlaxoSmithKline: definition of GlaxoSmithKline and synonyms .., http://dictionary.sensagent.com/GlaxoSmithKline/en-en/ (accessed July 22, 2013).
89. ^ "UK Corporate Citizenship rankings". Icharter.org. http://www.icharter.org/list/corporate_citizenship/index.html. Retrieved 18 April 2011.
90. GlaxoSmithKline: definition of GlaxoSmithKline and synonyms .., http://dictionary.sensagent.com/GlaxoSmithKline/en-en/ (accessed July 22, 2013).
91. ^ "Global 500 – Pharmaceuticals". Fortune. 20 July 2009. http://money.cnn.com/magazines/fortune/global500/2009/industries/21/index.html. Retrieved 19 August 2010 GlaxoSmithKline - List of Pharmaceutical Companies - Diseases .., http://www.diseases-diagnosis.com/virtual/GlaxoSmithKline (accessed July 22, 2013).
92. ^ a b c "Annual Report 2010" (PDF). http://www.gsk.com/investors/reps10/GSK-Annual-Report-2010.pdf. Retrieved 18 April 2011.
93. ^ "Company Profile for GlaxoSmithKline PLC (GSK)". http://zenobank.com/index.php?symbol=GSK&page=quotesearch. Retrieved 3 October 2008
94. ^ "FTSE All-Share Index Ranking". stockchallenge.co.uk. http://www.stockchallenge.co.uk/ftse.php. Retrieved 26 December 2011.

GlaxoSmithKline: definition of GlaxoSmithKline and synonyms ..,
http://dictionary.sensagent.com/GlaxoSmithKline/en-en/ (accessed July 22, 2013).
95. ^ a b c d e f g h i j k l m n o p q r s t "GSK History". Gsk.com.
http://www.gsk.com/about/history-noflash.htm. Retrieved 18 April 2011.
GlaxoSmithKline - List of Pharmaceutical Companies - Diseases ..,
http://www.diseases-diagnosis.com/virtual/GlaxoSmithKline (accessed July 22, 2013).
96. GlaxoSmithKline - The Full Wiki - Students, get citable ..,
http://www.thefullwiki.org/GlaxoSmithKline (accessed July 22, 2013).
97. Ibid.
98. Ibid.
99. Ibid.
100. Ibid.
101. Alliance for Human Research Protection - Stanford University ..,
http://www.ahrp.org/cms/content/view/340/148/ (accessed July 22, 2013).
102. Ibid.
103. Ibid.
104. Ibid.
105. Ibid.
106. Drug Makers Battle A U.S. Plan to Curb Rewards for Doctors ..,
http://www.nytimes.com/2002/12/26/us/drug-makers-battle-a-us-plan-to-curb-rewards-for-doctors.html (accessed July 22, 2013).
107. Robert Pear. Drug Makers Battle A U.S. Plan to Curb Rewards for Doctors. New York Times. Published: December 26, 2002. Drug Makers Battle A U.S. Plan to Curb Rewards for Doctors .., http://www.nytimes.com/2002/12/26/us/drug-makers-battle-a-us-plan-to-curb-rewards-for-doctors.html (accessed July 22, 2013).
108. Do doctors get a kickback or percentage of prescriptions they ..,
http://answers.yahoo.com/question/index?qid=20090901165436AAEIFg8 (accessed July 22, 2013).
109. Ibid.
110. Drug Makers Battle A U.S. Plan to Curb Rewards for Doctors ..,
http://www.nytimes.com/2002/12/26/us/drug-makers-battle-a-us-plan-to-curb-rewards-for-doctors.html (accessed July 22, 2013).
111. Financial Statement - Vaccine information,
http://www.vaccinetruth.org/finacial_statement.htm (accessed July 22, 2013).
112. Drug Makers Battle A U.S. Plan to Curb Rewards for Doctors ..,
http://www.nytimes.com/2002/12/26/us/drug-makers-battle-a-us-plan-to-curb-rewards-for-doctors.html (accessed July 22, 2013).
113. Financial Statement - Vaccine information,
http://www.vaccinetruth.org/finacial_statement.htm (accessed July 22, 2013).
114. Ibid.
115. Ibid.
116. Ibid.
117. Ibid.
118. Ibid.
119. Ibid.
120. Ibid.
121. Ibid.
122. Ibid.
123. Ibid.

124. Drug Makers Are Still Giving Gifts to Doctors, F.D.A .., http://www.globalaging.org/health/us/2005/gift.htm (accessed July 22, 2013).
125. Gardiner Harris. Drug Makers Are Still Giving Gifts to Doctors, F.D.A. Official Says. New York Times. March 4, 2005. Drug Makers Are Still Giving Gifts to Doctors, F.D.A .., http://www.globalaging.org/health/us/2005/gift.htm (accessed July 22, 2013).
126. Drug Makers Are Still Giving Gifts to Doctors, F.D.A .., http://www.globalaging.org/health/us/2005/gift.htm (accessed July 22, 2013).
127. Statement – Letter in response to Independent on Sunday .., http://www.abpi.org.uk/media-centre/newsreleases/2011/Pages/040711.aspx (accessed July 22, 2013).
128. Ibid.

Chapter eleven - Quackery - Top Health Frauds

How easily are we conned?

Anyone who suffers from cancer, or knows someone else who does, understands the fear and desperation of cancer sufferers. When so-called orthodox or Western medicine is no longer effective or fails there can be a great temptation to accept any alternative form of hope. People accept anything that appears to offer a chance for cure. No blame can be attached for this.

Medicinal products and devices used in the treatment of cancer must be approved by the Food and Drug Administration in the USA before they are marketed. This helps to ensure that these products are safe and effective. Other forms of cancer treatment, not regulated by the Food and Drug Administration, may not be safe or effective.

Health fraud is a cruel form of greed at the best of times but fraud involving cancer treatments can be particularly heartless. There are many companies selling bogus cancer "treatments". They may cause harm on their own but they may also cause indirect harm by delaying or interfering with proven beneficial treatments. These fraudulent "cancer treatments" are frequently sold as natural treatments or dietary supplements. They are widely advertised but are now offered on the Internet as well. Fraudulent information regarding these products can be provided in an instant and obtained immediately by accessing the Web, day or night. Many of these websites provide false hope for cancer sufferers.

An article in the *British Sunday Tribune* of 8th August 2004 by Kate Devlin quotes Professor Ernst, who warned[1] that the lives of thousands of cancer patients were at risk due to internet websites promoting bogus cures. He said that a flood of so-called "miracle cures" were available on the internet which were not clinically proven to be effective. These varied from powdered shark fin to a cyanide compound, laetrile, found in apricot kernels. The study found that not one of the multitudes of treatments or medications advocated could be proven to cure or prevent the onset of cancer and three sites were found to offer advice that was potentially harmful to cancer sufferers. A further 16 per cent of sites actively discouraged patients from continuing with conventional treatment as opposed to complementary therapies which implied a significant risk to cancer patients. "This was to us quite an eye-opener and pretty scary stuff," said Ernst. "Our conclusion was that a significant proportion of these websites was actually a risk to cancer patients" he added. "Not everything that is natural is risk free. People should use their common sense and think twice about the motives of these websites."

One of the "misleading" cures featured on the internet was Gerson's diet. It was this therapy which sparked an outcry in the scientific world when Prince Charles controversially praised it during a speech. "I think Prince Charles is doing a very good job in raising awareness of complementary medicines, but I very much regret his mention of Gerson's diet," said Professor Ernst. "There's no evidence at all to show that it helps anybody". Offering advice to patients, Profesor Ernst said, "If it sounds too good to be true, it probably is. Don't believe ridiculous promises and claims. Use your brain; take some reasonable and responsible advice." This, remember is from a Professor of "Alternative Medicine".

Richard Dawkins[2] quotes the results of a 2008 Gallup Poll showing that 44 per cent of Americans deny evolution totally. In Britain the figure is slightly less. Partly as a result of Charles Darwin's work, in Britain today, more people attend museums than attend church.[3] In the United Kingdom 1.6 million people are regular churchgoers and there are 47,000 churches. There are about 1,500 mosques.[4] Faith has been described as a "valuable ally in achieving a 'cure' and a dangerous enemy in assessing it."[5] No wonder then that a large proportion of people believe in "so-called" alternative medicine. The tooth fairy is alive and well.

In 1989 the Food and Drug Administration in the USA compiled a list of "Top Health Frauds".[6] Some categories were selected because they posed serious harm, others were chosen because people were being conned to part with their money having been given false hope. In many cases, having been given this false hope, patients stopped their conventional treatment with harmful results.

The top health frauds included unproven treatment for cancer, arthritis and AIDS, instant weight loss schemes, fraudulent sexual aids, quack baldness remedies and other appearance modifiers, false nutritional schemes, unproven use of muscle stimulators and candidiasis hypersensitivity. The FDA might just as well have added another thousand "quack" remedies. It's all about marketing and taking money from gullible people. Whatever happened to Snake Oil, Sanatogen, Carter's Little Liver Pills, Dr. MacKenzie's Veinoids, Salusa 45 and split ends?

Unfortunately people do become desperate and are willing to try any form of therapy. The unscrupulous quacks seize on this and make their money without any qualms of conscience.

There are thousands of "alternative" tests available to the gullible.[7] A small sample follows: AM-2, Amyloxine, Antimalignocyt (CH-23), Antineoplastons (Stanislaw Burzynski, MD), Anvirzel (FDA warning letter), Aveloz, Bemer 3000 , Bio-Ionic System (Evans Rapsomanikis), Biotech Cell Information, BioResonance Tumor Therapy, Bioterrain Management System, Bob Beck Protocol, Bryomixol and we have not even reached the C's.

There are 104 more "cancer cures" on a list provided by Quackwatch including such enticing names as Cat's Claw, Cellular Health™ from the notorious Matthias Rath, Chaparral, "Cure for All Cancers" (Hulda Clark), Forticel tea (with a Food and Drug Administration warning letter),

Galvanotherapy, Gerson Method, Health Restoration Program - Lorraine Day again, Holt microwave treatment, Whole body Hyperthermia, Immuno-Augmentative Therapy, Instinctotherapy (raw food diet), Issels Whole Body Therapy, Jason Winters tea, Laetrile, "Oxygenation therapies", Psychic surgery, Seasilver, Shark Cartilage, Two Feathers Healing Formula, Ultraviolet blood irradiation, Vitamin C, Wheatgrass and many, many more

Thousands of quack practitioners use "electrodiagnostic" devices[8] to help select their recommended treatment. Many claim to determine the cause of any disease by detecting the "energy imbalance" supposedly the cause of the problem. Some claim that the devices can detect whether someone is allergic or sensitive to foods, deficient in vitamins, or has defective teeth![9] Some claim they can tell whether a disease, such as cancer or AIDS, is not present. One Mexican clinic even claimed that a device they had could cure cancer.[10] The diagnostic procedure is most commonly referred to as Electroacupuncture according to Voll (EAV)[11] or electrodermal screening (EDS), but some practitioners call it bioelectric functions diagnosis (BFD), bio resonance therapy (BRT), bio-energy regulatory technique (BER), biocybernetic medicine (BM), computerised electrodermal screening (CEDS), computerised electrodermal stress analysis (CDCSA), electrodermal testing (EDT), limbic stress assessment (LSA), meridian energy analysis (MEA), or point testing. EAV devices are marketed by several companies, most of which also sponsor seminars.

The first Electroacupuncture according to Voll (EAV) devices were developed by Reinhold Voll, a West German physician who had been engaged in acupuncture practice in the 1950's.[12] In 1958, he combined Chinese acupuncture theory with galvanic skin differentials to produce his EAV system.[13] His first transistorised model was the Dermatron.[14] A few years later, one of his students (another German physician named Helmut Schimmel) simplified the diagnostic system, made small modifications to the equipment and created the first model of the Vegatest.15 Subsequent variants include the Accupath 1000, Asyra, Avatar, BICOM, Bio-Tron, Biomeridian, Computron, CSA 2001, Dermatron, DiagnoMètre, Eclosion, e-Lybra 8, ELAST, Interro, Interactive Query System (IQS), I-Tronic, Kindling, LISTEN System, MORA, Matrix Physique System, Meridian Energy Analysis Device (MEAD), MSAS, Oberon, Omega Acubase, Omega Vision, Orion System, Phazx, Prognos, Prophyle, Punctos III, Syncrometer, Vantage, Vegatest, Victor-Vitalpunkt Diagnose, Vistron, Vitel 618 and ZYTO.

Proponents claim that these devices measure disturbances in the body's flow of "electro-magnetic energy" along "acupuncture meridians"[16] but actually such devices are little more than fancy galvanometers that measure electrical resistance of the patient's skin when touched by a probe. The device emits a tiny direct electric current that flows through a wire from the device to a brass cylinder covered by moist gauze, which the patient holds in one hand. A second wire is connected from the device to a probe, which the operator touches to "acupuncture points" on the patient's other hand or a foot. This completes a low-voltage circuit and the device registers the flow of current. The information is then relayed to a gauge or computer screen that provides a numerical readout on a scale of 0 to 100.[17] According to Voll's theory; readings from 45 to 55 are normal or "balanced"; readings above 55 indicate inflammation of the organ "associated" with the "meridian" being tested; and readings below 45 suggest "organ stagnation and degeneration." However, if the moisture of the skin remains constant, as it usually does, the only thing that influences the size of the number is how hard the probe is pressed against the patient's skin.

A few of the devices are claimed to measure "vibrations" or "resonance" of body tissues and/or organs. In the earlier devices, the number was indicated by a needle that moved over a dial gauge. Later versions, such as the Interro make sounds and provide the readout on a computer screen.[18]

The treatment selected depends on the scope of the practitioner's practice and may include acupuncture, dietary change, and/or vitamin supplements as well as homeopathic remedies. Stephen Barrett says that in 1986, while investigating the homeopathic marketplace for *Consumer Reports* magazine, he underwent testing with the Interro device at The Nevada Clinic in Las Vegas, Nevada.[19]

When the doctor left the examining room he played with the device and found that the movement of the bar and the loudness of the noise were determined only by how hard the probe was pressed to his skin.[20]

Some EAV sellers make direct medical claims, some couch their claims in terms of correcting "imbalances," and some pretend that the device is used for "stress testing."[21] In addition some devices are claimed to help the practitioner make as well as select the recommended remedies.[22] The e-Lybra 8, for example, is said to provide "over 285,000 remedies at your fingertips" and to "make single or multiple remedies easily and quickly in any potency."[23]

Some devices are claimed to restore health by rendering signals that correct "imbalances." A 1997 patent application for the LISTEN device, for example, states: "By determining the electrical resistance at different points on a patient, it is possible to determine which organs are affected by a disease. In addition, a patient can be treated by providing a radiofrequency electrical signal which restores electrical conductance at specific points to normal levels."[24]

Some practitioners claim to use their device as aids to diagnosis rather than the sole basis for diagnosis but Stephen Barrett believes that they say this to make it harder for licensing boards to discipline them for nonstandard practice. Capital University of Integrated Medicine, a non-accredited postgraduate school offered a three-day course in "Electro Dermal Resistance Analysis."[25] The course was said to provide "assessment of health and the treatment of imbalances of the immune system through the resistance characteristics of specific acupuncture meridians on the body" and how to "locate the systemic roots of immune system weakness and to provide stimulation to strengthen the weakness." The school closed in 2005.

Phazx Systems told prospective device purchasers: "You will be able to create a new profit centre, because patients will be willingly paying for the services, as well as purchasing vitamins and supplements directly from you. Often the biofeedback testing can be billed and reimbursed through insurance companies or health plans, using biofeedback CPT codes."[26]

Phazx ceased operations after receiving an FDA warning letter. In a double-blind study, British researchers compared their results with a Vegatest device to those of conventional skin-prick testing in 30 volunteers, half of whom had previously reacted positively for allergy to cat dander or house dust mite.[27] Each participant was tested with six items by each of three operators in three separate sessions, a total of 54 tests per participant.[28] The researchers concluded that Vega testing does not correlate with skin prick testing and so should not be used to diagnose these allergies.[29] The authors estimated that more than 500 EDS devices were being used in the United Kingdom to assess sensitivity to potential allergens.[30]

The Australian College of Allergy concluded that "Vega testing is a technique of diagnosis without scientific basis."[31] In 1997, a biomedical engineer found that placing ampoules in the honeycomb of a Vegatest I device, a common practice in Vega testing, did not affect the device's readings.[32] This is not surprising, because glass is not an electrical conductor.The FDA in the USA classifies "devices that use resistance measurements to diagnose and treat various diseases" as Class III devices, which require FDA approval prior to marketing.[33]

In 1986, an FDA official informed Stephen Barrett that the FDA Centre for Devices and Radiological Health had determined that the Dermatron and Accupath 1000 were diagnostic devices that posed a "significant risk."[34] No such device can be legally marketed in the United States for diagnostic or treatment purposes. A few companies have obtained 510(k) clearance (not approval) by telling the FDA that their devices will be used for biofeedback or to measure skin resistance, but this does not entitle them to market the devices for other purposes.

According to Barrett, EAV devices are not biofeedback devices.[35]

Biofeedback is a relaxation technique that uses an electronic device that continuously signals pulse rate, muscle tension, or other body function by tone or visual signal. In biofeedback, the signal originates and is influenced by the patient. In EAV, the signal is influenced by how hard the operator presses the probe against the patient's skin. (Pressure makes the electric current flow more easily between the device to the patient's skin.) The now-defunct International Academy of Bioenergetic Practitioners encouraged device purchasers to bill insurance companies using biofeedback codes[36] but doing this could result in prosecution for insurance fraud.

The FDA has banned importation of EAV devices into the United States and warned or prosecuted a few marketers. Foreign and state regulatory agencies have also taken a few actions.[37] However, no systematic effort has been made to drive them from the marketplace. As a result, these bogus devices are being used by many chiropractors, acupuncturists, dentists, "holistic" physicians, veterinarians, self-styled "nutritionists," and various unlicensed individuals . The most common use is for prescribing homeopathic products. They are also used to determine "allergies," detect "nutrient deficiencies," and locate alleged problems in teeth that contain amalgam ("silver") fillings.

EAV devices pose several serious risks.[38] The transmittal of false or misleading health information can cause emotional harm, a false sense of security, or a false set of beliefs that can lead to unwise decisions. During the past ten years, more than 200 people have told Stephen Barrett about their experiences with EAV practitioners.[39] In most cases, they or someone they knew wasted hundreds (or even thousands) of dollars for the test and recommended treatment. In some cases, the person tested became very frightened and wound up undergoing expensive medical tests that showed that the diagnosed conditions were not present. Unnecessary follow-up procedures can also be a serious problem. Several patients had healthy teeth extracted after being misdiagnosed with an EAV device.[40] In another case, a man who consulted a physician about rectal bleeding and abdominal cramps was examined only with a Dermatron and told that his colon was fine. Unfortunately, the man had colon cancer which was not diagnosed until at least seven months later when he consulted another doctor. Two others had advanced cancers and were erroneously told they were cancer-free.[41] One of them was sold 33 products to get rid of "parasites" and other nonexistent problems. One victim who tried to get a refund was told that the products had been electrically specifically modified for her and could not be used for anyone else.

Many other "bioenergetic" devices have been claimed useful for diagnosing and/or treating health problems. They rely on detection and/or manipulation of either "vibrations" and/or a body "energy" system that have no scientific recognition.[42] The devices include the Quantum Medical Consciousness Interface (QMCI) System (also called the EPFX or SCIO), the Orion Bioscan, the Electro Interestitial Scanner (EIS), and various Rife frequency generators. The devices described by Stephen Barrett in his article, he says, are used to diagnose nonexistent health problems, select inappropriate treatment, and defraud insurance companies. He believes that EAV devices should be confiscated and that practitioners who use them are either delusional, dishonest, or both.[43] They should be reported to the practitioner's state licensing board, the state attorney general, the FDA, the Federal Trade Commission, the FBI, the National Fraud Information Centre, and any insurance company to which the practitioner submits claims that involve use of the device.

Magnetic wristbands are now the common craze – nearly all the English and South African cricket sides wear them. Professional golfers wear them. What publicity! What marketing! What gullibility!

The American Council on Exercise published the results of a study on Power balance bracelets. Three million of these bracelets were sold in three years. John Porcari and Rachel Hazuga [44]carried out a series of tests on 40 athletes half men and half women. One half of the group wore the power balance US $30 bracelet and the other half a placebo US $0.30 one. The researchers found that there was no significant difference in flexibility, balance, strength or vertical jump height between the Power Balance and placebo groups. Porcari stated that the bracelets simply do not work. "To me, it's an absolute scam", he said.

The Australian government took Power Balance to court because the company had no credible scientific evidence to back up the claims they made. As a result the maker of Power Balance in Australia was forced to make a public apology: "We admit that there is no credible scientific evidence that supports our claims. Therefore we engaged in misleading conduct". They offered a full refund.

A local golf teaching professional, Roger Baylis, bought a Power Balance magnetic wristband. The same evening he fell and dislocated his hip. While lying where he fell, he tore the wristband off and threw it away.

Johannes Nohl in his book *The Black Death* which described the great plague epidemics in Italy in 1345 and 1350 stated that a great many protective amulets were sold at that time in the belief that they protected against the plague.

These were sold not only by "quacks, old women and begging friars, but quite frequently by medical men". Not much has changed. People are still gullible.

Homemark, a South African company is often criticised by the South African Advertising Standards Authority for making claims about products that are not true.[45] In response, Homemark did what companies often do. They simply undertook to stop advertising the product. Usually the Advertising Standards Authority regards this as an acceptable solution but not on this occasion. The company admitted that it launches products without establishing if they actually do what they claim to do relying instead on the word of its "reputable suppliers" and that it effectively uses South African consumers to test the products. These admissions incensed the Advertising Standards Authority and, after considering Homemark's long history of having to withdraw adverts and the large number of rulings against it, the Advertising Standards Authority ordered Homemark to submit all its advertising to the Advertising Standards Authority for pre-clearance (i.e. for adjudication before use) for a period of six months. For a big advertiser like Homemark this will be inconvenient, expensive and downright humiliating.

The Food and Drug Administration and the United States Federal Trade Commission, in collaboration with other North American government agencies, announced a new drug safety initiative to prevent deceptive products from reaching consumers by removing potentially unsafe and unapproved drugs from the market. Gary Coody, [46]the National Health Fraud Coordinator and a Consumer Safety Officer with the United States Food and Drug Administration's Office of Regulatory Affairs, said that as part of the joint campaign, the Food and Drug Administration and the Federal Trade Commission had sent approximately 135 warning letters and two advisory letters to firms that marketed these products online. The initiative originated not only from consumer complaints, he said, but also from a Web surf for fraudulent cancer products by the Food and Drug Administration and members of the Mexico-United States-Canada Health fraud working group.

The new initiative included a final guidance titled "Marketed Unapproved Drugs -Compliance Policy Guide (CPG)." Prepared by the Centre for Drug Evaluation and Research (CDER) at the Food and Drug Administration it outlined its enforcement policies aimed at efficiently and rationally bringing all such drugs into the approval process. This Compliance Policy Guide provided official notice that any illegally marketed product was subject to Food and Drug Administration enforcement at any time. This enforcement included but was not limited to: requesting voluntary compliance, providing notice of action in a Federal register notice, issuing an untitled letter, issuing a warning letter, or initiating a seizure, injunction, or other proceeding. This guidance, did not establish legally enforceable responsibilities. Instead, it described the Food and Drug Administration Agency's current thinking and that the purpose of the guide should be viewed only as recommendations unless specific regulatory or statutory requirements were cited. The use of the word "should" meant that something was suggested or recommended, but not required. It was not stronger than that. They recognised that they were unable to take action immediately against all of the illegally marketed products and that they needed to make the best use of scarce

Agency resources. They had to prioritise their enforcement efforts and exercise enforcement discretion with regard to products that remained on the market.

The Food and Drug Administration defined health fraud[47] as the "deceptive promotion, advertisement, distribution or sale of articles... that are represented as being effective to diagnose, prevent, cure, treat, or mitigate disease (or other conditions), or provide a beneficial effect on health, but which have not been scientifically proven safe and effective for such purposes".[48] Of highest priority in this area were drugs that presented a direct risk to health. Indirect health hazards existed if, as a result of reliance on the product, the consumer was likely to delay or discontinue appropriate medical treatment.

On April 28th, 2010 Schwarz Pharma had to pay US $22 million to settle false claims allegations concerning reimbursement for unapproved drugs. On September 15th, 2010 the drug manufacturer Forest plead guilty and agreed to pay more than US $313 million to resolve criminal charges and false claims act allegations.

On March 2nd, 2011, the United States Food and Drug Administration issued a statement that it was taking action against companies that manufacture, distribute, or market oral agents that are not approved by the Food and Drug Administration. The drugs are prescribed for the treatment of coughs, colds, and allergies in the United States. On the same day Forest Pharmaceuticals were fined US $164 Million for Criminal Violations. On April 1st, 2011 the Food and Drug Administration filed a complaint against a Texas-Based firm, Healthpoint Ltd. under the false claims act.

The beauty specialist

Another class of quack to be considered is the beauty specialist. In the Cromwell era beauty was frowned upon. Beauty specialists fled to the continent. After Cromwell, women in Britain resumed taking pains with their complexions, attending to their figures, their hair, their skin and their nails. Beauty specialists returned from the continent. They set up consulting-rooms near Bond Street a part of London which their modern successors still favour. The advertisements issued by the beauty specialists of the two different times have not changed. [49] They advertised then, as they still do now, hair experts who "cut and curl Ladies' and Gentlemen's Hair extremely fine and after the Fashion". There were then, as there still are now, vendors of Beautifying Creams, Vanishing Creams, Spot Removers, Wrinkle Smoothers, Hair Restorers, Beauty Elixirs and the like.

They advertise their elixirs possessing virtues such that it "gives and restores to Nature what is wanting and takes away what is hurtful." One lady "understands thoroughly the secret of preserving Youth and Beauty and can even beautify without recourse to paint." My own favourite is, in recent years, the advertisements for the repair of "split-ends".

There is really nothing new in the modern art of selling cosmetics. Publicity methods have advanced but otherwise the quacks and the vendors of beauty parlour preparations remain very much the same. "The thing that hath been, it is that which shall be; and that which is done is that which shall be done: and there is no new thing under the sun. Is there anything whereof it may be said, See, this is new? It hath been already of old time, which was before us." (Ecclesiastes, I 10-11).[50]

Humanity is forever the same. Many things change but the essence of humanity remains unaltered. Quackery in olden times was very much the same as quackery is today.

Harriet Moore[51] reported on a Health and Food Fair she attended in Belfast which offered various cures for sale. The fair had been publicised in *The Belfast Telegraph*, with articles and a large colour photograph of an attractive female posing with some crystals in her hands. Admission was £2.50.

There were about 100 traders altogether representing a virtual A-Z of Alternative Medicine from Acupuncture to Zero Balancing. According to Moore, a vast array of non-science and only two or three stalls that could be described as representing anything conventional.

She collected many leaflets most including references to "arthritis", "cancer", "diabetes", "MS" and "healing." Claims included "may be effective", "has been shown to be useful for...", "is believed to assist in treating ...". References to treatments having an "exotic tradition", and "natural" being "good" appeared frequently. There was also a leaflet about Crystal Therapy which stated that this forgotten therapy had been re-discovered 150 years ago! She was not told nor did she read in any of the leaflets, advice to prospective clients to check with their family practitioner about their condition. The emphasis, Moore stated, was frequently anti-science, against fluoridation, against food preservatives, against medications and just occasionally anti-vaccination and, in one case, she saw a written statement that traditional Chinese Medicine could be used instead of conventional means for the successful reduction of fractures, this from Ri Fang Ho, Doctor of Chinese Medicine and Member of the British Acupuncture Council. Sums upwards of £15 were being paid for on-the-spot tests at various stalls.

There are regulations controlling the type of claims that can be made with regard to health treatments attempting to protect from ineffective or potentially dangerous purchases. These regulations do not appear to be effective.

Dr Thurstan Brewin attended a similar Health Show in Birmingham.[52] He describes how, when BBC television's magazine program, *Here and Now*, heard about a big Health Show in Birmingham they invited *HealthWatch* to send someone to walk round the stands, talk to sellers and buyers and comment.

They also decided to arrange a spoof exhibit of ordinary grass and to call it Indian Grass Therapy. According to Brewin "this aroused great interest among those attending the show. Unbelievably, nobody seemed to suspect for a minute that it might be completely bogus. The leaflet that went with it for all to read said "Keep for use in times of stress. Just open the bag of grass and inhale ... full of nature's own powerhouse ingredient, working holistically to give feelings of renewal... this is an innovative veganbiophysics product available without prescription." Available without prescription must have been a real selling point. Later the presenter interviewed the organisers and asked them how they could justify accepting something like this from someone who just walked in with no credentials whatever. They said that they usually expected membership of some organisation. A lame excuse.

Brewin said that he never saw the slightest indication that any of those flocking to this vast, popular exhibition; "hundreds and hundreds of them, nearly all women between the ages of 30 and 50 when I was there, were doing anything but trusting what they were being asked to trust. Perhaps some were allowing for a little exaggeration, but that's all. Every vestige of critical faculty, of healthy scepticism, of doubt or of humour seemed to have been left at the door when they entered the exhibition hall." He continued by saying that it was a different story with those who manned the stalls and exhibits. Some seemed very sincere about the supposed value of their product, but, he says "I soon found that others, whether men or women, did not need a lot of encouragement to make it privately crystal clear, perhaps with a nudge and a wink, that they knew perfectly well that it was all a bit of a joke, but if so many of their customers were happy to spend their money in this way, who were they to stop them?"

He continued; "It was the usual heady mixture of trendy jargon, pseudo science and ancient mysticism. Everybody was urged to 'power up their immune system'. And it seems that our atmosphere is now so loaded with pollutants that the need for high quality antioxidants is greater than ever before. Free radicals can destroy healthy tissues both internally and externally, but luckily the "Forever Young" brand of antioxidants can stop this. Did you know that 'research has shown' (a popular phrase at many stalls) that oxygen deficiency can be the single greatest cause of disease, that hostile microbes and viruses are unable to survive in the presence of oxygen, and that normal breathing definitely does not supply us with enough of it? No wonder we all need to take—two or three times a day for the rest of our lives—a solution containing "buffered and stabilised oxygen waiting to be released into a bioactive environment".

For £20 a month one could take "what they have been taking in India for thousands of years to improve their memory." For only £7 a simple hand-held massage machine consisting of six rotating balls also "used in the East for several thousand years" was selling well. A copper bracelet would not only help cleanse the body of toxins, it would also replace any copper loss in the body. A natural "age reversing miracle" was also available as well as several "stress busters." Brewin said that "osteopathy and homeopathy were nowhere to be seen. Perhaps they were wise enough to regard this exhibition as beneath their dignity. But acupuncture, reflexology, iridology, and 'healing astrology' were all there". Almost the only sign of mainstream medicine was a sensible stall manned by the National Pharmaceutical Association, and a London plastic surgeon advertising himself and his cosmetic surgery.

It has long been illegal to advertise remedies for cancer; yet quack cures abound and are frequently promoted in the small ads.[53] The Cancer Act was passed in Britain in1939.[54] Many of its provisions were replaced by legislation brought in at the time the National Health Service was introduced but Section 4 of the Act survives. Its essential wording is: "No person shall take any part in the publication of any advertisement containing an offer to treat any person for cancer or to prescribe any remedy therefore or to give any advice in connection with the treatment thereof." Breach of this provision is a crime for which the offender can be subject to a fine or to a maximum of three months' imprisonment, or both. In theory, if an offence is committed, it is the duty of local authorities to institute proceedings but, unfortunately, the Act is rendered almost toothless by the requirement that a prosecution can only be brought with the consent of the Attorney General or the Solicitor General. If a person or body is prosecuted for this offence, various defences are available. The main one is that the advertisement was published only so far as necessary to bring it to the notice of MPs, local councillors, or members of the medical profession, including nurses and pharmacists, or persons training for those professions. It is also a defence that the publication was in a technical journal. Finally, it is a defence if you published the advertisement in such circumstances that you did not know, and had no reason to believe, that you were taking part in its publication. In addition, the Act does not apply to advertisements published by a local authority or the governing body of a voluntary hospital, or to someone acting with the sanction of the Minister for Health.

The defence that you did not know the advertisement was being published has been tested in various cases that have come before the Courts. If you shut your mind to the obvious, you are deemed to have knowledge of what is going on but you would not be guilty if you "neglected to ascertain what could have been found out by making reasonable enquiries." There is clearly a great deal of room for argument about what someone's actual state of knowledge might have been! If the accused did not mention cancer in the original advertisement but sent a follow-up letter claiming to provide a treatment or medicine which could cure cancer, then an offence under the Act would be committed. The need to obtain consent before starting a prosecution and the various defences available mean that, in practice, not much use has been made of the Act.

There was earlier legislation of a similar nature applying to advertisements for treating venereal disease and, more recently, the UK government has taken powers under the Health and Medicines Act 1988, restricting not only the advertisement but also the sale of kits used to detect HIV.

In reviewing the position of the Cancer Act, Malcolm Brahams in a *HealthWatch Newsletter* was struck with the fact that Acts of Parliament dealing with medical matters were relatively few before the Second World War compared with the substantial body of legislation that has been passed since 1945.[55] All of this was, no doubt, for our protection as patients and consumers Brahams says but he suspects that whatever the law says there will always be people out there advertising "quack" remedies for cancer.[56]

References:

1. K. Schmidt and E. Ernst. Assessing websites on complementary and alternative medicine for cancer. Annals of Oncology number 15, pp. 733-742, 2004. http://annonc.oupjournals.org/cgi/content/full/15/5/733 . The Deadly Hazards of Cancer-Cure - CTM Home, http://campaignfortruth.com/Eclub/240804/CTM%20-%20deadly%20hazards%20of%20cancer%20cure.htm (accessed July 22, 2013).
2. Richard Dawkins. "The Greatest Show on Earth". The Evidence for Evolution. Transworld Publishers. London. Bantam Press. 2009.p 429.
3. Fifty things you need to know SKY News. 11.01.12.
4. www.MuslimsInBritain.org
5. Michael O'Donnell. A Sceptic's Medical Dictionary. BMJ publishing. 1997.

6. Top Health Frauds. www.quackwatch.com/01QuackeryRelatedTopics/fdatopfraud... 5 Apr 1999 – Top Health Frauds.
7. www.quackwatch.com
8. Stephen Barrett, M.D. "Quack 'Electrodiagnostic' Devices." Revised on August 24, 2011. Webglimpse Search Results - Quackwatch, http://www.quackwatch.com/search/webglimpse.cgi?ID=1&query=electrodermal+screening (accessed July 22, 2013).
9. Webglimpse Search Results - Quackwatch, http://www.quackwatch.com/search/webglimpse.cgi?ID=1&query=electrodermal+screening (accessed July 22, 2013).
10. Stephen Barrett S. BioResonance tumor therapy. Quackwatch, Nov 6, 2004. Webglimpse Search Results - Quackwatch, http://www.quackwatch.com/search/webglimpse.cgi?ID=1&query=electrodermal+screening (accessed July 22, 2013).
11. Webglimpse Search Results, http://www.quackwatch.com/search/webglimpse.cgi?ID=1&query=voll (accessed July 22, 2013).
12. The EAV history and roots (original method). Institute for ElectroAcupuncture & ElectroDiagnostics Web site, March 8, 1999.
13. Quack "Electrodiagnostic" Devices, http://www.quackwatch.org/01QuackeryRelatedTopics/electro.html?__hstc=200813169.8bb9743d9baee45731125e4f7569f60a.1364562260312.1364562260312.1364562260312.1&__hssc=200813169.1.1364562260313 (accessed July 22, 2013).
14. Ibid.
15. Terjebak Penipuan Pengobatan Terapi ala Rumah Sakit Holistik .., http://www.desentralisasi-kesehatan.net/index.php?option=com_content&view=article&id=574:t.. (accessed July 22, 2013).
16. American Association of Acupuncture and Bio-Energetic Medicine. Basic explanation of the electrodermal screening test and the concepts of bio-energetic medicine. AAABEM Web site, 1998. Eric Rentz DO, Hyping Homeopathic Health Huckster .., http://debunktionjunction.net/archives/344 (accessed July 22, 2013).
17. Voll scale. BioMeridian Web site, accessed Sept 4, 2007. Terjebak Penipuan Pengobatan Terapi ala Rumah Sakit Holistik .., http://www.desentralisasi-kesehatan.net/index.php?option=com_content&view=article&id=574:t.. (accessed July 22, 2013).
18. Quack "Electrodiagnostic" Devices, http://www.quackwatch.org/01QuackeryRelatedTopics/electro.html?__hstc=200813169.8bb9743d9baee45731125e4f7569f60a.1364562260312.1364562260312.1364562260312.1&__hssc=200813169.1.1364562260313 (accessed July 22, 2013).
19. Eric Rentz DO, Hyping Homeopathic Health Huckster .., http://debunktionjunction.net/archives/344 (accessed July 22, 2013).
20. Stephen Barrett. My visit to the Nevada Clinic. Nutrition Forum 4:6-8, 1987. Wikileax.net: Eric Rentz DO, http://wikileaxnet.blogspot.com/2011/06/bad-year-for-alternative-medicine-and.html (accessed July 22, 2013).

21. Quack "Electrodiagnostic" Devices, http://www.quackwatch.org/01QuackeryRelatedTopics/electro.html?__hstc=200813169.8bb9743d9baee45731125e4f7569f60a.1364562260312.1364562260312.1364562260312.1&__hssc=200813169.1.1364562260313 (accessed July 22, 2013).
22. Ibid.
23. Brewitt B. Methods for treating disorders by administering radio frequency signals corresponding to growth factors. U.S. Patent Number 5,626,617, May 13, 1997. Patent Number 5,629,286 contains additional information.
24. Information for e-Lybra 8. World Development Systems Web site, accessed September 4, 2007. Eric Rentz DO, Hyping Homeopathic Health Huckster .., http://debunktionjunction.net/archives/344 (accessed July 22, 2013).
25. Quack "Electrodiagnostic" Devices, http://www.quackwatch.org/01QuackeryRelatedTopics/electro.html?__hstc=200813169.8bb9743d9baee45731125e4f7569f60a.1364562260312.1364562260312.1364562260312.1&__hssc=200813169.1.1364562260313 (accessed July 22, 2013).
26. Ibid.
27. Ibid.
28. Ibid.
29. Ibid.
30. Lewis GT and others. Is electrodermal testing as effective as skin prick tests for diagnosing allergies? A double blind, randomised block design study. British Journal of Medicine 322:131-134, 2001.
31. Katalaris CH and others. Vega testing in the diagnosis of allergic conditions. Medical Journal of Australia 155:113-114, 1991. Quack "Electrodiagnostic" Devices, http://www.quackwatch.org/01QuackeryRelatedTopics/electro.html?__hstc=200813169.8bb9743d9baee45731125e4f7569f60a.1364562260312.1364562260312.1364562260312.1&__hssc=200813169.1.1364562260313 (accessed July 22, 2013).
32. Mosenkis R. Examination of a Vegatest device. Quackwatch, Sept 4, 2001. Quack "Electrodiagnostic" Devices, http://www.quackwatch.org/01QuackeryRelatedTopics/electro.html?__hstc=200813169.8bb9743d9baee45731125e4f7569f60a.1364562260312.1364562260312.1364562260312.1&__hssc=200813169.1.1364562260313 (accessed July 22, 2013).
33. Quack "Electrodiagnostic" Devices, http://www.quackwatch.org/01QuackeryRelatedTopics/electro.html?__hstc=200813169.8bb9743d9baee45731125e4f7569f60a.1364562260312.1364562260312.1364562260312.1&__hssc=200813169.1.1364562260313 (accessed July 22, 2013).
34. Rollings JN. Letter to Stephen Barrett, M.D., November 28, 1986. Quack "Electrodiagnostic" Devices, http://www.quackwatch.org/01QuackeryRelatedTopics/electro.html?__hstc=200813169.8bb9743d9baee45731125e4f7569f60a.1364562260312.1364562260312.1364562260312.1&__hssc=200813169.1.1364562260313 (accessed July 22, 2013).
35. Quack "Electrodiagnostic" Devices, http://www.quackwatch.org/01QuackeryRelatedTopics/electro.html?__hstc=200813169.

8bb9743d9baee45731125e4f7569f60a.1364562260312.1364562260312.1364562260 312.1&__hssc=200813169.1.1364562260313 (accessed July 22, 2013).
36. Bioenergetics - Space age technology available today. IABP Web site, archived Nov 8, 1999. Eric Rentz DO, Hyping Homeopathic Health Huckster ..,
http://debunktionjunction.net/archives/344 (accessed July 22, 2013).
37. Barrett S. Regulatory Actions Related to EAV Devices. Quackwatch, Sept 5, 2007.
38. Quack "Electrodiagnostic" Devices,
http://www.quackwatch.org/01QuackeryRelatedTopics/electro.html?__hstc=200813169.8bb9743d9baee45731125e4f7569f60a.1364562260312.1364562260312.1364562260312.1&__hssc=200813169.1.1364562260313 (accessed July 22, 2013).
39. Eric Rentz DO, Hyping Homeopathic Health Huckster ..,
http://debunktionjunction.net/archives/344 (accessed July 22, 2013).
40. Quack "Electrodiagnostic" Devices,
http://www.quackwatch.org/01QuackeryRelatedTopics/electro.html?__hstc=200813169.8bb9743d9baee45731125e4f7569f60a.1364562260312.1364562260312.1364562260312.1&__hssc=200813169.1.1364562260313 (accessed July 22, 2013).
41. Webglimpse Search Results - Quackwatch,
http://www.quackwatch.com/search/webglimpse.cgi?ID=1&query=eav (accessed July 22, 2013).
42. Ibid.
43. Eric Rentz DO, Hyping Homeopathic Health Huckster ..,
http://debunktionjunction.net/archives/344 (accessed July 22, 2013). Quack "Electrodiagnostic" Devices,
http://www.quackwatch.org/01QuackeryRelatedTopics/electro.html?__hstc=200813169.8bb9743d9baee45731125e4f7569f60a.1364562260312.1364562260312.1364562260312.1&__hssc=200813169.1.1364562260313 (accessed July 22, 2013).
44. Sean Bell. The Boabwe. Issue 9. April 2011.
45. Noseweek.
Issue 23. 1st January 2010.
46. Gary Coody. Beware of Online Cancer Fraud FDA's Consumer Updates page. Updated: September 18, 2008.
www.fda.gov/ForConsumers/ConsumerUpdates/ucm048383.h.8 Dec 2011
47. Quackery-Related Definitions - National Council Against ..,
http://www.ncahf.org/pp/definitions.html (accessed July 22, 2013).
48. Ibid.
49. The Story of Medicine. Kenneth Walker. Arrow Books. London. 1959 p. 311.
50. The New Thing - iBibleStudies.com: Free Online Sermons and ..,
http://ibiblestudies.com/auth/huntington/the_new_thing.htm (accessed July 22, 2013).
51. Harriett Moore. HealthWatch 'Health & Food Fair'.
52. Dr Thurstan Brewin. Healthwatch. Meeting Report. Indian Grass Therapy.
53. Malcolm Brahams. Law: Advertising remedies for cancer. HealthWatch Newsletter no 21: April 1996HealthWatch Newsletter no 21, http://www.healthwatch-uk.org/newsletters/nlett21.html (accessed July 22, 2013).
54. HealthWatch Newsletter no 21, http://www.healthwatch-uk.org/newsletters/nlett21.html (accessed July 22, 2013).
55. Ibid.
56. Ibid.

CHAPTER TWELVE - EVIDENCE-BASED MEDICINE

In the book "Bad Science", Ben Goldacre[1] traces what he calls a "natural crescendo, from the foolishness of quacks via the credence they are given in the mainstream media, through the tricks of the £30 billion food supplements industry, the evils of the £300 billion pharmaceuticals industry, the tragedy of science reporting and on to cases where people have wound up in prison, derided or dead simply through the poor understanding of statistics and evidence that pervades our society."

He goes on to say that at school we are taught nothing about death, risk, statistics and the science of what will kill or cure one. He says the "hole in our culture is gaping". This is evidence-based medicine, the ultimate applied science. According to Goldacre evidence-based medicine "contains some of the cleverest ideas from the past two centuries, it has saved millions of lives, but there has never once been a single exhibit on the subject in London's Science Museum".[2]

The term "Evidence based medicine" was first coined in 1990 by G. H. Guyatt[3]. It may be defined as "the conscientious, judicious and explicit use of current best evidence in making decisions about the care of an individual patient". Guyatt's contribution to quality of life research, randomised trials and meta-analysis has been considered groundbreaking. He has been a leading exponent of evidence-based approaches to clinical practice.

How many times during lectures and other conversations have we heard the words "It has been shown", "we have seen", "it has been demonstrated", "They say" or, my favourite "It's a well known fact!" When asked the results of his latest piece of research one doctor apparently replied "33.3 per cent of the patients did well, 33.3 per cent did poorly and the third patient failed to return for follow up". This is hardly acceptable research with only three patients. One researcher is said to have encountered several "methodological challenges" and as a result his findings were inconclusive! Another of my favourites is that someone has had "all the tests" done. What tests and who has determined the limit on these tests? I read somewhere that a piece of scientific work had been described as "Half cocked cobbled together piece of nonsense". It was Andrew Lang (1844-1912) who in the early part of the 20th Century said, of a colleague, "He uses statistics as a drunken man uses lamp-posts ... for support rather than illumination".

Apparently Brooks Brothers have made suits for every American president since Abraham Lincoln. Lincoln was wearing one of their suits when he was shot dead in 1865. Statistically, therefore, you are more likely to be assassinated if you are wearing a Brooks Brothers suit rather than, say, a Saville Row one. The Brooks Brothers public relations department sensibly prefers to promote the fact that you're more likely to be elected president if you are wearing one of their suits. The saying "There are three kinds of lies: Lies, damned lies and statistics", although popularised in the United States by Mark Twain in "Chapters from My Autobiography", has been attributed to Disraeli although the phrase is not found in any of Disraeli's works and the earliest known appearances were years after his death. Statistics, like facts, can be, and often are, twisted and utilised in any way one wants to.

Experience is another term I have difficulty with. When a doctor tells me that he has been doing something the same way for the last twenty years I do become slightly anxious. I liken this to a golfer who has had the same golf swing for the last 20 years. His swing might always have had the same faults or he may have developed a fault over time. This fault may be able to be corrected by one or two lessons from the local golf professional. The doctor may have been performing a procedure the same way for the past 20 years. There may be a newer technique for the procedure. He may have been giving the same medicine for a certain condition for the past 20 years. The appropriate treatment for the condition may have changed. The doctor may have always done the procedure in a less than perfect way or he may have developed a fault in technique which he has been unable to recognise. By reading the literature, attending courses, talking to colleagues and keeping up to date any doctor can improve in much the same way that a golfer can. Experience is extremely valuable as long as one is prepared to learn and "change" if necessary. A golfer obtaining help from his local golf professional has the advantage of listening to only one source of information and help. Doctors, on the other hand, have to wade through truly mountains and mountains of information. About 5,000 medical journals are published every month. Many of these journals will contain contradictory claims. How do we choose which ones are reliable? When we discuss evidence-based medicine, what do we mean by "evidence"? What is good evidence? Science needs evidence. So does medicine.

One of the earliest ever clinical trials took place in 1747, when James Lind successfully treated twelve ships passengers with a mixture containing, among other ingredients, oranges and lemons, and compared the effects with those passengers who were given a different concoction recommended by the ship's surgeon. The success of the treatment containing the oranges and lemons led to the provision of lime juice to all sailors, thereby eliminating scurvy from the navy and, incidentally, leading to the term "limey".

Even before that time a medical trial of sort took place and is quoted in the Old Testament; Daniel 1: 1-16.[4] Daniel was arguing with King Nebuchadnezzar's chief eunuch over the Judaean captives' rations. Their diet was rich in food and wine, but Daniel wanted his own soldiers to be given only vegetables and water. The eunuch was worried that they would become worse soldiers if they didn't eat their rich meals. Daniel suggested the first ever clinical trial. He suggested to the guard that his own soldiers would eat and drink only vegetables and water for ten days. They would then be compared with the young men who lived on the food assigned by the King. At the end of ten days Daniel's soldiers apparently looked healthier and were better nourished than all the other young men.

The origin of modern epidemiology is often traced to John Snow, who, in 1854, demonstrated that cholera was being spread from contaminated water from the Broad Street Pump in London's Golden Square. He analysed the rates of cholera among the citizens who obtained their water from this pump and he arrested the further spread of the disease simply by removing the pump handle.[5]

The editors of *The New England Journal of Medicine* in their Editorial of January 6th 2000[6] chose eleven of what they considered to be the most important medical developments of the past thousand years. One was the Application of Modern Statistics to Medicine. In 2007, the *British Medical Journal* had an international election for the most important contributions to healthcare. Evidence-based medicine came seventh. It was considered even more important than the advent of the computer.

Randomised controlled trials were first introduced in the United Kingdom in 1948 by the Medical Research Council and were adopted by the National Institutes of Health in the United States in the early1960s. How often does one hear a "statement of fact" from one individual based on his or her own personal experience; "It works for me. Therefore it must be effective". Scientists or doctors, who are scientists, cannot accept this. A series of one! One swallow does not make a summer. One cannot reason from one individual's own personal experience especially when that individual has been selected out to make a point. We cannot base beliefs on the experience of a mere handful of individuals either.

Clinical trials are aimed at finding out how different treatments compare with each other. Many illnesses get better even when no treatment is given. Control groups are used to ensure that any differences in outcome between the test group and the control group can be attributed to the test treatment.[7]

Everything else about the two groups should be as near as possible the same. The most reliable way to ensure this is to randomise the groups but even this is not always enough to eliminate bias. In double-blind trials neither the investigators nor the trial participants know which treatment is given to which participant.

The strength of medicine is the controlled clinical trial. Such trials differentiate that which works in medicine from charlatanism. Although randomised controlled trials became the "gold standard" of research based evidence, it is now recognised that in searching for the best possible evidence, they take second place to the systematic review. Systematic reviews are an essential element of evidence based medicine. In a systematic review one tabulates the characteristics of each study one is investigating, ideally being blind to the results of the study. One measures the methodological quality of each study to see how fair it is. Alternatives are compared, and then a critical, weighted summary is given. Iain Chalmers and others established the Cochrane Collaboration in Oxford in 1992. This collaboration, named in honour of Archie Cochrane, has become the world's largest source of systematic reviews. The Cochrane Reviews are designed to facilitate the choices that practitioners, consumers, policy- makers and others face in health care. In July 2010 Richard Horton, the editor of *The Lancet* advised users of the medical literature to start paying more attention to the *Cochrane Database of Systematic Reviews* and less attention to some better known competitors." They have said that: "The Cochrane Collaboration is an enterprise that rivals the Human Genome Project in its potential implications for modern medicine.[8]

The best available evidence may not always be obtained only from systematic reviews however; sometimes the best available evidence is obtained from a combination of studies of different types including systematic reviews. On one occasion I was trying to exhort clinicians to become familiar with the concept of the "randomised controlled trial" and explaining how valuable it was. One doctor mentioned that he would not volunteer as a participant in a randomised controlled trial if the subject was parachute packing!

As men get older they often have difficulty passing urine or micturating especially in the mornings. This is due to an enlarged prostate gland and can be a considerable problem. I have spoken to some of my elderly friends as well as to urologists about this and some of us agree that sex before one gets up to micturate alleviates this problem to a large degree. This fact is not mentioned in any medical book that I have read and I do not know of any randomised double blind trial that has been carried out on this subject! The investigation of the problem and the results would both be interesting. By writing this I might have started a trend. Imagine all the elderly men now approaching their wives every morning! In the film *The Bucket List,* Jack Nicholson might have been totally correct after returning from a liaison with a pretty stewardess in an aeroplane he described the liaison as "medicinal".

Doctors and medical administrators know that patients want to and should be more involved in decisions regarding their own health. Questionnaires, focus groups and patient panels have been shown to be effective in gaining an understanding about what patients think. Patients are no longer shy about demanding effective care from clinicians. They can be strong advocates for change. Evidence based medicine has moved on to "evidence-based patient choice".

There is an opposing point of view. The Honorary Secretary of the Royal College of Obstetricians and Gynaecologists, Richard Warren, in his newsletter to all Members and Fellows of the College[9] quite rationally said that he agreed, in principle, with the concept of "patient choice" but he believed that healthcare changes in the United Kingdom at the time were restricting rather than enhancing choice. He then asked whether choice was truly beneficial to an individual and or healthcare system.

He said that it was easy to support the concept of choice, the option of choosing one's preferred medical facility, preferred clinician or personalised treatment, but it was very difficult for the National Health Service to make provision to match the expectation. Not every local medical facility could have the facilities for expensive, state of the art treatment and how would a patient know the attributes that allow a considered, fully informed, choice? In the U.K. despite a woman and her specialist having considered all the issues, the final decision on treatment often lies with administrators whose priority puts finance before choice.[10]

Richard Warren questions a woman's choice to request a caesarean section when she is fully informed but there is no medical justification? Both medical and financial arguments may exist and the doctor may counsel but the patient may choose to the contrary, perhaps following a previous bad birth experience.[11]

The result is a patient population with high expectation of choice but increasingly being told what care they will receive and, unfortunately, it is the doctors who have to explain such limitations. Warren also mentions the issue of surgery without medical justification. Does a patient have the right to demand treatment or a doctor the right to refuse?[12]

What are the arguments for and against these "rights" and how is it best to handle the dilemma in an all too common clinical situation? These are all very valid points. Does patient choice override the financial considerations of a health service?

The book *Effective Care in Pregnancy and Childbirth*[13] is a book for consumers or patients. In the appendix of the second edition of this book there is a very clear classification of the different forms of care.[14] It divides care into six different forms; beneficial, likely to be beneficial, with a known trade off between beneficial and adverse effects, of unknown effectiveness, unlikely to be beneficial and likely to be ineffective or harmful. This, together with the regularly updated electronic database of systematic reviews, the *Cochrane Pregnancy and Childbirth Database*[15], enables patients to make their own choices, as to how they are cared for in pregnancy, based on evidence and not on hearsay.

This is not always acceptable to some doctors. Guidelines are most necessary if clinical practice is to improve but there has been a very slow process of acceptance. We do, however, need medicine to change. It has become a business. It has to follow the principles of business. This has been forced upon doctors by others. We need to become efficient rather than just providing "tender loving care". It demands a change in attitude.

Home births

Home births have long been a controversial subject in midwifery. During the 1920s in the United Kingdom approximately one-fifth of mothers were delivered in hospital.[16] By 1954 this figure had reached almost 64 per cent. By 1972 it had increased to 92 per cent and by 1991 approximately 99 per cent of women were delivered in maternity institutions. In the Netherlands, however 35 per cent of births occurred at home.[17] A Commons Health Committee in the United Kingdom advised in 1992 that, for low-risk mothers, there should be a return to births at home, in general practitioner or in midwifery units. In response the Royal College of Obstetricians and Gynaecologists pointed to a 51.7 per 1000 perinatal mortality from such a system in the Netherlands. The delivery of twins carries added risks but I know of a family practicioner who delivered twins at the patient's home.

J. R. Wax and others[18] published a paper in the *American Journal of Obstetrics and Gynecology* in 2010 which stirred up a hornet's nest. By means of a meta-analysis they showed that planned home births were associated with fewer maternal interventions including epidural analgesia, electronic fetal heart rate monitoring, episiotomy, and operative delivery, all of which, one would expect.

Facilities for these procedures are not available at patient's homes. The patients delivered at home were less likely to experience lacerations, haemorrhage, and infections but patients selected to deliver at home are usually the low risk patients who are less likely to experience these complications. Newborn babies born at home were less frequently premature, of low birth weight or needed assisted ventilation. This would also be expected. The neonatal mortality rates were significantly elevated in those patients having planned home births. Wax et al concluded that less medical intervention during planned home birth was associated with a tripling of the neonatal mortality rate.

Largely on the basis of this meta-analysis new guidelines outlining recommendations for women who were planning home births were issued by the American College of Obstetricians and Gynecologists' Committee on Obstetric Practice.[19] This committee explained that although the absolute risk is low, planned at-home births are associated with a 2 to 3 fold risk for neonatal death compared with hospital births. The committee stated that "it respects the right of a woman to make a medically informed decision about delivery." To reduce the risks, they recommended that "women who choose at-home birth should be informed about appropriate candidates for home birth; have at hand a certified midwife, certified nurse-midwife, or physician; have consultation access; and ensure timely transport to a nearby hospital if needed". They believed that "the hospital, including a birthing centre within a hospital complex ... or freestanding birthing centers ... is the safest setting for labor, delivery, and the immediate postpartum period." The statement continued "although the group acknowledges a woman's right to make informed decisions regarding her delivery, the American College of Obstetricians and Gynecologists does not support programs or individuals that advocate for or provide home births".

Eugene Declercq, Professor of Maternal and Child Health at the Boston University School of Public Health in Massachusetts, explained that the committee's opinion was based on "what I think is a flawed study. It's a concern," he said.[20]

Much more severe criticism of Wax's paper came from Carl A. Michal and others.[21] They pointed out that the statistical analysis upon which the author's conclusion was based was "deeply flawed". They stated that "despite the publication of statements and commentaries querying the reliability of the findings, this faulty study now forms the evidentiary basis for an American College of Obstetricians and Gynecologists Committee Opinion meaning that its results are being presented to expectant parents as the state-of-the-art in home birth safety research". They concluded that "the debate over the safety of home birth is deeply divided and emotionally charged. Reliable information is required to allow productive debate and informed decisions. In an era of evidence-based medicine, it is incomprehensible that medical society opinion can be formulated on research that does not hold to the most basic standards of methodological rigor".

The United Kingdom press was not far behind. *The Weekly Telegraph* of July 7-13th 2010 published an article stating that "Home Birth Raises Risk for Baby. Researchers say that less medical intervention is to blame for an increased risk of fatalities attributed to respiratory distress and failed resuscitation". The paper supposedly is allowed some licence. What the researchers actually said was that "less medical intervention during planned home birth was associated with a tripling of the neonatal mortality rate".[22] Being "associated with" is totally different from "to blame". *The Weekly Telegraph* said that the findings of the research did appear to question accepted thinking that home births were a safe option for women in low risk categories.

The study by Wax and others also drew criticism from major associations for midwives: the National Association of Certified Professional Midwives and the American College of Nurse-Midwives (ACNM).[23, 24,25,26,27] In a prospective cohort study investigators in Britain[28] found no significant differences in the odds of morbidity for births planned in any non-obstetric unit setting compared with those planned in obstetric units. They did observe a significantly higher incidence of morbidity for planned home births than for planned obstetric unit births among nulliparous women. They suggested that the low incidence of adverse events suggests that women with low-risk pregnancies should be provided a choice of birth setting.

If patients want to deliver their babies in a home environment and if safety is an essential requirement, which it most certainly is, then surely it is incumbent upon the medical authorities to provide hospitals and clinics that are more like homes. Pastel colours rather than clinical white. Delivery by qualified midwives with instantly available medical back-up. Unlimited visiting hours. Freedom for husbands or partners to be present whenever they want. Other members of the family able to visit and many other items of the patient's choice. The admission of fathers and other supporters to the labour wards was one of the major advances starting in British hospitals in 1962. If the hospital administrators do not make hospitals more like homes then I personally would acquiesce to patient's demands for home deliveries in selected low risk patients provided that there was a type of "flying squad" service readily available.

Hormone replacement therapy

Moving on from home births, another example of controversial medical research is that of hormone replacement therapy.

In 1968 Robert Wilson wrote a book titled *Feminine Forever*[29] in which he promoted the beneficial effects of estrogens. The word estrogen became synonymous with the Venus Pill".

Even before that time and for more than 60 years, hormone therapy has been used in the treatment of menopausal symptoms, such as hot flushes and vaginal dryness.[30] In the mid-1980s, the Food and Drug Administration in the United States approved estrogen (ET) for the treatment of osteoporosis. Estrogen given in this way is known to produce thickening and can cause cancer of the endometrium, the inner lining of the uterus. The addition of progesterone to the estrogen prevents this. A patient whose uterus is still in situ should always be given progesterone together with the estrogen. Estrogen given together with progesterone is termed hormone replacement therapy (HRT). Observational studies in the 1980's suggested that estrogen might prevent heart disease. The groups of women in these studies who used estrogen had about half the number of heart attacks as those who did not use estrogen.[31]

Estrogen was also shown to lower levels of the "bad" low density lipoprotein (LDL) cholesterol and raise levels of the "good" high density lipoprotein (HDL) cholesterol in postmenopausal women. Lower LDL cholesterol levels are associated with a reduced risk of heart disease.[32] Other research had also suggested that HRT might help prevent the onset of Alzheimer's disease.

Because so many questions about HRT and ET remained unanswered, The National Institutes of Health in the United States decided in 1993 to look for definitive answers. This body is responsible for giving medical researchers tens of billions of dollars every year. They conducted a randomised controlled study involving a total of 161,809 women known as the Women's Health Initiative (WHI).[33] The results of this study carried much weight because of the sheer number of study participants; it was designed to take place over many years, the time it takes for hormones to show any effect, and it was a blinded controlled study.

In May 2002, the Women's Health Initiative stopped one arm of the study. This included more than 16,608 women aged 50-79 years whose uterus was intact when the study began and who were on both estrogen and progesterone.[34] This part of the WHI was supposed to be of eight years duration but after an average of 5.2 years of follow-up it was stopped. The study data showed increases in the risk of breast cancer, heart disease and stroke, but decreased risk of colon and rectal cancer, uterine cancer, hip fracture, and death from other causes. The researchers concluded that the risks for the study group on HRT outweighed the benefits. Although the risks were small, they were outside the safety standards set for the study and this resulted in the early termination of this arm of the study.

The only statistically significant findings from the study, however, were the reduced risks of fracture and colon and rectal cancer. There was no effect seen on the overall risk of cancer, deaths from cancer, or death from any other cause. Nevertheless, this caused total panic. Many doctors worldwide stopped prescribing estrogen alone (ET) which had not been incriminated in the arm of the study which was stopped as well as estrogen and progesterone (HRT) which had been incriminated in that arm. Millions of patients stopped their treatment resulting in the resumption of their symptoms. The arm of the study in which the women took only estrogen (ET) was left ongoing by the researchers but doctors and millions of patients all over the world stopped all forms of estrogen treatment such was their panic.

The WHI trial results were reported primarily in terms of relative risk. The absolute risk of harm to an individual woman was very small: Among 10,000 women taking the combined HRT for a year, there would be seven more coronary heart disease events, eight more invasive breast cancers, eight more strokes, and eight more pulmonary emboli, but six fewer colorectal cancers and five fewer hip fractures. When counting all events over the 5.2 years of the trial, the excess number of "events" in the group taking HRT was 100 per 10,000 (or 1 in 100 women). Although these figures in absolute terms are very small one must consider that if one million patients used HRT they would have approximately 2,000 adverse events annually or 20,000 events over a 10 year period.

Conclusions drawn from the WHI data are controversial. They have been, interpreted in various ways. The average age at which women in this study began taking HRT, for example, was 63.2 years, far beyond the age at which women typically begin hormone replacement therapy and most of the WHI study participants had no menopausal symptoms. In addition, because the study lasted only 5.2 years, and based on our knowledge of the rate of growth of breast cancer, almost all the breast cancers would have been pre-existing. The average body mass index (BMI) of participants was 28.5. (34.1 per cent had BMIs of over 30 kg per square metre), one third were hypertensive and half the women in the study smoked. 6.8 to 6.9 per cent were on statins. 1.6 to 1.9 per cent had a previous history of myocardial infarction and 15 to 16 per cent had a family history of breast cancer. Only 17 per cent were within five years of their menopause.

The participants in the WHI study were certainly not representative of the average patient starting hormonal treatment. Many other issues regarding this study have also been raised in scores of letters to the editors and additional articles in the medical literature.

In spite of the panic caused by the cessation of part of the study, another part of the WHI, involving 11,000 healthy postmenopausal women who were using estrogen alone, continued for two more years.[35] Early in 2004, that arm of the study was also halted. Researchers discovered that ET did not prevent cardiovascular disease and appeared to increase the risk of stroke at about the same rate as HRT did.[36] That is, women using ET had about 12 more strokes per year for every 10,000 women than did those who took a placebo.[37]

The NIH believed that an increased risk of stroke was not acceptable in healthy women in a research study[38] This was especially true if estrogen alone did not affect (either increase or decrease) heart disease, as appeared to be the case in the current study. ET also increased the risk of deep venous thromboses. It did not appear to increase or decrease a woman's risk of breast cancer during the seven years the women took it and the women on ET had a lower risk of hip fractures.[39]

The Food and Drug Administration in the USA issued a press release on March 4, 2004 emphasising that when estrogen-containing products are used for relief of postmenopausal symptoms such as hot flushes, they should be used only when the symptoms are moderate to severe.[40] They also recommended that healthcare providers used the lowest dose and the shortest treatment duration needed to achieve treatment goals.*[41] The South African Menopause Society* (SAMS) interpreted the WHI findings in a slightly different way. They revised their previous guidelines[42]saying: "In the five years since the American study ended, new information has emerged around the use of hormone therapy (HT) in relation to cardio-vascular disease, cancer and osteoporosis. When one of the trials in the study was suspended in 2002 because the health risks appeared to outweigh the benefits, it triggered a panicky rejection of HT by many women and their healthcare providers.[43]

However the latest scientific response to the data reflects a shift back to a middle ground of HT use for younger menopausal women. An important factor in understanding this shift in attitude is to realise that the original WHI study was a study on women whose average age was 63 years. In the study, women were being started on hormone therapy in their mid and late 60's and in their 70's. This is completely unlike the real life situation where HT is started in the early 50's when symptoms are most severe. The new guidelines follow reanalysis of the results of those studies looking at the effects on different age groups particularly those patients between 50 and 59 years who are the most likely group who will need HT. When the estrogen only (ET) and estrogen plus progestin (EPT) arms of the WHI study were analysed together, researchers found a 30 per cent lower mortality rate in the women using hormones.[44] In this group the overall incidence of heart disease events was significantly decreased in users of HT. One of the main elements in the latest guidelines has to do with the use of ET compared with EPT. In the estrogen only arm of WHI, no increase in breast cancer was seen over the seven plus years of the study.[45] In addition, the younger patients (between 50 and 59) who took part in this trial showed a decrease in overall cardiac events. This has lead to a "window of opportunity theory" which suggests that early use of estrogen is beneficial to blood vessels.[46] However, if ET is delayed and used in older women in whom vascular damage has already occurred, the effect could be detrimental. HT in relation to osteoporosis also gets a nod of approval. The new SAMS position is that "hormone use should be considered a first line of treatment for younger menopausal women with osteoporosis".[47] They also said "Research into the use of plant estrogens and herbal formulations has not produced results from which SAMS can make confident recommendations about treating menopausal symptoms.[48] No published data is available on the use of traditional African medicine". They continued: "One of the crucial elements in deciding whether a woman should use HT is the beneficial effect on quality of life which can only be judged by each individual woman.[49] Undertaking HT must be a joint decision between the healthcare provider and an informed woman, based on relevant clinical factors and ongoing scientific evidence".

The North American Menopause Society (NAMS) weighed in, publishing a position statement in 2010.[50] NAMS is a nonprofit scientific organisation and they had published previous position statements on the role of menopausal hormonal therapy (HT) in 2002, 2003, 2004, 2007 and 2008. They collaborated with other interested societies and after considering all the evidence, they provided the recommendations, which were reviewed and approved by the NAMS 2009- 2010 Board of Trustees as an official NAMS position statement. They stated that estrogen therapy (ET), with or without a progestogen, is the most effective treatment for menopause-related vasomotor symptoms (i.e. hot flashes and night sweats) and their potential consequences (e.g. Diminished sleep quality, irritability and reduced quality of life). (In the USA the vasomotor symptoms are referred to as "hot flashes" whereas in Britain and South Africa the term used is "hot flushes").

NAMS continued to say that there was no statistically significant difference in mean weight gain or body mass index that had been demonstrated between women who used hormone therapy and those who did not. Patients have often told me that hormonal replacement therapy has made them put on weight. NAMS made the point that most observational and pre-clinical studies supported the potential benefits of systemic hormone therapy in reducing the risk of coronary heart disease. Most randomised controlled trials did not. They went on to say that it is now understood that the characteristics of women participating in the observational studies were markedly different from those of woman enrolled in randomised controlled trials, and that some of these demographic or biological differences, or both, influenced baseline cardiovascular risks and might modify the effects of HT on cardiovascular risk. They said that the disparity in findings between observational studies and randomised controlled trials may be related in part to the timing of initiation of the HT in relation to age and proximity to the menopause. Most women studied in observational studies of coronary heart disease risk were younger than 55 years at the time HT was initiated and within two to three years of menopause. On the other hand women enrolled to date in randomised controlled trials with clinical cardiovascular endpoints were an average of 63 to 64 years old and more than 10 years beyond menopause. When analysed by age and time since menopause at initiation of HT, the ET arm of the WHI is in general agreement with observational studies indicating that ET may reduce coronary heart disease risk when initiated in younger and more recently post-menopausal woman. These findings suggested that ET initiated by recently postmenopausal woman may slow the development of calcified atherosclerotic plaque. They concluded that there was emerging evidence that initiation of ET in early post-menopause may reduce coronary heart disease risk.

In the WHI, the increase in breast cancer risk was limited to those who had used combined estrogen and progesterone treatment before enrollment because there was no increased risk of breast cancer in women who had not previously used hormone treatment. Women in the estrogen only arm of the WHI demonstrated no increase in risk of breast cancer after an average of 7.1 years of use, with six fewer cases of invasive breast cancer per 10,000 women per year of estrogen only use. This was not statistically significant. Fewer breast cancers with localised disease were diagnosed in the estrogen treatment group than in the placebo group and a similar reduction was found for ductal carcinomas. This reduction in risk was statistically significant. A larger significant reduction was observed in a six-month follow-up when the women were no longer using estrogen treatment.[51] When the estrogen treatment was extended beyond 10 to 15 years in observational studies, the breast cancer risk seemed to have increased.

NAMS also stated that the association between ovarian cancer and hormone treatment beyond five years, if any, would fall into the rare or very rare category. They stated too, that although the Women's Health Initiative Memory Study (WHIMS) of women between 65 and 79 years of age reported an increase in dementia incidence with hormone therapy use, a number of observational studies have reported associations between hormonal therapy and reduced risk of developing Alzheimer's disease. Hormone therapy exposure in observational studies is more likely to involve use by younger woman closer to the age of menopause then by woman eligible for the WHIMS trial.

They emphasised the point that all women with an intact uterus who use systemic estrogen therapy should also be prescribed adequate progestogen. Incidentally, the level of progesterone in one's body cannot be measured by testing saliva. The Food and Drug Administration have stated this and it directly contradicts statements to this effect often quoted by the sellers of "natural progesterone". NAMS reiterated this in their position statement.

NAMS also emphasized the necessity of pretreatment evaluation. They stated that "hormonal treatment should be considered only when an indication for therapy has been clearly identified, contraindications ruled out, and the potential individual benefits and risks adequately discussed with each woman so that an informed decision can be made". Before initiating hormonal therapy, a comprehensive history and physical examination are essential. They also recommended assessment of risk factors for stroke, coronary heart disease, venous thromboembolism, osteoporosis and breast cancer and discussion of these results with each woman before initiating therapy. Mammography should be performed according to national guidelines and age but preferably within the twelve months before starting hormonal treatment. Other specific examinations, such as bone densitometry, may be considered on a case by case basis. NAMS stated that "Each woman is unique, having her own risk profile and preferences. When hormone treatment is desired by patients, individualisation of therapy is the key to providing health benefits with minimal risks, thereby enhancing the quality of life".

When considering duration of use of hormone treatment, The NAMS statement emphasised that data from large studies such as The Women's Health Initiative (WHI) and the Heart and Estrogen/progestin Replacement Study (HERS) should not be extrapolated to symptomatic postmenopausal women who initiate hormone therapy younger than age 50 as these women were not studied in those trials. WHI and HERS involved predominantly asymptomatic postmenopausal women aged 50 and older (with mean ages of 63 and 67 respectively), most of whom were 10 years or more beyond menopause; and HERS was conducted solely among women with known coronary heart disease. Like must be compared with like.

The NAMS position statement concluded that recent data supported the initiation of hormone therapy around the time of menopause to treat menopause-related symptoms; to treat or reduce the risk of certain disorders, such as osteoporosis or fractures in select postmenopausal woman; or both.[52] The benefit-risk ratio for menopausal HT is favourable for women who initiate HT closer to menopause but decreases in older woman and with time since menopause in previously untreated woman.

NAMS published its updated 2012 position online in *Menopause* on 27th February 2012.[53] They re-iterated that the most effective treatment for menopausal vasomotor symptoms and associated quality of life is ET or EPT but stressed that the decision to use HT should still be individualised and patient-specific, based on the patient's priorities regarding health and quality of life, as well as on specific risk factors for thrombosis, cardiovascular disease, stroke, and breast cancer.

The symptoms of the climacteric do not always have to be as severe as the example I once saw on the rear window of a car which read "I'm out of estrogen and have a gun!" but they can be life disturbing.

In the WHI investigation the long-term effects of combined estrogen and progesterone hormone therapy on breast cancer and other outcomes, including incidence and mortality rates, were uncertain. More recent WHI data present a clearer picture of breast cancer outcomes after nearly 11 years of follow-up.[54] The incidence of breast cancer as well as the rate of death from breast cancer was increased in the estrogen plus progestin group but not in the estrogen alone group.

The duration of follow-up was 11 years: 5.6 years of treatment and then several years post-intervention. In terms of the absolute rates, the risk of breast cancer mortality was low. In the women receiving placebo, there were 1.3 deaths from breast cancer per 10,000 women per year, and in the women using combined estrogen and progesterone, there were 2.6 deaths from breast cancer per 10,000 women per year. In relative risk terms the risk is doubled! Sounds terrifying but that is in reality only 1.3 extra deaths from breast cancer per 10,000 women per year attributable to hormone therapy. The excess deaths from breast cancer should not be downplayed, but no health outcome can be considered in isolation. Some effects of hormone therapy appear to be favourable, and most medications involve a complex balance of benefits and risks.

In terms of all-cause mortality, there was no evidence, during the 5.6 years of treatment with estrogen and progesterone, that overall mortality rates were increased in the active treatment group compared to placebo. Moreover, in younger women aged 50-59 years, overall mortality rates appeared to be slightly reduced with hormone therapy.

It is planned to continue following the Women's Health Initiative participants for at least five more years, and hopefully even longer. They will continue to be monitored for the risk of breast cancer, breast cancer mortality, all-cause mortality, and risks and benefits related to a variety of other health outcomes.

One of the key findings of the WHI study was that estrogen-alone therapy was associated with a significant reduction in risk for invasive breast cancer; overall about a 23 per cent reduction in risk for breast cancer. Important differences were found by age group. The women who were in their 50s at the time of enrollment appeared to have a much more favorable benefit-risk profile than the women who were in their 70s and more distant from menopause. The younger women had about a 40-50 per cent lower risk for coronary events and myocardial infarction (MI) and about a 27 per cent lower risk for all-cause mortality, whereas the women in their 70s had a pattern of increased risk for MI and all-cause mortality.

In terms of absolute risk, for every 10,000 women per year using estrogen-alone therapy, women who were in their 50's had 12 fewer heart attacks and 13 fewer deaths with estrogen therapy compared with placebo. However, women in their 70s experienced 16 extra heart attacks and 19 extra deaths.

Overall, the bottom line of this WHI report is that estrogen-alone therapy, in contrast to estrogen plus progestin, may be related to a reduced risk for breast cancer.

The findings also provide powerful and compelling evidence that younger women have a more favorable benefit-risk profile with estrogen therapy than older women, and this is supportive of the timing hypothesis. The results provide reassurance to younger women with hysterectomy and moderate-to-severe hot flushes and other menopausal symptoms, who may choose to be on estrogen therapy, that treatment would have an overall favorable benefit-risk profile. When considering the overall effect of estrogen and progesterone therapy, on the other hand, we must consider the balance of benefits and risks of the therapy for the individual woman. The absolute rates of adverse events in younger women are quite low, and for some, the benefits of hormone therapy far outweigh these risks.

The most up to date opinion on estrogen therapy, although this is probably far from being the finished word comes from the International Menopause Society. Their recommendations on menopausal hormone therapy and their Global Consensus Statement on Menopausal Hormone Therapy have recently been published.[55,56]

The global consensus statement was to be published simultaneously in the journals *Climacteric*[57] and *Maturitas* on behalf of the International Menopause Society and The European Menopause and Andropause Society, respectively. The statement was endorsed by The American Society for Reproductive Medicine, The Asia Pacific Menopause Federation, The Endocrine Society, The European Menopause and Andropause Society, The International Menopause Society, The International Osteoporosis Foundation and The North American Menopause Society.

It read: "The past 10 years saw much confusion regarding the use of menopausal hormone therapy (MHT). New evidence challenged previously accepted clinical guidelines, especially on aspects of safety and disease prevention. This led to many women unnecessarily being denied the use of MHT. Detailed revised guidelines were published and regularly updated by the major regional menopause societies. The confusion was initially escalated by significant differences amongst published guidelines. In recent revisions, the differences have become much less. In view of this, The International Menopause Society took the initiative to arrange a round-table discussion, in November 2012, between representatives of the major regional menopause societies to reach consensus on core recommendations regarding MHT. The aim was to produce a short document in bullet-point style, only containing the points of consensus. It is acknowledged that, in view of the global variance of disease and regulatory restrictions, these core recommendations do not replace the more detailed and fully referenced recommendations prepared by individual national and regional societies. This document serves to emphasize international consensus regarding MHT and is aimed at empowering women and healthcare practitioners in the appropriate use of MHT. MHT is the most effective treatment for vasomotor symptoms associated with menopause at any age, but benefits are more likely to outweigh risks for symptomatic women before the age of 60 years or within 10 years after menopause. MHT is effective and appropriate for the prevention of osteoporosis-related fractures in at-risk women before age 60 years or within 10 years after menopause. Randomized clinical trials and observational data as well as meta-analyses provide evidence that standard-dose estrogen-alone MHT may decrease coronary heart disease and all-cause mortality in women younger than 60 years of age and within 10 years of menopause. Data on estrogen plus progestogen MHT in this population show a similar trend for mortality but in most randomized clinical trials no significant increase or decrease in coronary heart disease has been found. Local low-dose estrogen therapy is preferred for women whose symptoms are limited to vaginal dryness or associated discomfort with intercourse. Estrogen as a single systemic agent is appropriate in women after hysterectomy but additional progestogen is required in the presence of a uterus.

The option of MHT is an individual decision in terms of quality of life and health priorities as well as personal risk factors such as age, time since menopause and the risk of venous thromboembolism, stroke, ischemic heart disease and breast cancer. The risk of venous thromboembolism and ischemic stroke increases with oral MHT but the absolute risk is rare below age 60 years. Observational studies point to a lower risk with transdermal therapy. The risk of breast cancer in women over 50 years associated with MHT is a complex issue. The increased risk of breast cancer is primarily associated with the addition of a progestogen to estrogen therapy and related to the duration of use. The risk of breast cancer attributable to MHT is small and the risk decreases after treatment is stopped. The dose and duration of MHT should be consistent with treatment goals and safety issues and should be individualized. In women with premature ovarian insufficiency, systemic MHT is recommended at least until the average age of the natural menopause.

The use of custom-compounded bioidentical hormone therapy is not recommended.

Current safety data do not support the use of MHT in breast cancer survivors.

These core recommendations will be reviewed in the future as new evidence becomes available."

Jenny Hope[58] voiced her opinion on the panic caused by the WHI investigation more strongly. She termed the debacle "A wasted decade".

She explained how thousands of women have had a 'wasted decade' of suffering since the HRT scare, quoting the international panel of experts who wrote the recent series of articles published in *Climacteric,* the *Journal of the International Menopause Society.* This panel included clinicians from the US National Institutes of Health who worked on the original Women's Health Initiative study. These articles showed that many of the conclusions reached by the 2002 study, including the raised risk of breast cancer, "have now been overturned". She suggested that this major reassessment of the WHI research had concluded that "menopausal women were the victims of 'mass fear' generated by the WHI findings. An estimated one million women in the UK stopped taking their hormone treatment. This was roughly half the number who were using it when the scare started.

The *Climacteric* joint editor-in-chief Dr Nick Panay, who is also chairman of the British Menopause Society said that the consensus was now that the absolute risks for a woman taking HRT in her 50s is "extremely low". He claimed that the benefits of HRT far outweigh the risks and pointed out "This has been a wasted decade for thousands of women whose quality of life could have been improved. The big scandal is their risk of osteoporosis could have been reduced" and he added that the absolute risks of breast cancer for women using HRT were low. Around one extra case occurs per 1,000 women taking HRT for one year and the risk only starts rising after seven years of use. Dr Panay said "HRT is safe for women who need it in their late 40s and early 50s'. He said that mass fear had been generated among women and doctors. Overgeneralising the results of the research led to needless suffering and lost opportunities. One of the original WHI researchers, Professor Matthew Allison, of the University of California, San Diego, was quoted as saying "Being obese, not exercising or excess alcohol consumption confer higher absolute risks for breast cancer than HRT use."

Unfortunately authors like Dr. Paul Offit and others unknowingly "added fuel to the fire".[59] They uncritically accepted the initial WHI findings causing further anxiety. Offit in his otherwise excellent book *Killing Us Softly The Sense and Nonsense of Alternative Medicine* states that estrogens "came with a price". He states that the study was cut short when the researchers "noticed a dramatic increase in breast cancer. And it wasn't only breast cancer; replacement hormones also increased the risk of heart disease, strokes, and blood clots. As a consequence, hormone replacement therapy became something doctors began to fear, not embrace".

Coronary heart disease (CHD) represents the leading cause of death in women in the United States. Findings from the Women's Health Initiative and the Nurses' Health Study have suggested that timing of initiation of hormone therapy (HT) profoundly affects its cardiovascular safety.

Diana Petitti [60] in an article titled "Hormone Replacement Therapy and Heart Disease Prevention" pointed out that three different meta-analyses had concluded that estrogen replacement therapy decreased the risk of coronary heart disease by 35 per cent to 50 per cent. The predicted increase in life expectancy in hormone users, based on estimates of the risk of CHD in users of ERT derived from observational studies, was two to three years. In another recent report from a large prospective cohort study of female California teachers,[61] investigators assessed the effects of age at current HT use on CHD mortality. Current HT use was associated with a 16 per cent lower risk for CHD-related death. This risk reduction was most pronounced in current HT users younger than 60 years of age, in whom a 62 per cent risk reduction was noted. As the age of users increased, this apparent protection against fatal CHD attenuated. Results were similar with use of estrogen-alone or combination estrogen-progestin HT. The findings from this important observational, California-based study reinforce a large body of evidence in women and in non-human primates, which in aggregate provide robust reassurance about the cardiovascular safety of HT when it is used by recently menopausal women for management of bothersome symptoms.

Peter Kovacs chose the effects of hormone therapy on mortality and ischemic heart disease as one of his "game changers" in obstetrics and gynaecology in 2011.[62] He pointed out that for a long time estrogen therapy had been used to prevent heart disease. It became standard practice to initiate hormone therapy once a woman entered menopause. This practice was challenged by randomised trials[63,64] and women stopped taking estrogen.

The known beneficial lipoprotein effects and the direct effects of estradiol on arteries supported the concept that estrogen was of benefit. Estrogen, however, also has prothrombotic effects (a tendency to clotting of blood) and the progestin used in the combined form as HRT also reduces the beneficial effects of estradiol. After the WHI results menopausal women, according to Kovacs, can no longer be regarded as a single group. When deciding on hormone therapy a woman's age must now be considered. Younger women with less atherosclerosis approaching the menopause may still enjoy the beneficial cardiovascular effects of hormone therapy. In older women hormone therapy may lead to plaque rupture and an increase in heart disease.

Chrisandra Shufelt, reported for *Medscape* on a newsletter from the *North American Menopause Society*[65] which described a paper by O'Donnell and others[66] showing the increase on atherosclerosis or "hardening of the arteries" associated with low estrogen blood levels. A low estrogen level is a characteristic of abnormal function of the hypothalamus (FHA) in premenopausal women. A common and reversible form of FHA is exercise associated amenorrhea (EAA). O'Donnell and others studied both original and review articles from 1974 to 2011 regarding cardiovascular changes in women with FHA and particularly women with EAA. Despite regular exercise, women with low estrogen levels who had exercise associated amenorrhea showed unexpected cardiovascular changes, including endothelial dysfunction, which is related to atherosclerosis. The evidence suggested that the beneficial vascular effects of exercise were nullified by low estrogen levels. In the opinion of the authors, exogenous estrogen therapy or restoration of endogenous estrogen restores vascular function in premenopausal women.

T. Yoshida and others from Japan[67] described the "Impact of surgical menopause on lipid and bone metabolism". They showed that patients who had both ovaries removed at the time of hysterectomy with consequent loss of estrogen production had a significant elevation in their level of "bad" low density lipoprotein (LDL) cholesterol compared with the baseline level.

The bone mineral density (BMD) was also significantly decreased by as much as 6.7 per cent at 12 months in the same patients. They concluded that bilateral oophorectomy seemed to cause dyslipidemia and serious loss of bone mineral density within only one year. This is presumably due to the sudden lack of estrogen in these patients.

As stated previously after the initial Women's Health Initiative (WHI) trial publication, millions of women across the globe abruptly discontinued postmenopausal hormone therapy. In the United States hormone therapy prescription rates declined by 46 per cent between July 2002 and December 2002.[68] Another report showed a 44 per cent decline between 2001 and 2003. A similar magnitude of decline in hormone therapy prescriptions was also observed around the world. Hormone therapy conclusively protects against osteoporosis. The hip fracture risk, which is associated with a 25 per cent case-fatality rate, increased in the post-WHI era. Women who discontinued postmenopausal hormone therapy had a significantly increased risk of hip fracture compared with women who continued taking the treatment. The protective association of hormone therapy with hip fracture disappeared within two years of cessation of hormone therapy.[69] Similar findings were reported at the North American Menopause Society 21st Annual Meeting in October 2010. Women were said to be making decisions to stop hormones based on Women's Health Initiative findings, which were basically based on cardiovascular and other outcomes but hormones were known to be beneficial for hip fracture.[70]

Bone fracture is a large public health issue with major medical and economic consequences. The cost of medical care associated with osteoporotic fractures is estimated to be more than US$18 billion annually in the United States alone. Hip fractures result in a greater cost, disability, and mortality than all other osteoporotic fractures combined. Within the first year of a hip fracture, there is an approximate 25 per cent increase in mortality. The negative impact worldwide of the cessation of hormone therapy is not to be underestimated.

The polycystic ovary syndrome

Yet another example of controversial research and its effect on patients is that of the polycystic ovary syndrome (PCOS). This is a distressing problem in many young patients causing subfertility and an assortment of other symptoms such as acne, hirsutism and alopecia. There is a considerable difference of opinion as to whether insulin sensitising agents such as Metformin and other similar drugs should be used in the treatment of the polycystic ovary syndrome or not.[71]

In these patients weight loss can be effective in regulating menses and restoring ovulation[72] but because weight loss is not easy to sustain, insulin sensitising agents such as Metformin have been used in the management of both reproductive and metabolic disturbances. Although it is used by many gynaecologists for this purpose, the efficacy of Metformin in the treatment of subfertility caused by the PCOS is unproven. Its use in patients with impaired glucose tolerance or frank diabetes is not questioned.

There have been over 500 publications on the subject of Metformin since the mid 1990s.[73] Many of these publications have reported improvement in menstrual regularity, ovulation rates and fertility, with and without additional Clomiphene treatment, but, according to Stephen Franks it is "only in the last few years that we have seen adequately powered, double-blinded, randomised controlled studies (RCTs) with the appropriate endpoints".[74]

He goes on to say "Perhaps the most impressive results from the earlier studies, including RCTs, have been reports of increased frequency of menstruation and rates of ovulation amongst women with PCOS, especially in those who were overweight. Indeed an early meta-analysis concluded that this medication was an effective means of management of infertility in PCOS.[75] Results from the most recent, and most definitive, studies, including a very large RCT and an updated meta-analysis have, however, led to rather different conclusions.[76]

Compared with Clomiphene treatment alone, when Metformin was used as an adjunct to Clomiphene treatment, ovulation and pregnancy rates were improved. The live birth rate, however, was unaffected by the addition of Metformin. Whilst Metformin on its own may marginally improve the rate of ovulation compared with placebo, it is not clear whether this effect is independent of attendant weight loss.[77]

There is no clear evidence that Metformin treatment, either alone or in combination with Clomiphene improves fertility in women with PCOS. In conclusion and despite its enormous use, the author states that questions remain about the efficacy of Metformin in the management of women with PCOS. Changes in diet and lifestyle remain the primary choice of management of reproductive and metabolic sequelae in overweight and obese women with PCOS.[78,79,80]

Calcium supplementation

Osteoporotic fractures are frequent in elderly populations, especially in women, and are associated with considerable suffering as well as high healthcare costs. As the population ages the burden of osteoporotic fractures on society will increase in the coming years and the prevention of these fractures is therefore a major public health issue.[81] The importance and optimal level of calcium intake to compensate for skeletal calcium losses and for the prevention of osteoporosis and fractures have been much debated and remain unclear. There is, in fact, considerable debate as to whether calcium supplements are advantageous or even harmful.

There is also debate as to the recommended dose of calcium. The Institute of Medicine in the United States (IOM) released dietary guidelines for calcium earlier in 2011, and their recommended dietary allowance for calcium from a combination of diet plus supplements was set at 1,000 mg a day for adult women until age 50 years and 1,200 mg a day for women older than 50 years of age. There is a wide range of daily calcium recommendations however. For individuals older than 50 years in Britain it is 700 mg,[82] 800 mg in Scandinavia,[83] 1200 mg in the United States,[84] and 1300 mg in Australia and New Zealand.[85]

The IOM also set a tolerable upper intake level of about 2,000 mg a day for women in these age groups because of concern about kidney stones and other health risks when calcium intake is very high. In Zimbabwe and probably in many other hot countries there is a high incidence of kidney stones and this may be increased further by calcium supplements.

The Women's Health Initiative Calcium/Vitamin D Supplementation Study[86] linked calcium supplements to an increased risk for cardiovascular events, vascular calcification and kidney stones while only providing a modest benefit in preserving bone mass and preventing hip fractures. There was a 17 per cent increase in kidney stones; 34 cases per 10,000 per year compared with 29 cases per 10,000 per year in those ladies not on calcium and Vitamin D supplements. The daily dose of the calcium carbonate supplement given was 1,000 milligrams combined with 400 IUs of vitamin D. They concluded that for every 10,000 women treated for one year, two hip fractures would be prevented and five cases of kidney stones would be caused.

Other authors in a reanalysis of the Women's Health Initiative Limited Access Dataset updated the meta-analysis of calcium supplements and cardiovascular risk.[87] They concluded that calcium supplements with or without vitamin D modestly increased the risk of cardiovascular events, especially myocardial infarction, a finding obscured in the WHI Study by the widespread use of personal calcium supplements. They advocated a reassessment of the role of calcium supplements in osteoporosis management.

The same authors had previously reported increases in rates of cardiovascular events in women given calcium supplements.[88,89] The size of this increase is modest, but, because of the widespread use of calcium supplements even small increases in cardiovascular disease incidence may translate to a substantial population burden of disease, particularly in older age groups. Serum calcium concentrations are thought to be positively associated with carotid artery plaque thickness, aortic calcification, incidence of myocardial infarction, and mortality.

A large prospective study from Sweden[90] indicated that even when it comes to bone health, "more is not better" for calcium intake. This was a very large study of more than 61,000 women, followed for 19 years overall. They had a total of more than 14,000 incident fractures and more than 3,800 incident hip fractures.

The study suggested that it was only the women who had the lowest intake of calcium, below about 750 mg a day, who had an increased risk for fracture, and then with increasing intake of calcium, evidence of further benefit for bone health and fracture reduction was very limited.[91] The women who had the highest intake of calcium (above 1,100 mg a day) actually had a hint of increased risk for hip fracture.[92] More moderate levels of calcium intake were best for bone health and more was not better. Nearly every day there are advertisements on the television for calcium supplements advocating a minimum dose of 1,400mg a day. Maybe extra calcium is not necessary and may even be harmful.

The *British National Formulary* states that a number of lifestyle factors affect bone mass. Measures such as ensuring adequate calcium intake in the diet, exercise and abstinence from smoking are likely to have a favourable influence on fracture risk. According to the Formulary, hormone replacement therapy forms the mainstay of osteoporosis prevention and prevention is likely to be the best means of dealing with osteoporosis since the bone structure once lost is only restored with difficulty. Bone mass is rapidly lost however when therapy is discontinued and recent data suggest that prolonged therapy is required if any beneficial effect is to persist into later life. Even, once established, osteoporosis patients may benefit from treatment to preserve bone mass. In post-menopausal women, hormone replacement therapy is the treatment of choice. Other treatments may be useful when hormone replacement therapy is unacceptable or inappropriate.

The value of calcium supplementation itself is therefore controversial. Calcium supplements do not prevent the profound loss of bone mass which occurs at menopause and no controlled study has shown a decrease in fracture rate after treatment with calcium. The American College of Obstetricians and Gynecologists Task Force Report on Hormone Therapy issued in October 2004 stated "To protect their bones, all peri- and postmenopausal woman should be sure to consume 1,200 to 1,500 mg. of calcium per day, a multi-vitamin containing vitamin D, and engage in regular weight bearing exercise such as walking".

If calcium supplements are taken it should be noted that not just "any old calcium" will do. There are many different over-the-counter calcium supplements that have their own pros and cons. For example, calcium carbonate is a supplement that needs to be taken with food because it requires an acidic environment for it to be absorbed. In contrast calcium citrate may be taken at any time of the day.

At the American Society for Bone and Mineral Research 2011 Annual Meeting,[93] Richard Prince, from Perth, Australia, argued that calcium supplementation was safe, effective, and necessary in a society where the majority of people did not get enough calcium. He said that concerns of potential cardiovascular risks related to supplementation were based on somewhat inconclusive data. Portraying an opposing point of view was Roger Francis, from the Institute for Aging and Health at Newcastle University in the United Kingdom. He argued against calcium supplementation and he managed to change more audience members' minds and ultimately prevailed in the debate, earning the society's "Golden Femur" award. An audience survey taken at the beginning and end of the session showed that support for the pro-calcium argument shifted substantially from an overwhelming 80 per cent before the arguments to just 55 per cent after the two debaters' talks. This according to the author showed the eroding of support for calcium supplementation.

Unfortunately many clinicians tend to base their knowledge and practices on "standards of practice" generated by other clinicians; standards that are often at odds with the scientific evidence.[94] In one study 76 per cent of physicians surveyed were aware of the concept of evidence-based practice but only 40 per cent believed that evidence was very applicable to their practice, only 27 percent were familiar with methods of critical literature review, and, faced with a problem, most would consult a colleague rather than the evidence.[95] Clinicians' insufficient knowledge of evidence is compounded by the fact that new information on efficacy and risks keeps emerging. A moving target demands more reading.[96]

Clinicians are also turning to the Internet, where medical chat lines are full of misinformation on efficacy and risks with no control of validity.[97]

When all is said and done however, medical advice and evidence based medicine are of absolutely no consequence whatsoever if people still elect to smoke.

References:

1. Ben Goldacre. Bad Science. Fourth Estate. Harper Collins Publishers. London.2009. Introduction p ix
2. Ibid. Introduction p x.
3. Guyatt GH, Oxman AD, Schünemann HJ, Tugwell P, Knottnerus A. GRADE guidelines: A new series of articles in the Journal of Clinical Epidemiology. J Clin Epidemiol. 2011 Apr:64(4):380-2.
4. Ben Goldacre. Bad Science. Fourth Estate. Harper Collins Publishers. London.2009. Introduction p 42 .
5. Ibid. p105.
6. Looking Back on the Millennium in Medicine. The New England Journal of Medicine. Editorial of January 6th 2000. Vol. 342 No. 1 p 44.
7. Drugs and other treatments to prevent and control nausea and .., http://www.nvp-volumes.org/p1_20.htm (accessed July 22, 2013).
8. Lancet. 2005 May 7-13;365(9471):1657-61.
http://www.sciencedirect.com/science/article/pii/5014067369592969X

9. Richard Warren. A Letter from Sussex Place. Royal College of Obstetricians and Gynaecologists. August 2011.http://www.rcog.org.uk/what-we-do/membership/fellows-members/rcog-scanner/-letter-sussex-place-august-2011 (accessed July 22, 2013).
10. A Letter from Sussex Place - August 2011 | Royal College of .., http://www.rcog.org.uk/what-we-do/membership/fellows-members/rcog-scanner/-letter-sussex-place-august-2011 (accessed July 22, 2013).
11. Richard Warren. A Letter from Sussex Place - August 2011 | Royal College of .., http://www.rcog.org.uk/what-we-do/membership/fellows-members/rcog-scanner/-letter-sussex-place-august-2011 (accessed July 22, 2013).
12. Ibid.
13. M Enkin, M J Kierse, M Renfrew, J Neilson. Effective Care in Pregnancy and Childbirth. Oxford University press, 1989.
14. Ibid.
15. The Cochrane Pregnancy and Childbirth Database. Cochrane Collaboration. web@cochrane.org.
16. "The History of Obstetrics and Gynaecology" by the Michael J O Dowd and Elliot E. Philipp.
The Parthenon publishing group. New York.
London. 1994. p 27.
17. Ibid p 25.
18. Wax J R, Lucas F L, Lamont M, Pinette M G, Cartin A, Blackstone J. Maternal and newborn outcomes in planned home birth vs planned hospital births: a meta-analysis. Am J Obstet Gynecol. 2010;203.
19. College of Obstetrics and Gynecologists. Committee on Obstetric Practice, Committee Opinion. Planned Home Birth. Obstet Gynecol. 2011;117:425-428.
20. Kling, Jim. Medscape Medical News in email correspondence with Eugene Declercq, PhD, Professor of Maternal and Child Health at the Boston University School of Public Health in Massachusetts. Planned home vs hospital birth: A meta-analysis gone wrong .., http://midwifery.ubc.ca/2012/06/12/planned-home-vs-hospital-birth-a-meta-analysis-gone-wrong/ (accessed July 22, 2013).
21. Carl A. Michal, PhD; Patricia A. Janssen, PhD; Saraswathi Vedam, SciD; Eileen K. Hutton, PhD; Ank de Jonge, PhD Planned Home vs Hospital Birth: A Meta-Analysis Gone Wrong Medscape Ob/Gyn & Women's Health © 2011. Posted on April 1st 2011.
22. Planned home vs hospital birth: A meta-analysis gone wrong .., http://midwifery.ubc.ca/2012/06/12/planned-home-vs-hospital-birth-a-meta-analysis-gone-wrong/ (accessed July 22, 2013).
23. Keirse M J. Home birth: gone away, gone astray, and here to stay. Birth. 2010;37:341-346.
24. Gyte G, Newburn M, Mcfarlane A. Critique of a meta-analysis by Wax and colleagues which has claimed that there is a three-times greater risk of neonatal death among babies without congenital anomalies planned to be born at home. July 7, 2010. Available at: http://www.scribd.com/doc/34065092/Critique-of-a-meta-analysis-by-Wax Accessed March 28, 2011.
25. American College of Nurse-Midwives. The American College of Nurse-Midwives expresses concerns with recent AJOG publication on home birth. Available at: http://www.medscape.com/viewarticle/725382 Accessed March 28, 2011.

26. Simkins G. Letter. RE: Maternal and newborn outcomes in planned home birth vs. planned hospital births: a meta-analysis. July 6, 2010. Available at: http://mana.org/pdfs/MANA-Response-AJOG-Article-7-6-2010.pdf.
27. National Association of Certified Professional Midwives. Press release. July 6, 2010. Available at: http://www.nacpm.org/documents/070610-NACPM-Press-Release-Wax-etal.pdf Accessed March 28, 2011.
28. Joe Barber Jr., PhD Medscape Medical News. The Birthplace in England Collaborative Group. Home Birth Adverse Events Rare in Low-Risk Pregnancies published online November 24 in the British Medical Journal.
29. Robert A. Wilson. M. D. "Feminine Forever" 1968. Pocket Book. First Printing Edition. ASIN B000J00XN0.
30 Women's Health Information at Bayside Gynecology, http://baysidegyn.com/health%20information.htm (accessed July 22, 2013).
31. Ibid.
32. Ibid.
33. Fletcher SW, Colditz GA. Failure of estrogen plus progestin therapy for prevention. JAMA 288:366 368, 2002.
34. Writing Group for the Women's Health Initiative Investigators. Risks and benefits of estrogen plus progestin in healthy postmenopausal women: Principal results from the Women's Health Initiative Randomized Controlled Trial. JAMA 288:321 333, 2002.
35. Women's Health Information at Bayside Gynecology, http://baysidegyn.com/health%20information.htm (accessed July 22, 2013).
36. Ibid.
37. Ibid.
38. NIH Asks Participants in Women's Health Initiative Estrogen .., http://www.nhlbi.nih.gov/news/press-releases/2004/nih-asks-participants-in-womens-health-initiative-estrogen-alone-study-to-stop-study-pills-begin-follow-up-phase.html (accessed July 22, 2013).
39. Women's Health Information at Bayside Gynecology, http://baysidegyn.com/health%20information.htm (accessed July 22, 2013).
40. Estrogen-Alone Therapy, http://www.preventivehealthtoday.com/alerts/fda_estrogen-alone_040302.html (accessed July 22, 2013).
41. Ibid.
42. The South African Menopause Society. www. menopause. co.za. ADSA - New guidelines - This will soon be the new home of the .., http://www.adsa.org.za/new-guidelines/ (accessed July 22, 2013).
43. ADSA - New guidelines - This will soon be the new home of the .., http://www.adsa.org.za/new-guidelines/ (accessed July 22, 2013).
44. Ibid.
45. Ibid.
46. Ibid.
47. Ibid.
48. Ibid.
49. Ibid.
50. Menopause: The Journal of The North American Menopause Society. Vol 17, No. 2 pp 245-255. Estrogen and progestogen use in postmenopausal women: 2010 .., http://www.ncbi.nlm.nih.gov/pubmed/20154637 (accessed July 22, 2013).

51. Estrogen, progestogen and cancer. | POGOe - Portal of ..,
http://www.pogoe.org/content/4214 (accessed July 22, 2013).
52. Estrogen and progestogen use in postmenopausal women: 2010 ..,
http://www.ncbi.nlm.nih.gov/pubmed/20154637 (accessed July 22, 2013).
53. Menopause: The Journal of The North American Menopause Society.
2012;19:257-271. Published online.
54. Journal of the American Medical Association (JAMA) 2011:305:1305-1314,
1354-1355
55. T. J. de Villiers, A. Pines, N. Panay, M. Gambacciani, D. F. Archer, R. J. Baber,
S. R. Davis, A. A. Gompel, V. W. Henderson, R. Langer, R. A. Lobo, G. Plu-Bureau,
D. W. Sturdee. Updated 2013 International Menopause Society recommendations on
menopausal hormone therapy and preventive strategies for midlife health. Climacteric
Jun 2013, Vol. 16, No. 3, Pages 316-337.
56.T. J. de Villiers , M. L. S. Gass, C. J. Haines , J. E. Hall , R. A. Lobo , D. D.
Pierroz and M. Rees . Global Consensus Statement on Menopausal Hormone
Therapy.April 2013, Vol. 16, No. 2 , Pages 203-204
(doi:10.3109/13697137.2013.771520).
57. CLIMACTERIC 2013;16:203–204. © 2013 International Menopause Society and
Elsevier Inc. DOI: 10.3109/13697137.2013.771520.
58. Jenny Hope HRT: A wasted decade' How one HRT scare has 'caused thousands of
women 10 years of needless suffering'- IOL Lifestyle | IOL.co.za.
www.iol.co.za/lifestyle/hrt-experts-slam-wasted-decade-1.1314968. Jun 8, 2012.
59. Dr. Paul Offit. Killing Us Softly.The Sense and Nonsense of Alternative
Medicine. Fourth Estate. London. ISBN 978-0-00-749172-8. p 115.
60. Diana B. Petitti, Hormone Replacement Therapy and Heart Disease Prevention.
JAMA. 1998;280(7):650-652. doi: 10.1001/jama.280.7.650.
61. Stram DO, Liu Y, Henderson KD, et al. Age-specific effects of hormone therapy
use on overall mortality and ischemic heart disease mortality among women in the
California Teachers Study. Menopause. 2011;18:253-261.
http://www.medscape.com/viewarticle/738092 Accessed November 15, 2011.
62. Peter Kovacs, MD, PhD. Game Changers in Obstetrics & Gynecology: 2011:
Effects of Hormone Therapy on Mortality and Ischemic Heart Disease. Medscape
Ob/Gyn > Viewpoints. Posted: 11/23/2011
63. Manson JE, Hsia J, Johnson KC, et al. Estrogen plus progestin and the risk of
coronary heart disease. N Engl J Med. 2003;349:523-534.
64. Hemminki E, McPherson K. Impact of postmenopausal hormone therapy on
cardiovascular events and cancer: pooled data from clinical trials. BMJ.
1997;315:149-153.
65. From The North American Menopause Society (NAMS) © 2011 First to Know e-
newsletter released November 22, 2011. http://www.menopause.org/news.aspx
66. Ovarian Disruption and CVD. O'Donnell E, Goodman JM, Harvey PJ.
Cardiovascular consequences of ovarian disruption: a focus on functional
hypothalamic amenorrhea in physically active women. J Clin Endocrinol Metab 2011
Sept 28.
67. T Yoshida,
K. Takahashi , H. Yamatani , K. Takata , H. Kurachi Climacteric 2011;
68. Karim, Roksana MBBS, PhD; Dell, Richard M. MD; Greene, Denise F. RNP,
MS; Mack, Wendy J. PhD; Gallagher, J. Christopher MD; Hodis, Howard N. MD Hip
Fracture in Postmenopausal Women After Cessation of Hormone Therapy.

Menopause. 2011;18(11): 1172-1177. © 2011 The North American Menopause Society Posted: 11/22/2011.
69. Yates J, Barrett-Connor E, Barlas S, Chen YT, Miller PD, Siris ES. Rapid loss of hip fracture protection after estrogen cessation: evidence from the National Osteoporosis Risk Assessment. Obstet Gynecol. 2004 Mar;103(3):440-6.
70. Roksana Karim, Hip Fractures Soar When Hormone Therapy Stops. North American Menopause Society. 21st Annual Meeting: Abstract S-1. Presented October 8, 2010. Fran Lowry reporting for Medscape Medical News.
71. Stephen Franks. Clin Endocrinol. 2011;74(2):148-151.
© 2011 Blackwell Publishing. Institute of Reproductive & Developmental Biology, Imperial College London, Hammersmith Hospital, London, UK. When should an insulin sensitizing agent be used in the .., http://onlinelibrary.wiley.com/doi/10.1111/j.1365-2265.2010.03934.x/full (accessed July 22, 2013).
72. Moran, L.J., Pasquali, R., Teede, H.J. et al. (2009) Treatment of obesity in polycystic ovary syndrome: a position statement of the Androgen Excess and Polycystic Ovary Syndrome Society. Fertility and Sterility, 92, 1966–1982.
73. When should an insulin sensitizing agent be used in the .., http://onlinelibrary.wiley.com/doi/10.1111/j.1365-2265.2010.03934.x/full (accessed July 22, 2013).
74. Lord, J.M., Flight, I.H. & Norman, R.J. (2003) Metformin in polycystic ovary syndrome: systematic review and meta-analysis. BMJ, 327, 951–953. When should an insulin sensitizing agent be used in the .., http://onlinelibrary.wiley.com/doi/10.1111/j.1365-2265.2010.03934.x/full (accessed July 22, 2013).
75. Tang, T., Lord, J.M., Norman, R.J. et al. (2010) Insulin-sensitising drugs (metformin, rosiglitazone, pioglitazone, D-chiro-inositol) for women with polycystic ovary syndrome, oligo amenorrhoea and subfertility. Cochrane Database of Systematic Reviews, Issue 1. Art.No.: CD003053. DOI:10.1002/14651858.
76. Stephen Franks. Clin Endocrinol. 2011;74(2):148-151.
© 2011 Blackwell Publishing. Institute of Reproductive & Developmental Biology, Imperial College London, Hammersmith Hospital, London, UK.
77. When should an insulin sensitizing agent be used in the .., http://onlinelibrary.wiley.com/doi/10.1111/j.1365-2265.2010.03934.x/full (accessed July 22, 2013).
78. Moll, E., Bossuyt, P.M., Korevaar, J.C. et al. (2006) Effect of clomifene citrate plus metformin and clomifene citrate plus placebo on induction of ovulation in women with newly diagnosed polycystic ovary syndrome: randomised double blind clinical trial. BMJ, 332, 1485.
79. Legro, R.S., Barnhart, H.X., Schlaff, W.D. et al. (2007) Clomiphene, metformin, or both for infertility in the polycystic ovary syndrome. New England Journal of Medicine, 356, 551–566.
80. Tang, T., Glanville, J., Hayden, C.J. et al. (2006) Combined lifestyle modification and metformin in obese patients with polycystic ovary syndrome. A randomized, placebo-controlled, double-blind multicentre study. Human Reproduction, 21, 80–89. When should an insulin sensitizing agent be used in the .., http://onlinelibrary.wiley.com/doi/10.1111/j.1365-2265.2010.03934.x/full (accessed July 22, 2013).

81. Cashman KD. Diet, nutrition, and bone health. J Nutr 2007;137(suppl 11):2507-12S. High Calcium Intake No Better for Bone Health - full text pdf .., http://www.natap.org/2011/HIV/052511_03.htm (accessed July 22, 2013).
82. NHS Choices. Vitamins and minerals: calcium. www.nhs.uk/conditions/vitamins-minerals/pages/calcium.aspx
83. Anonymous. Nordic nutrition recommendations 2004. Integrating nutrition and physical activity. 4th ed. Nordic Council of Ministers, 2004.
84. Yates AA, Schlicker SA, Suitor CW. Dietary reference intakes: the new basis for recommendations for calcium and related nutrients, B vitamins, and choline. J Am Diet Assoc 1998;98:699-706.
85. Department of Health and Ageing (Australia), National Health and Medical Research Council (Australia), Ministry of Health (New Zealand). Nutrient reference values for Australia and New Zealand, including recommended dietary intakes. 2006. www.nhmrc.gov.au/_files_nhmrc/file/publications/synopses/n35. High Calcium Intake No Better for Bone Health - full text pdf .., http://www.natap.org/2011/HIV/052511_03.htm (accessed July 22, 2013).
86. The Women's Health Initiative Trial of the Effect of Calcium Plus Vitamin D Supplementation on Risk of Fractures and Colorectal Cancer. The New England Journal of Medicine. 16th February 2006. Calcium and Vitamin D Supplements: Still Modestly Beneficial .., http://www.albertfuchs.com/blog/?p=14 (accessed July 22, 2013).
87. Bolland M. J., Andrew Grey; Alison Avenell; Greg D Gamble; Ian R Reid. Calcium Supplements With or Without Vitamin D and Risk of Cardiovascular Events. British Medical Journal. Posted: 05/10/2011; BMJ 2011; 342:d1473.
88. Bolland M. J., Barber, P. A., Doughty R. N., Mason B., Horne A., Ames R. et al. Vascular events in healthy older women receiving calcium supplementation: randomised controlled trial. BMJ 2008;336:262-6.
89. Bolland M. J., Avenell A, Baron J A, Grey A, MacLennan G S, Gamble GD, et al. Effect of calcium supplements on risk of myocardial infarction and cardiovascular events: meta-analysis. BMJ 2010;341:c3691.
90. Eva Warensjö; Liisa Byberg; Håkan Melhus; Rolf Gedeborg; Hans Mallmin; Alicja Wolk; Karl Michaëlsson. Dietary Calcium Intake and Risk of Fracture and Osteoporosis. BMJ 2011; 342:d1473.
BMJ 316: 365–66.Study spanned 19 years for less calcium supplement .., http://www.inspire.com/groups/national-osteoporosis-foundation/discussion/study-spanned-19-years-for-less-calcium-supplement/ (accessed July 22, 2013).
91. Study spanned 19 years for less calcium supplement .., http://www.inspire.com/groups/national-osteoporosis-foundation/discussion/study-spanned-19-years-for-less-calcium-supplement/ (accessed July 22, 2013).
92. Ibid.
93. Nancy A. Melville. Medscape Medical News. The American Society for Bone and Mineral Research. Annual Meeting. September 19, 2011 (San Diego, California).
94. Wagner, M. 1998. The public health versus clinical approach to maternity services: the emperor has no clothes. J Public Health Policy 19: 25–35. Choosing Caesarean Section - by Marsden Wagner, MD, http://www.midwiferytoday.com/articles/ChoosingCaesarean.asp (accessed July 22, 2013).
95. Olatunbosun, O.A., Edouard, L. & Pierson, R.A. 1998. British physicians' attitudes to evidence based obstetric practice.
96. Choosing Caesarean Section - by Marsden Wagner, MD, http://www.midwiferytoday.com/articles/ChoosingCaesarean.asp (accessed July 22, 2013).
97. Ibid.

CHAPTER THIRTEEN - CHANGE

Kenneth Walker in his book *The Story of Medicine*[1] states that one of the lessons of watching the slow growth of medical theories is that no medical discovery can ever be made until the world is ready to receive it. A striking example of this was the "germ theory of disease". The Italian nobleman Fracastoro first formulated this theory during the middle ages but it was looked upon at that time as being nothing more than a fantastic dream in the mind of a poet. Several centuries had to elapse before Leeuwenhoek and Pasteur helped Fracastoro's idea to be considered as a possible approximation to the truth. A theory, like a man of destiny, must make its entry at the right psychological moment if it is to be accepted. Timing is everything.

As I write this in 2013, change is the "buzz word" in politics. In Britain, in the Middle East and in many other parts of the world, change is happening. It should also be the "buzz word" in medicine but medicine lingers behind politics and business. Marcus Aurelius in *Meditations*, advocated change and he died in AD 180! He said: "We shrink from change; yet is there anything that can come into being without it?[2] What does nature hold dearer, or more proper to herself? Could you have a hot bath unless the firewood underwent some change? Could you be nourished if the food suffered no change? Is it possible for any useful thing to be achieved without change? Do you not see then, that change in yourself is of the same order, and no less necessary in nature?"

A colleague in Bahrain told me his definition of "Change". He said "It is a natural, inevitable, constant, dynamic, and sometimes assisted process during which there is alteration or transformation to something different, or substitution of one thing for another, or passing from one stage to another".

The Royal College of Obstetricians and Gynaecologists in the United Kingdom, in mid 2011, published a report "High Quality Women's Health Care: A proposal for change". They said that the move to reform the National Health Service and the financial and workforce pressures faced, meant that urgent change was needed. This was set against the backdrop of the rise in the birth rate, increasing complexity of cases and an ageing population. Their motives, in publishing the report, were to "drive up quality and improve outcomes". For this to happen, they said "radical change is needed", including finding different ways of working.

Change, however, should never be undertaken merely for the sake of change. The process of change may induce feelings of tension and anxiety or even fear. Change involves the risk of loss of identity or of producing emotions of denial, anger or depression. Resistance to change, that is to say, opposing, obstructing, or blocking movement in the change process is either active or passive. It may be active by refusing, opposing or attacking the proposed change or it may be passive by avoidance, delay, apathy, silence or detachment from the proposed change

On the other hand there may be a sense of need to change, a feeling of hope, a search for something better, acceptance and the positivity of adjustment. New goals may be set. There may be a renewed commitment to these goals. A beneficial change in behaviour may result.

Change also needs to be followed by periods of stability and consolidation. If change is rapid, equilibrium must be restored before one can move ahead again. After change too, there will be feedback, whether positive or negative, and this will bring further ideas, needs, and renewal of the process. In business, once a change has been made a PDCA (plan–do–check–act) is often used to assess the effects of the change. PDCA was made popular by Dr. W. Edwards Deming[3] who is considered by many to be the father of modern quality control; however he always referred to it as the "Shewhart cycle" after Walter Andrew Shewhart. It is known as either the Deming or the Shewhart cycle.[4,5,6] It is a successive cycle which begins as a small sample to test potential effects on processes but then gradually leads to larger and more targeted change. Later in Deming's career, he modified PDCA to "Plan, Do, Study, Act" (PDSA) so as better to describe his recommendations.

The concept of PDCA is based on the scientific method, as developed from the work of Francis Bacon (Novum Organum, 1620).[7] The scientific method can be written as "hypothesis"–"experiment"–"evaluation" or plan, do and check. A fundamental principle of the scientific method and PDSA is iteration - once a hypothesis is confirmed (or negated), executing the cycle again will extend the knowledge further. PDCA should be repeatedly implemented in spirals of increasing knowledge of the system that lead to the ultimate goal, each cycle closer than the previous.[8] With the improved knowledge after each cycle the goal may be refined or altered.

The work of Dr Joseph Juran is well known to most quality scholars. With a starting salary of $27 per week he worked at the Western Electric Hawthorne plant in Cicero, Illinois, USA, from 1924 to 1941. There, he was influenced by Shewhart and Deming. The three are considered to be the key founders of the quality improvement movement.

Mark Best and Duncan Neuhauser[9] described Juran's contributions to management and his attempts to overcome resistance to change. Amongst other contributions Juran described the Pareto Chart and the Juran Trilogy. The Pareto Chart is named after the 19th century Italian economist, Vilfredo Pareto. Pareto stated that 80 per cent of the wealth of the country was held by approximately 20 per cent of the population. In 1937, Juran stated that this principle also applied to defects, so that 80 per cent of the problems are caused by 20 per cent of the defects, which meant that if you focused on that 20 per cent, you could have a big effect with minimal effort. Juran called this the Pareto Principle. The Pareto chart is used to prioritise problems or processes that require an input of resources to improve. It separates the "vital few" from the "useful many".

Less well known, but described by Best and Neuhauser, is that half a block away from the Hawthorne plant in Cicero, Illinois, on 22nd Street was the headquarters of Al Capone's gang. Capone was the most famous of America's prohibition gangsters. He helped give Chicago the reputation it holds to this day. Juran remembered reports of rival gang members driving down 22nd Street passing the Hawthorne buildings with guns blazing as they battled for criminal supremacy. At Capone's nearby gambling establishment, "The Shop", Juran observed that one of Capone's workers was so inept and so repetitive in running the roulette wheel that Juran collected and analysed data about this dealer's behaviour and was able to win $100 as a result. In those days $100 was equal to several weeks of Juran's pay.[10] Juran was wise enough not to win too much, to avoid the close attention of Capone's thugs.

The Juran trilogy linked finance and management to quality improvement. The three trilogy components[11] were quality planning, quality control and quality improvement. Juran saw "organisational inertia" as a major obstacle to change. He viewed resistance to change as taking place in the context of cultural resistance. Change had to be tailored to the values, norms and customs of the organisation. He felt that overcoming cultural resistance in organisations was the key to making quality management philosophy and principles work by allowing implementation and practice.

Juran also stated in his memoirs: "To those whose careers are in the field of managing for quality, thank your lucky stars. Your field will grow extensively during your lifetime, especially in three of our giant industries - health, education and government. There will be exciting opportunities for innovation and service to society."[12] It is interesting that he mentioned health.

Are doctors prepared to accept these exciting opportunities for innovation? Are doctors prepared to change? Charles D. Shaw wrote an editorial in the *International Journal for Quality in Health Care* titled; "Changing Clinical Practice and Perceptions".[13] In this editorial he praised the Leeds University Maternity Audit Project[14] for throwing "new light" on the complexity of change. The Audit Project identified four accessible markers of compliance – with available evidence-based guidelines and applied them to existing records in 20 maternity units in the United Kingdom in 1988 (before the evidence was widely published) and again in 1996 to show how practice had changed. There was a massive and appropriate shift in clinical practice but there were also notable pockets of resistance. Donald Berwick has said that "It is usually easier to defend the status quo than to change it, and in this lies the dominant professional response".

The authors of the Audit Project gave reasons for the uptake of research findings as well as for the resistance. Since April 1991, all hospital doctors in the National Health Service had been required to participate in systematic medical audit.[15,16] Shaw said that Hospitals had set up audit committees, appointed audit assistants, and organised audit meetings. Some professional associations and Royal Colleges provided training and guidelines on clinical practice and audit. The *British Medical Journal* ran a regular section on "how to do it"; doctors were given the opportunity, the incentives, and the instructions to audit systematically and to improve their own performance against valid published criteria. These were among the reasons for the uptake of the research findings. The resistance was not associated with aversion to the published guidelines. Most respondents thought they were a "good thing" but, according to Shaw, at least three essential elements were missing at that time. "Firstly doctors did not know how to compare patterns of practice against standards: the use of evidence, guidelines, audit, and measurement were not taught in medical school, in speciality training or in the working environment. Secondly, the power of systematic reviews and meta-analysis had yet to illuminate many contentious areas of clinical practice. Thirdly, the extent and mechanisms of doctor's accountability to the public and to managers was unclear both ethically and legally. The public inquiry into paediatric surgery in Bristol[17] documented many of the failings of medical audit and management in the early 1990s, and pointed out that these were not unique to Bristol or to cardiac surgery, or even to that era; most of its messages could be usefully considered in any country, any town and any speciality".

A major change since 1996 was that health service managers, regardless of their professional background were held statutorily accountable not only for finance but also for clinical performance.[18] Another was the development of guideline methodology and dissemination, especially electronically, in the National Health Service in Britain and worldwide. Shaw concluded that maybe these changes, combined with the passage of time, would overcome the pockets of resistance. In an ideal world, he said, the findings from the Leeds University Maternity Audit Project would sound clarion alarms and pose questions in every maternity unit: "Do we have local guidelines on these four topics? Are they consistent with current evidence? When did we last audit our performance against them? How would we score now, or in 1996, or in 1985? And for those who are not in the regular business of babies, what are the equivalent markers of our compliance with best practice? Routine examination of diabetic feet, hand-cleansing between patients, timely thrombolytics in myocardial infarction, prophylactic anticoagulation in surgery. The maternity study is a good example of a simple criterion-based audit, using data culled by non-clinicians from existing records to quantify current practice in common conditions against evidence-based standards; and the next step, delegated to whoever reads this, is to define and implement an action plan, and repeat the audit to demonstrate the improvement". Shades of the PDSA cycle.

Shaw then deviated a little from his praise for the Maternity Audit Project to criticise the media. He quoted a report about the same paper on the Leeds study published in a national Sunday broadsheet newspaper.[19] "Birth ward errors kill 200 babies: overstretched doctors and midwives are providing substandard care, admits official report" were the headlines that drew his anger. He suggested that perhaps one way medicine can build the public faith in health care and the doctors own faith in quality improvement is to celebrate achievements, rather than "bemoan the residual bad apples, tail-enders, and outliers. He pointed out that in 1985, in the 20 maternity units described in the article, the median value for giving steroids to pre term babies was zero but by 1996 it had risen to 82%, reducing mortality for those treated from 18 to 7.2%; If all pre term babies had been treated, a further 200 would have been saved". He pointed out that the *Observer,* rather than saying "Birth ward errors kill 200 babies" could have said, "shift in practice saves 850 babies a year; improvements following introduction of evidence-based guidelines and clinical audit are set to continue".

The press in the United Kingdom have a lot to answer for. The "hacking" scandal is in the news. *The News of the World* is now no more and I have just observed a journalist informing viewers of *Sky News* that it is justifiable to pay policemen for information!

Medicine has changed even in the limited time that I have been a doctor. Mike Standish-White an orthopaedic colleagues of ours once told me the story of the 30 year old medical registrar who complained that his 60 year old consultant never listened to him. He wrote a letter and lodged it with his bank manager to remind him when he reached 60 years not to do the same. On reading the letter 30 years later he remarked that people of 30 years of age wrote remarkable rubbish.

When I first entered private practice the doctor would never charge a fellow doctor's family or a nurse he might have treated. Doctors and nurses had an altruistic attitude and financial matters were relegated to the back burner. Medicine was not a business like it is today. This has been brought about largely by the Medical Insurance companies. It must be remembered that these are insurance companies and their primary interest, unlike doctors and nurses, is to provide financial insurance for the patients. The doctor's primary interest, on the other hand, is to provide a service for his or her patient and financial rewards are secondary. A very good friend of mine, Dr. Cahi needed to have an operation in a clinic in Johannesburg. On the morning he was due to be discharged from the clinic the matron told him that he would not be charged for his treatment. She explained that he had obviously helped many people in Rhodesia and Zimbabwe and had refused payment from them. They wanted to do the same. This was a very kind gesture for the clinic to make. It is not commonly known that many doctors see patients and treat them without charging. Doctors are not allowed to advertise these facts but I have seen it on numerous occasions. Obviously you do get some doctors who are very mercenary. When Fiona, my wife, consulted a general surgeon in London he charged us £180. I have never charged a fellow doctor's wife. Unlike the managerial staff of big conglomerates doctors do not get too many perks but treating one's colleagues and their families free is one I would like to see continue. An orthopaedic colleague of mine in Harare charged me £4,000 to repair my torn Achilles tendon. Yes, £4,000. I have not erred in the number of noughts.

My own vision of medical practice would be to have something like, what I call the "Robin Hood" effect. Some sort of equitable arrangement should be found where the wealthier subsidise the treatment for the poorer. At Groote Schuur Hospital in Cape Town in 1965, when I qualified, the two main medical wards were A1 and A5. These were divided on racial grounds at the time but patients received equal treatment regardless of their colour. They were seen by the same doctors, received the same excellent nursing care, underwent the same laboratory and other investigations and there was no preferential drug or other treatment. A similar arrangement but this time on a financial rather than racial basis might work. Unfortunately the idea of a "means test" is not socially acceptable as it is deemed not to be "politically correct".

Duke Khuu, writing in *Dermatology*[20] outlined some issues that might be useful to doctors running their own practice. The first was efficient staff. Friendly, reliable, and resourceful staff was a must. The second issue was choosing the right billing infrastructure. He said that insurance companies and their "games" are a nightmare. I have always believed that to be successful in private medical practice one has to adhere to the principle of the four A's of private practice. These are Ability, Affability, Availability and Affordability. One does not necessarily need "the right billing structure".

Are we changing in medicine? Do we really need to change? Should doctors become involved in politics? A few facts of life:

1.2 billion people across the world are hungry. Seven out of ten of them are women and girls. Millions of children start school but eventually drop out leaving school without basic literacy and numeracy skills.[21]

Women hold 18 per cent of seats in parliament in the UK. On Sky news on the 26th September 2011 it was reported that Saudi Arabia was giving the vote to women for the very first time but they will still not be allowed to drive.

Every year, 536,000 women and girls die as a result of complications of pregnancy.[22] Ninety-nine per cent of them occur in developing countries. Two thirds of people living with HIV are in sub-Saharan Africa. Most of them are women. 1.2 billion people lack access to basic sanitation. The vast majority of them live in rural areas. Aid to the poorest countries falls far short of the 2010 target.

If the causes of such illnesses as malnutrition, rheumatic fever and tuberculosis are political then, according to Chris Ellis, the treatment must be political.[23] Should doctors try to promote individual and collective methods of improving the patient's health by socio political means. We do not have to encourage protest marches but we could teach increased awareness and educate doctors in orthodox socio political activity with the sole purpose being to help patients. According to Ellis there are several arguments against the medical profession taking a political role even in this limited way. The first is that it is not a legitimate area for us to be in and does not concern us by tradition or profession. He then says that this is not strictly true. The early medical professions and traditional healers in many societies had political roles in addition to the medical ones. Another argument, he says, comes from the "grain of sand" school. This is based on the feeling that we are but a grain of sand on the beach. It is a sense of powerlessness. An individual doctor's work does not affect society. This is not strictly true either. Many thousands of doctors treating patients on a one to one basis do have an effect. We can, should and do educate the public and politicians on health matters. One of the original roles of the "Doctor" comes from the Latin *docere,* to teach. Can we teach others to change? Can we effect change ourselves by doing so?

In the preparation for the International Conference on Population and Development (Cairo 1994), an alliance of women's groups (Women's Voices 1994) prepared a list of reproductive health principles[24] which included; Women must be subjects not objects, of any development policy; Population policies must be based on the principle of respect for the sexual and bodily integrity of girls and women; Women have a right to information and services; Men also have a personal and social responsibility for their own sexual behaviour; Sexual and social relationships between women and men must be governed by principles of equality, non-coercion, mutual respect and responsibility; Fundamental sexual and reproductive rights of women cannot be subordinated, against a woman's will, to the interest of partners and family members. This list preceded the Millenium Declaration. This Declaration, endorsed by 189 world leaders at the United Nations in September 2000, is a commitment to work together to build a safer, more prosperous and equitable world.[25]

The Declaration set out eight time-bound and measurable goals to be achieved by 2015. Known as the Millennium Development Goals (MDGs) they are supposed to provide concrete, numerical benchmarks for tackling extreme poverty in its many dimensions. The MDGs provide a framework for the entire international community to work together towards a common end, making sure that human development reaches everyone, everywhere. If these goals are achieved, world poverty will be cut by half, tens of millions of lives will be saved, and billions more people will have the opportunity to benefit from the global economy.

The eight listed goals[26] are to eradicate extreme poverty and hunger, to achieve universal primary education, to promote gender equality and empower women, to reduce child mortality, to improve maternal health, to combat HIV/AIDS, malaria and other diseases, to ensure environmental sustainability and to develop a global partnership for development.

A decade after the Millennium Declaration, there have been noticeable reductions in poverty globally,[27] significant improvements in enrolment and gender parity in schools, reductions in child and maternal mortality and increasing HIV treatments. Steps have been taken towards ensuring environmental sustainability and developing countries are incorporating the goals into their development strategies. Despite this the challenges facing the goals are numerous. While the share of poor people is declining, the absolute number of the poor in South Asia and in sub-Saharan Africa is increasing.[28]

Rapid reductions in poverty are not necessarily addressing gender equality and environmental sustainability. Lack of progress in reducing HIV is curtailing improvements in both maternal and child mortality. The expansion of health and education services is not being matched by quality.

Progress towards the MDGs is also threatened by the combination of high food prices and the impact of the international financial and economic crisis.[29] Sustained poverty and hunger reduction is at risk because of vulnerability to climate change, particularly in the area of agricultural production. Weak institutional capacity in conflict and post-conflict countries also slows MDG progress, and rapid urbanisation is putting pressure on social services.

Progress across the MDGs is being achieved where strong government leadership, effective policies and institutional capacity for expanding public investments are complemented by financial and technical support from the international community.

The 2010 Millennium Development Goals Summit, ten years after the original Millennium Declaration focussed on the pragmatic steps that can be taken in the next five years, to develop an acceleration framework drawing on the past decade's evidence base.

The Government of Zimbabwe also produced an MDG Status Report in 2010[30] in which they highlighted the. challenges in the attainment of the MDGs in Zimbabwe and provided proposed intervention strategies. According to Robert Mugabe, the Government was determined to realise the Millennium Development Goals by the year 2015.

Of the eight Millennium Development Goals (MDGs), the Government of Zimbabwe identified the eradication of extreme poverty and hunger, the promotion of gender equality and empowerment of women and the combat of HIV/AIDS, malaria and other diseases as their three national priorities. The 2010 report acknowledged that reliable and new data was a major problem in Zimbabwe. Nevertheless it formed the basis of a national "MDG Action Plan" aimed towards accelerating MDG-related achievements in Zimbabwe.

From 2000 to 2008, Zimbabwe's economy had suffered a severe decline. By 2003, the population living below the total consumption poverty line (TCPL) stood at 72 per cent. Estimates in 2010 suggested a figure of up to 80 per cent Notwithstanding the poor performance of the economy, Zimbabwe had been able to make significant progress in a number of key areas of the MDGs, such as universal primary education and a gradual decline in HIV and AIDS. Unemployment and under-employment remained a persistent challenge.

Zimbabwe, once the food basket for the southern African region, became a net importer of food and Zimbabwe is unlikely to meet the proposed target of eradication of extreme poverty and hunger by 2015.

The MDG Status Report of 2010 felt that it was possible for Zimbabwe to attain universal primary education by 2015. They felt that the target of increasing the participation of women in decision-making in all sectors, and at all levels, to 50:50 by 2015 was seriously "off-track " and would be difficult to achieve. It was also unlikely that the under-five mortality rate would be reduced by the target of two-thirds, before 2015. The provision of a safe water supply and good sanitation are major contributory factors to positive childcare. At present, Zimbabwe is unable to provide clean water for all rural and urban areas. Of the total population, 33 per cent still rely on the bush toilet for sanitation.[31]

The maternal mortality ratio (MMR) has worsened significantly over the past 20 years, the leading cause being AIDS related illnesses. Despite this only 5.4 per cent of pregnant women in Zimbabwe know their HIV status before pregnancy, and just 34% of pregnant women were tested for HIV during pregnancy. The MDG target is to reduce the maternal mortality ratio by three-quarters between1990 and 2015 but it is unlikely that Zimbabwe will meet this target as the capacity of the healthcare system has deteriorated significantly. The proportion of births attended by skilled health personnel has also fallen over the past 20 years. The target aimed at is universal access to skilled attendance at delivery by 2015.[32]

A real positive is that, according to the MDG Status Report, the target set for universal access to contraception is likely to be achieved by 2015. Zimbabwe has continued to register a gradual decline in HIV prevalence. The decline has been attributed to behaviour change, including delayed sexual debut, decrease in the number of sexual partners, and increased condom use. Similar declines are evident in the HIV prevalence rate for pregnant women. These trends show that great achievements have been made in this area and indicate that Zimbabwe is likely to attain the MDG target of 9 per cent for HIV prevalence in pregnant women aged between 15 and 24 by 2015.

Malaria was the third leading cause of hospital admissions in Zimbabwe in 2009.[33] Controlling malaria is one of the government's main priorities. In 2000, the Government of Zimbabwe signed the Abuja Declaration, agreeing to try to meet the target of reducing malaria cases by 50 per cent between 2000 and 2010, and by 75 per cent by 2015.[34] The incidence of malaria in Zimbabwe has been in decline since 2005. According to the Abuja targets, Zimbabwe was aiming for an incidence rate of 68 per 1,000 by 2010, a rate the country has already achieved.

Zimbabwe currently ranks 17th out of the world's 22 high-burden tuberculosis countries.Its tuberculosis incidence rates significantly increased during the last decade, rising from 97 per 100,000 people in 2000 to 411 per 100,000 people in 2004 and to 782 per 100,000 in 2007.[35] This increase is attributed to the high incidence of HIV and AIDS and it is estimated that 72 per cent of all tuberculosis patients are co-infected with HIV.

Zimbabwe has experienced several cholera out-breaks since the early 1970s, but since 1998, cholera has become a yearly occurrence.[36] While previous outbreaks were relatively quickly contained by emergency approaches supported by a sound health delivery system, the most recent outbreak was the severest on record. The breakdown of medical services and poor maintenance of water and sanitation infrastructure provides a major challenge towards halting and reversing the incidence of diarrhoeal diseases by 2015. In addition to the cholera, a recent outbreak of typhoid indicated the continued challenges to the provision of clean water and good sanitation, especially in high-density urban areas. There is also a shortage of essential medicines and equipment for treatment. Cholera and other diarrhoeal disease outbreaks will continue to occur until the water and sanitation situation improves. Both urban and rural areas are now at risk.

As the economic crisis in Zimbabwe deepened between 2000 and 2008 a significant proportion of the population was forced to rely more heavily on natural resources for their livelihood.[37]

These resources included firewood, bush meat, traditional medicines, and wild fruits and vegetables, and caused biodiversity loss. The sporadic power cuts that began in 2007, coupled with inaccessibility of paraffin (the main energy source for low-income urban-dwellers), led to significant deforestation, particularly in peri-urban areas. Estimates suggest that between 100,000 and 320,000 hectares of forest cover per annum were lost during this time.

References:

1. Kenneth Walker. The Story of Medicine. Arrow Books. London. 1959. P15.
2. Quotes on It Is The Right Thing To Do :: Finest Quotes, http://www.finestquotes.com/quotes/on/It_Is_The_Right_Thing_To_Do/6 (accessed July 23, 2013).

3. PDCA - Wikipedia, the free encyclopedia, http://en.wikipedia.org/wiki/Demming_cycle (accessed July 23, 2013).
4. Shewhart, Walter Andrew (1939). Statistical Method from the Viewpoint of Quality Control. New York: Dover. ISBN 0-486-65232-7.
5. Deming, W. Edwards (1986). Out of the Crisis. MIT Center for Advanced Engineering Study. ISBN 0-911379-01-0.
6. Shewhart, Walter Andrew (1980). Economic Control of Quality of Manufactured Product/50th Anniversary Commemorative Issue. American Society for Quality. ISBN 0-87389-076-0. PDCA Term Definition - Manufacturing Terms, http://www.manufacturingterms.com/PDCA.html (accessed July 23, 2013).
7. SIP Project for MDL - Amit - Scribd, http://www.scribd.com/doc/21575115/SIP-Project-for-MDL-Amit (accessed July 23, 2013).
8. PDCA Term Definition - Manufacturing Terms, http://www.manufacturingterms.com/PDCA.html (accessed July 23, 2013).
9. Best M and Neuhauser, D. Joseph Juran: Overcoming Resistance to Organisational Change. Qual Saf Health Care 2006;15:380-382 doi:10.1136/qshc.2006.020016
10. Stephen AB, Orville BR. Manufacturing the future: a history of western electric. Cambridge: Cambridge University Press, 1999:161.
11. Juran Institute. www.juran.com. UpFront: The Legacy of J.M. Juran, http://asq.org/quality-progress/2008/04/basic-quality/upfront-the-legacy-of-jm-juran.html (accessed July 23, 2013).
12. Juran JM. Architect of quality: the autobiography of Dr. Joseph M. Juran. New York: McGraw-Hill, 2003.
13. Shaw, Charles D. International Journal for Quality in Health Care. Editorial. 2002. Vol. 14. No 3. p 173.
14. Wilson R, Thornton J G, Hewison J et al. The Leeds University Maternity Audit Project. Int. J. Qual. Health Care 2002; 14: 175-181.
15. Department of Health, Medical Audit in the Hospital and Community Health Services. Health Care (91)2. London. Department of Health 1991.
16. Health Circular Resulting from the Government White Paper "Working for patients: London. HMSO. 1989.
17. The Bristol Royal Infirmary Inquiry (proceedings, submissions and report), UK: http://www.bristol-inquiry.org.uk. Accessed 15 March 2002.
18. Health Bill, 1999. London, UK: http:///www.hmso.gov.uk/legislation.
19. Ahmed K. Birth ward errors kill 200 babies. The Observer 2002. 24 February p.7
20. The new era of private practice. Duke Khuu, MD, Dermatology, General, 02:57AM Jan 31, 2011. Board Certified Dermatologist, Khuu Dermatology, California.
21. Seattle U.N. association looks at development goals .., http://crosscut.com/2010/10/21/social-services/20271/Seattle-UN-association-looks-at-development-goals/ (accessed July 23, 2013).
22. Seattle U.N. association looks at development goals .., http://crosscut.com/2010/10/21/social-services/20271/Seattle-UN-association-looks-at-development-goals/ (accessed July 23, 2013).
23. Chris Ellis. The Soft Edges Of Family Practice. Premier book publishers (Pty) Ltd. Sloane Park 2152. South Africa p 61.
24. WOMEN'S DECLARATION ON POPULATION POLICIES, http://www.users.interport.net/i/w/iwhc/wd.html (accessed July 23, 2013).

25. Millennium Development Goals (MDGs)- All You Need To Know, http://www.naijafinder.com/threads/675813-Millennium-Development-Goals-(MDGs)-All-You-Need-To-Know (accessed July 23, 2013).
26. WHO | Millennium Development Goals (MDGs), http://www.who.int/topics/millennium_development_goals/about/en/index.html (accessed July 23, 2013).
27. Millennium Development Goals (MDGs)- All You Need To Know, http://www.naijafinder.com/threads/675813-Millennium-Development-Goals-(MDGs)-All-You-Need-To-Know (accessed July 23, 2013).
28. Diocese of Bath and Wells | Reflection and sharing, http://www.bathandwells.org.uk/faithandmission/reflection-and-sharing/ (accessed July 23, 2013).
29. Ibid.
30. 2010. Millennium Development Goals Status Report. Zimbabwe. UNDP-MDG-report. 17/9/10
31. MILLENNIU M MILLENNIUM DEVELOPMENT GOALS - UN in Zimbabwe http://www.zw.one.un.org/sites/default/files/Zimbabwe%20MDGR%20%202010.pdf (accessed July 23, 2013).
32. Ibid.
33. Ibid.
34. WHO, Malaria Report, 2009. MILLENNIU M MILLENNIUM DEVELOPMENT GOALS - UN in Zimbabwe .., http://www.zw.one.un.org/sites/default/files/Zimbabwe%20MDGR%20%202010.pdf (accessed July 23, 2013).
35. WHO, Global Tuberculosis Control: Surveillance, Planning, Financing, 2009 WHO/HTM/ TB/2009.411).
36. MILLENNIU M MILLENNIUM DEVELOPMENT GOALS - UN in Zimbabwe http://www.zw.one.un.org/sites/default/files/Zimbabwe%20MDGR%20%202010.pdf (accessed July 23, 2013).
37. Goal 7 - Ensure Environmental Sustainability - UNDP Zimbabwe, http://www.undp.org.zw/millennium-development-goals/goal-even-environmental-sustainability?3a1ed061a28f8a5e62fd4865066ea7fa= (accessed July 23, 2013).

CHAPTER FOURTEEN – MANAGEMENT

Quality has many definitions. The electrical company Philips defined it in 1994 as "Quality is when the customer comes back, not the product". Zink, in 1993, defined it as: "Quality is the fulfilment of (agreed) requirements to the customer's lasting satisfaction" and Thender Heuss in 1962 defined it as "Quality is simply what is right and decent".

Abraham Maslow described five hierarchical levels of needs. The lowest was basic needs, food and shelter and the highest was self esteem and self actualisation. In the last century doctors have seen their status and level of hierarchical need fall from the highest level of self actualisation to the lowest of basic physiological needs. This "Maslowian fall" is a result of increasing scarcity of funding, inadequate resourcing, greater accountability, litigation awareness and general "malaise" within the profession. Physicians must now see themselves as a part of the solution and not just a part of the problem. We must put the "WOW" factor back into medicine; but how?

We have to change. Medicine has to learn management principles from industry. Glenn Laffel and David Blumenthal[1], as long ago as in 1989, published an inspiring article titled "The Case for Using Industrial Quality Management Science in Health Care Organisations". I recommend this paper to anyone involved in management in medicine. Their conclusion stated: "The focus of most quality assurance programs in health care remains the technical expertise and interpersonal skills of physicians. Their ability to mobilise the resources of complex health care organisations remains unassessed. Health care organisations themselves contribute to overall quality in ways that have yet to be measured. In addition, regulatory and legal demands to define standards of care encourage or force physicians to pursue conformance rather than the possibility that continuous improvement is possible. Industrial quality science appears to offer solutions to these conceptual problems. It includes the use of statistics to analyse production and service provision processes. It is based on the assumption that employees and top leadership, should continuously strive to improve these processes. It stresses interdepartmental cooperation, training and experimentation. These techniques have been associated with improved product quality in many Japanese and American industries, but they have yet to be widely implemented in health care. It is an appropriate time for the health care industry to begin experimentation with these techniques."

The traditional approach to quality in medicine has been that of measuring the performance of the individual caregiver involved and ensuring that the performance conforms to set standards. When standards are not met we try to improve that performance. The contributions of other non-physicians and organisational processes generally may not be considered. Healthcare administrators and physicians must now consider the involvement in patient care of many other stakeholders other than the individual. Other family members, funders of healthcare, referring doctors, laboratories, ancillary staff, X-ray departments and a multitude of other services must all be considered as part of a process although the patient, of course, remains paramount. In medicine "process" refers to the "set of activities that go on within and between practitioners and patients." Any event or process over which the physician may or may not have control may be involved. Until now most health care organisations do not routinely analyse the performance of such processes. They still search for the "rotten apples" in the theory of that name. In those organisations that do, the process may be perceived to be less important than evaluation of the individual physician's performance. Processes, not individuals, should be the objects of quality improvement.

In industry, continuous performance improvement is recognised as being far preferable to conforming to set standards. Conforming to standards means that some rate of poor outcomes is acceptable. If standards are set too low, according to Laffel and Blumenthal, quality assurance programs may breed complacency and contribute to poor quality. If they are set unrealistically high, they may alienate or frustrate providers. Other aspects of a physician's performance may also have a bearing on quality. His organisational skills, interpersonal relations, attention to detail, or ability to utilise resources may all contribute to the overall quality of care. These facets may be overlooked when only judging the technical expertise of the doctor.

In industrial settings, control charts have been used for 60 years to understand patterns and types of variation and to provide a rational framework on which to formulate and evaluate quality improvement efforts. They must be used more in medicine. In addition to control charts, quality experts recommend a set of managerial principles aimed at improving quality. These principles include continuous improvement of quality, a focus on processes as the objects of improvement, the elimination of unnecessary variation and revised strategies for personnel management. Health care organisations should adopt these principles from industry and pursue an ethic of continuous improvement in the quality of care and service.

The elimination of unnecessary variation in clinical practice may also contribute to the improvement of quality care. Allied health personnel would become familiar with the procedures and protocols that physicians expect them to perform. The lesser quality caused by unnecessary variation in practice is justification to develop consensus about "best practices" and to encourage adherence to these practices.

I had been a consultant obstetrician and gynaecologist for approximately 26 years before I learned anything about management in medicine. It was during my stay in Bahrain that I learned a lot from, of all people, a dentist Zbys Fedorowicz. He introduced me to medical management principles and the names of Shewhart, Deming, Juran, Berwick and others. He stimulated my interest in evidence based medicine, evidence based patient choice, policy and procedure guidelines, change, continuous performance improvement, accreditation and many other management principles especially those applicable to medicine. He stressed the importance of improvement in the quality of healthcare. Zbys taught me a lot and I have attempted to learn many of the principles of management that he outlined to me. I owe him a great deal. I still know very little but I am totally convinced that this is the way that medicine has to go. We have to learn from industry.

Zbys introduced me to the Joint Commission on Accreditation of Healthcare Organizations (JCAHO) now called The Joint Commission (TJC) and the Joint Commission International (JCI). JCAHO and TJC have been at the forefront of patient safety in the United States since JCAHO was established in 1951. Today, it accredits nearly 18,000 hospitals, nursing homes, home health agencies, outpatient clinics, surgery centers, behavioral health programs, laboratories and managed care organizations nationwide.

The Joint Commission (TJC) is a not-for-profit organisation which accredits over 19,000 health care organisations and programs in the United States.[2] In 1910 Ernest Codman, proposed an "end result system of hospital standardisation." Codman proposed that hospitals track patients to determine if treatment was effective. If not, steps could be taken to insure that similar patients in the future would receive improved treatment. The American College of Surgeons (ACS) was founded in 1913 with Codman's system as one of their objectives.[3]

In 1918, the ACS began a process of voluntary hospital, on-site inspections to promote hospital reform and from which the Joint Commission has evolved. The survey process grew over the next thirty years. In 1951, several organisations, including the American Hospital Association, joined with the ACS to create the Joint Commission on Accreditation of Hospitals (JCAH) as a non-profit organisation.[4]

In later years, JCAH became JCAHO, The Joint Commission for the Accreditation of Healthcare Organizations. In 2007, the name was changed again to simply the Joint Commission. Joint Commission International (JCI) was established in 1997 as a division of Joint Commission Resources to improve the quality of patient care by assisting international health care organisations, public health agencies, health ministries and others evaluate, improve and demonstrate the quality of patient care and enhance patient safety in more than 60 countries outside the United States of America.[5]

With the advent of medical tourism, international health care accreditation of hospitals located in countries around the world has increasingly grown in importance. Joint Commission International is one of the groups providing international healthcare accreditation services to hospitals around the world. Accreditation is not cheap. JCI currently accredits hospitals in Asia, Europe, the Middle East and South America[6] and charges an average fee of $46,000 for a full hospital survey[7] in addition to reimbursement for their surveyors' travel, their living expenses and accommodation.

These days, healthcare stakeholders such as purchasers, payers and patients are demanding documentary evidence of efficient high quality care. They are looking to see that hospitals manage costs well, that the patient's are satisfied and that the outcomes are desirable. The Institute of Medicine in the United States has reported that there are 90,000 deaths per annum in the United States due to hospital error!

In the 1980s efforts to measure, assess and improve healthcare received a "jumpstart'. Industry, especially in the United States, had seen increasing competition from overseas, principally Japan. It had moved away from "inspection" to a system of "doing the right thing right first time." Providers of health care followed the examples of industry. They looked to improve outcomes and to survive in an increasingly competitive market.

Many physicians objected to this "managed healthcare". In general physicians assume a leadership role and are not suited to "collaborative work". If they are not involved they probably will not co-operate with implementation or adherence. They may see quality improvement as a managerial function and may be unable to accept that clinical actions are related to processes. Some physicians have what Joseph Juran described as an "immune reaction" to quality improvement even in "normal" organisations. I have heard it said that by opposing quality processes in healthcare physicians may well prove to be the "killer lymphocytes" of the system.

Walter Andrew Shewhart, mentioned in the previous chapter with regard to the Shewhart cycle, was an American physicist, engineer and statistician. Sometimes known as the father of statistical quality control, Shewhart joined the Western Electric Company Inspection Engineering Department at the Hawthorne Works in Illinois in 1918. Engineers had been working to improve the reliability of their transmission systems at Bell's Telephones but because their amplifiers and other equipment had to be buried underground, whenever failures occurred and repairs were needed, considerable time and effort were required to repair them. There was a need to reduce the frequency of failures and repairs. Industrial quality at that time was limited to inspecting finished products and removing defective items. In 1924 Shewhart introduced a schematic control chart.[8] He also pointed out the importance of reducing variation in a manufacturing process and brought about the understanding that continual process-adjustment in reaction to non-conformance actually increased variation and degraded quality. His ideas were accepted with great success. His charts were adopted by the American Society for Testing and Materials (ASTM) in 1933 and advocated to improve production during World War II in American War Standards

Shewhart and Deming met in 1927 and began a long collaboration that involved work on productivity during World War II and led to Deming's championing of Shewhart's ideas in Japan from 1950 onwards.[9]

Deming was an American statistician, professor, author, lecturer and consultant best known for his work in Japan. He made a significant contribution to Japan's later reputation for innovative high-quality products and its economic power.[10] He is regarded as having had more impact upon Japanese manufacturing and business than any other individual not of Japanese heritage. Rafael Aguayo described how Deming's teachings and philosophy were best illustrated by examining the results they produced when they were adopted by Japanese industry. He describes how the Ford Motor Company was simultaneously manufacturing a car model with transmissions made in Japan and the United States.[11] Soon after the car model was on the market, Ford customers were requesting the model with Japanese transmission over the USA-made transmission, and they were willing to wait for the Japanese model.[12]

As both transmissions were made to the same specifications, Ford engineers could not understand the customer preference for the model with Japanese transmission. Finally, Ford engineers decided to take apart the two different transmissions. The American-made car parts were all within specified tolerance levels. On the other hand, the Japanese car parts were virtually identical to each other, and much closer to the nominal values for the parts - e.g., if a part was supposed to be one foot long, plus or minus 1/8 of an inch - then the Japanese parts were all within 1/16 of an inch. This made the Japanese cars run more smoothly and customers experienced fewer problems. Engineers at Ford could not understand how this was done until they met Deming.[13]

Deming taught statistical process control methods to Japanese business leaders, returning to Japan for many years to consult and to witness economic growth that he had predicted would come as a result of application of techniques learned from Walter Shewhart at Bell Laboratories.[14] Deming saw that Shewhart's ideas of statistical control of processes and the related technical tool of the control chart could be applied not only to manufacturing processes but also to the processes by which enterprises are led and managed.[15] This key insight made possible his enormous influence on the economics of the industrialised world after 1950.[16]

Shewhart's idea of common and special causes of variation led directly to Deming's theory of management. The message that Deming gave to Japan's chief executives was that improving quality would reduce expenses while increasing productivity and market share. A number of Japanese manufacturers applied his techniques widely and experienced theretofore unheard-of levels of quality and productivity.[17]

The improved quality combined with the lowered cost created new international demand for Japanese products. In recognition of his contribution to Japan's industrial rebirth and its worldwide success, Deming was awarded Japan's Order of the Sacred Treasure, Second Class in 1960.[18] He was largely unknown and unrecognised in the United States until, in 1980, he was featured prominently in an NBC documentary titled *"If Japan can... Why can't we?* about the increasing industrial competition the United States was facing from Japan. The demand for his services increased dramatically as a result of the broadcast. He continued consulting for industry throughout the world until his death at the age of 93.[19]

Deming's philosophy has been summarised as follows: "Dr. W. Edwards Deming taught that by adopting appropriate principles of management, organizations can increase quality and simultaneously reduce costs (by reducing waste, rework, staff attrition and litigation while increasing customer loyalty). The key is to practice continual improvement and think of manufacturing as a system, not as bits and pieces."[20]

Deming's advocacy of the Plan-Do-Check-Act cycle, his "System of Profound Knowledge" and his "Seven Deadly Diseases" have had tremendous influence outside of manufacturing and have been applied in many other arenas.[21]

He brought about considerable change for the better by these means and they should be used in medicine too. Anyone doubting that change in medicine is necessary should read Deming's "Some Notes on Management in a Hospital".

The "Notes" describe how he was once injured and had to spend several days in hospital.[22] During this time he required a blood transfusion and intensive nursing care. He commented that the *"nurses were working as hard as they could"*. They were well educated, but discouraged and defeated by the broken system they had to work in. Why were registered nurses making beds? The patient's shower was badly designed. Good food was served on cheap plates. Delays were the norm. Treatments given varied from treatment prescribed. Deming recognised that the healthcare system had flaws but did not blame the people working in it. The design of this system to reduce unwanted variation in care could only be improved by a leadership that was obviously lacking.[23] As a patient he saw that the nurses and doctors could not work any harder, but the broken systems they were forced to work in defeated their best efforts and robbed them of joy in work.[24]

Deming relentlessly pursued increased performance and joy in working, criticism of unemployment or underemployment and advocacy of waste reduction. He was one of the first to teach that a system gets the results that it gets due to its design, and that workers in the system are not to blame.[25] Leaders must have a vision and managers must implement the steps necessary for redesigning the system to improve quality, job satisfaction, and reduce waste. Deming stated: "Management's job is to optimise the whole system".

Doctors must change. We must link our professional knowledge with improvement knowledge. Improvements in the healthcare we provide obviously depends on our professional knowledge of the subject be it gynaecology, surgery, ophthalmology, psychiatry or any other speciality.

During the last century this professional knowledge was the driving force behind improvement in healthcare. A second body of knowledge that of improvement knowledge allows us to make more improvement of a different kind. It was first described by Deming as a "system of profound knowledge" and includes knowledge of a system, knowledge of variation and knowledge of psychology.

Knowledge of the organisation as a system entails being able to answer three basic questions.

Related to industry these are how we make what we make, why we make what we make and how we improve what we make? In medicine they may be regarded as how do we do what we do, why do we do what we do and how can we improve what we do?

Knowledge of variation is essential before a system can be improved. Variation is always present. Intended variation is acceptable and merited. Unintended variation is wasteful. It was divided by Deming into common cause and special cause. A certain amount of variation always occurs because of the collective influences of multiple causes. A stable system is said to exist if there is only common cause variation such as the diurnal variation in one's body temperature. When the temperature rises outside the normal range, when caused by an infection for example, this is called special cause variation. Improvement in common cause variation will require a fundamental change in the process.

Improvement of special cause variation requires correction of the "special cause" rather than improvement of the process. Distinguishing the type of variation is critical for quality improvement.

Errors are of two types. The first is reacting to common cause variation as if it were special cause and the second is reacting to special cause variation as if it were common cause. The first type is most common in health care. Reacting to each individual common cause variation only causes more variation. This type of interference is called tampering. If, for example, we measure a patient's prothrombin time and, as a result, we change the anticoagulant dose. The prothrombin time is measured again and the dose again altered in response to the result. This could be repeated again and again. It is the classical "knee-jerk" response which in turn can produce wild swings in variation. 85 per cent of process problems are due to common cause variation.

In the second type of error, that of reacting to a special cause variation as if it were a common cause variation, fundamental process changes may be introduced when they are not necessary and this, in turn, produces instability in the system. Reduction in special cause variation is the responsibility of people working in the process if they have been given the necessary authority.

Employees work in a system. The manager works on a system to improve it with the employees help. Knowledge of a certain amount of psychology of individuals, groups, learning and change is important when practicing medicine. Individuals have a need to learn, a need to be part of a group, a need to be respected and a need to avoid fear of punishment. Managers and physicians, who are also managers, must recognise and understand these tenets. Groups facilitate problem solving and collaborative or synergistic team work. This also fulfils the individuals need to be part of a group.

Not everyone agrees that Deming's ideas are applicable to medicine. Patwardhan and Patwardhan[26] felt that, although Deming's approach was successfully implemented in the manufacturing industry it is questionable whether it can be applied to manage quality in the health care sector. They felt that the consumer demand-led environment posed a threat to the health and social care system. It was expected to keep the sanctities for human values but also provide "quality for cost" services as in any other commercial organisation. In their opinion the structural complexity of health care services and their unique professional and human element of management made it difficult to bring about change by applying any one "magic approach".

They said that Deming's "total quality improvement" approach had not achieved much success or satisfaction when adapted to medicine and they analysed the rationale for this non-transferability. They questioned if the management tools that were basically designed for the manufacturing and commercial industries were adapted to a service industry like health care inappropriately in the first place? Maybe, according to them these tools might not have been applied with sufficient understanding or given enough time before evaluating their suitability? They felt that there was a need for discussion as to why and which part of Deming's approach is and is not transferable to a health and social care setting. Adjustments may be needed either in the approach or the systems to be successful.

"Such is Life" is a story about four people named everybody, somebody, anybody and nobody. There was a very important job which had to be done and EVERYBODY was told to do it. EVERYBODY hoped that SOMEBODY would do it. ANYBODY could have done it, but NOBODY did it. SOMEBODY got angry because it was EVERYBODY's job. EVERYBODY hoped that ANYBODY would do it, but NOBODY realized that EVERYBODY wouldn't do it. It all ended with EVERYBODY blaming SOMEBODY when NOBODY did what ANYBODY could have done.

In a centre with a functioning quality management system and correct management of personnel Everybody, Somebody, Anybody and Nobody all have specific names and know their area of work very precisely. This is proper management. Other questions to be asked of the level of training of staff in the medical establishment are whether all staff members are able to use plan B. Does the patient receive the same quality of care at any given point? How great is the degree of specialisation? Does the system for organising stand-ins and holiday planning work?

A basic principle of management is that the quality management system is not in place for punishment of the staff. It is an instrument for continually improving performance and this fact should always be stressed to the staff.

Are policy and procedure guidelines necessary in medicine? David A. Bergman,[27] talking about paediatrics, described how practice guidelines and other methods have been used to improve quality, principles and perspectives. This purpose had been broadened to include cost reduction, standardisation of practice, and reduction of medical liability but, he says, this has led to both confusion and distrust.

Clinical practice guidelines have a long and distinguished tradition in paediatrics.[28] The American Academy of Paediatrics has developed more than 15 practice guidelines and more than 250 clinical policy statements, outcome and performance measures that provide feedback to clinicians and allow for modification of the guidelines to meet the needs of the local patient population.[29]

The development of evidence-based practice guidelines, however, does not insure that it will have a major impact on physician practice. Implementation and audit are the challenges.

With the advent of managed care and managed care organisations,[30] there have been huge efforts to reduce the cost of care, programs to reduce the variability of clinical practice, increased malpractice litigation, and greater involvement of patients in clinical decision-making and treatment. As a result of these changes, the traditional role of practice guidelines as a means to disseminate new knowledge has been broadened to include such goals as decreasing clinical variability and increasing the standardisation of care, cost reduction, patient education, and protection against medical litigation.

The role of practice guidelines has become so complex that some goals such as the reduction of costs and the improvement of quality may run at cross-purposes.[31] All this has led to considerable confusion and distrust about practice guidelines on the part of the patient and practitioner.

In and of themselves, guidelines do not provide a model for improvement.[32] When used in conjunction with models such as rapid cycle improvement, however, they can become important tools for changing clinical practice and improving the outcomes of care.[33] They also provide a means to rapidly disseminate new knowledge into clinical practice.

In Zimbabwe policy and procedure guidelines are not taken seriously. At a combined meeting of Harare obstetricians and gynaecologists and paediatricians I was asked to prepare policy and procedure guidelines for induction of labour. I spent a total of 60 hours doing this. Policy and procedure guidelines are not written by one person. They are arrived at by consensus. Aiming at this consensus, I sent the draft guidelines to all relevant parties asking for their comments. I did not receive one reply. This was a sad state of affairs that seemed to be indicative of an unwillingness to learn and improve. Maybe it was merely resistance to change.

I was requested to write policy and procedure guidelines for the labour ward of the Avenues Clinic in Harare. This is a private medical clinic, which I was instrumental in building.

Tragically the request to write guidelines came too late in one particular case. One of the first guidelines I wrote had to do with communication. One of the major points in this particular guideline is how to contact the relevant doctor when he or she is needed. A tragedy occurred recently when a doctor was unable to be contacted and his patient died following a postpartum haemorrhage. I sincerely hope that due attention will be paid to these guidelines.

Despite my many protestations the Avenues Clinic, until very recently, still held perinatal mortality meetings. They were reluctant to accept change and to adopt principles of clinical risk management. Pleasingly they have now changed and hold audit meetings. I have accomplished this at last. It is a major achievement.

My final point under management should always be remembered. It is that "the customer is King", or in this case "the patient is King" - always.

It is my hope that maybe, just maybe, with correct observance of evidence based medicine, the willingness to change, better management and the avoidance of "quackery" medicine may yet improve.

References:

1. Glenn Laffel, MD, David Blumenthal, MD. The Case for Using Industrial Quality Management Science in Health Care Organisations (JAMA. 1989;262:2869 2873)
2. American Society for Healthcare Engineering.
http://www.ashe.org/ashe/codes/jcaho/ background.html. ASHE: Joint Commission Background - ASHE - American Society ..,
http://www.ashe.org/advocacy/organizations/TJC/background.html (accessed July 23, 2013).
3. ASHE: Joint Commission Background - ASHE - American Society ..,
http://www.ashe.org/advocacy/organizations/TJC/background.html (accessed July 23, 2013).
4. Ibid.
5. "Joint Commission Changes Its Name and Logo". American Association for Respiratory Care. February 28, 2007.
http://www.aarc.org/headlines/jcaho/change.cfm. Retrieved 2007-07-17.

6. "National Patient Safety Goals". The Joint Commission. http://www.jointcommission.org/PatientSafety/NationalPatientSafetyGoals/npsg_intro.htm
7. http://www.achs.org.au/
8. Shewhart, Walter Andrew (1939). Statistical Method from the Viewpoint of Quality Control. New York: Dover. ISBN 0-486-65232-7.
9. Deming, W. Edwards (1986). Out of the Crisis. MIT Center for Advanced Engineering Study. ISBN 0-911379-01-0.
10. Colin Power - What is Quality?, http://colinenergy.com/WhatisQuality.html (accessed July 23, 2013).
11. PRODUCCIÓN Y SEGURIDAD INDUSTRIAL: HISTORY OF W. EDWARDS DERMING, http://produccinyseguridadindustrial.blogspot.com/2010/11/hitory-of-w-edwards-derming.html (accessed July 23, 2013).
12. Boeing's mistakes are lessons to learn from, maybe SOX .., http://www.greenm3.com/gdcblog/2013/1/25/boeings-mistakes-are-lessons-to-learn-from-maybe-sox-conflic.html (accessed July 23, 2013).
13. Aguayo, Rafael (1991). Dr. Deming: The American Who Taught the Japanese About Quality. Fireside. pp. 40–41.
14. PRODUCCIÓN Y SEGURIDAD INDUSTRIAL: HISTORY OF W. EDWARDS DERMING, http://produccinyseguridadindustrial.blogspot.com/2010/11/hitory-of-w-edwards-derming.html (accessed July 23, 2013).
15. W. Edwards Deming - Wikipedia, the free encyclopedia, http://en.m.wikipedia.org/wiki/W._Edwards_Deming (accessed July 23, 2013).
16. A Brief History of Dr. W. Edwards Deming British Deming Association SPC Press, Inc. 1992. W. Edwards Deming - Wikipedia, the free encyclopedia, http://en.m.wikipedia.org/wiki/W._Edwards_Deming (accessed July 23, 2013).
17. The Doug Williams Group, http://www.thedougwilliamsgroup.com/NewsAndPublications/TakingAction/id/90/read/Dr-William-Edwards-Deming-Remembered-Part-1/ (accessed July 23, 2013).
18. Thiébaud, Jean-Marie (December 2007). "L'Ordre du Trésor sacré (The Order of the Sacred Treasure)" (in French). L'Harmattan. http://www.editions-harmattan.fr/index.asp?navig=catalogue&obj=article&no=8245. W. Edwards Deming: Map (The Full Wiki) - Google Maps meets .., http://maps.thefullwiki.org/W._Edwards_Deming (accessed July 23, 2013).
19. W. Edwards Deming - Wikipedia, the free encyclopedia, http://en.m.wikipedia.org/wiki/W._Edwards_Deming (accessed July 23, 2013).
20. Dr. Deming's Management Training. Accessed: 2006-06-18. W. Edwards Deming - Wikipedia, the free encyclopedia, http://en.m.wikipedia.org/wiki/W._Edwards_Deming (accessed July 23, 2013).
21. W. Edwards Deming - Wikipedia, the free encyclopedia, http://en.m.wikipedia.org/wiki/W._Edwards_Deming (accessed July 23, 2013).
22. Deming WE. Some notes on management in a hospital. J Soc Health Systems, Vol 2 No 1, Spring 1990. Reprinted in, Neuhauser D, McEachern E, Headrick L, eds. Clinical CQI: a book of readings Oakbrook Terrace, IL, Joint Commission on Accreditation of Healthcare Organizations Press 1995:183–6. W Edwards Deming: father of quality management, patient and .., http://qualitysafety.bmj.com/content/14/4/310.full (accessed July 23, 2013).
23. Best M. and Neuhauser, D. Heroes and martyrs of quality and safety. Qual Saf Health Care 2005;14:310-312 doi:10.1136/qshc.2005.015289. W Edwards Deming:

father of quality management, patient and ..,
http://qualitysafety.bmj.com/content/14/4/310.full (accessed July 23, 2013).
24. W Edwards Deming: father of quality management, patient and ..,
http://qualitysafety.bmj.com/content/14/4/310.full (accessed July 23, 2013).
25. Ibid.
26. Patwardhan, A. And Patwardhan, D.
How Transferable is Deming's Approach to a Health and Social Care Setting? Journal of Health Management. Dec 2007. Vol 9. No. 3. P 443-457.
27. David A. Bergman, M.D. Evidence Based Guidelines and Critical Pathways for Quality Improvement. PEDIATRICS Vol. 103 No. 1 January 1999 225
28. Evidence-Based Guidelines and Critical Pathways for Quality ..,
http://www.pediatricsdigest.mobi/content/103/Supplement_E1/225.full (accessed July 23, 2013).
29. Ibid.
30. Ibid.
31. Ibid.
32. Ibid.
33. Ibid.

Index

A

A Menace to Science, The Guardian, 166
A Shot in the Dark, 100
A wasted decade, 303
A.A.F, 241
Ability, Affability, Availability and Affordability, 320
Abraham of Groningen, Dr., 13
Abuja Declaration, 323
Academic Committee of Shandong University, 198
Academic Misconduct Literature Check (AMLC), 201
Académie de Médecine, 106
Academy of Medical Royal Colleges (AoMRC), 268
Academy of Medical Sciences, 46
Accreditation, 328
Accupath 1000, 277, 279
Acne, 306
Act of Parliament, 48
Acts of Parliament, 285
Acubase, 277
Acupressure, 132
Acupuncture, 30, 45, 56, 123, 133, 169, 278, 283, 284
Acupuncture and migraine headaches, 138
Acupuncture and osteoarthritis of the knee, 139
Acupuncture and related interventions for smoking cessation., 137
Acupuncture and rheumatoid arthritis, 139
Acupuncture and surgery, 126
Acupuncture during labour, Swedish trial, 138
Acupuncture meridians, 277
Acupuncture to manage pain in labour, 137
Acupuncture, adverse effects, 140
Acupuncture, Risks of, 140
Acupuncture, technique of, 126
Acupuncture: The Ancient Chinese Art of Healing, 142
Acupuncturists, 279

Adam and Eve, 128
Advanced Allergy Elimination, 169
AdvancePCS, 267
Advertising Standards Authority, 14, 166
Advisory Council, 38
Advisory Council of the Alternative Medicine Center at Columbia University's College of Physicians and Surgeons, 61
African medicine, 298
African National Congress, 175
Aguayo, Rafael, 329
Aguilar, Nancy, 45
AIG, 14
ALA, 238
Albert Einstein College of Medicine in New York, 214
Allergies, 229
Alliance for Natural Health (ANH), 239
Allied Health Professions Council of South Africa (AHPCSA), 106
Allison, Professor Matthew, 304
Allopathic products, 91
Al-Mufti and colleagues, 181
Alopecia, 306
Alternative Medicine Center at Columbia University's College of Physicians and Surgeons, 61
Alternative Medicine Resolution in June 2006, 35
Alzheimer's disease, 231, 299
Alzheimer's disease, 27, 296
AM-2, 276
Amarant, 24
Amenorrhoea, exercise associated, 305
American Academy of Paediatrics, 333
American Association of Clinical Endocrinologists, 27
American Association of Nutritional Consultants, 165
American Cancer Society, 27
American College of Nurse-Midwives (ACNM), 295
American College of Obstetricians and Gynecologists, 27, 294
American College of Obstetricians and Gynecologists (ACOG) District VIII and IX Meeting - August, 2000, 181

American College of Obstetricians and Gynecologists Committee Opinion, 294
American College of Obstetricians and Gynecologists Task Force Report on Hormone Therapy, 308
American College of Obstetricians and Gynecologists' Committee on Obstetric Practice, 294
American College of Obstetrics and Gynecology Task Force, 25
American College of Surgeons (ACS), 328
American Council on Exercise, 280
American Dietetic Association, 15
American Holistic College of Nutrition, 166
American Hospital Association, 328
American Institute of Nutrition, 15
American Journal of Clinical Hypnosis, 186
American Journal of Obstetrics and Gynecology, 293
American Medical Association, 27, 34, 130, 268
American Medical Association Council on Scientific Affairs, 142
American Medical College deans, 54
American Medical Writers Association, 206
American Pain Society/American College of Physicians, 133
American Physical Society, 170
American Society for Reproductive Medicine, 302
American Society for Testing and Materials (ASTM), 329
American Society of Clinical Nutrition, 15
Amish, 99
Amsterdam Medical Disciplinary Tribunal, 95
Amyloxine, 276
Androgens, 21
Andrographis, 33
Angell, Dr. Marcia, 31
Angell, M., 31
Angell, Marcia, 205, 257
Angiostatin, 14
Angley, Ernest, 69
Annals of Improbable Research (AIR), 14
Annals of Oncology, 55
Anthracinum, 61
Anthrax, 61
Anthroposophicals, 91
Antimalignocyt (CH-23), 276

Antineoplastons, 276
Antioxidants, 167, 229
    Lisa Melton's list - Cranberry capsules. Green tea extract. Effervescent vitamin C. Pomegranate concentrate. Beta carotene pills. Selenium. Grape seed extract. High-dose vitamin E. Pine bark extract. Bee spit., 167
Anvirzel, 276
Appleby, Dr John, 43
Application of Modern Statistics to Medicine, 291
Arkansas, 32
Arnica, 47, 48, 89, 104
Arnica Gel, 47
Aromatherapy, 30, 91
Arsenic, 23
Artemisia vulgaris (mugwort), 123
Ascencao, Maria, 21
Asda's Healthy wholegrain bread, 238
Asia Pacific Menopause Federation, 302
Asian Academic Journal, 203
Aspirin, 23, 232
Assistant Director of the Office of Compliance in the Food and Drug Administration's Center for Drug Evaluation and Research, 27
Assisted ventilation, 294
Association of British Pharmaceutical Industry (ABPI), 109
Association of the British Pharmaceutical Industry (ABPI), 268
Astrology, 57
Asyra, 277
At the American Society for Bone and Mineral Research 2011 Annual Meeting, 309
Atherosclerosis, 246
Atherosclerotic plaque, 299
Atrogel, 47
Atrogel Gel, 47
Attorney General, 285
Auckland District Court, 265
Aurelius, Marcus, 315
Aurignacian age, 11
Australasian Society of Clinical Immunology and Allergy (ACAI), 169
Australia, 307
Australian Anti-fat Miracle, The, 241
Australian College of Allergy, 279

Australian Council Against Health Fraud, 89
Australian Drug Regulatory Authorities, 22
Australian government, 280
Australian Menopause Society (Amarant), 22
Australian oncologists, 165
Austria, 104
Authors, Ghosts, Damned Lies and Statisticians, 52
Autism, 187
Autogenous urine therapy, 169
Avatar, 277
Aveloz, 276
Avenues Clinic, 334
Ayurvedic, 37
AZT, 230

B

B.Sc. degrees in Black Magic and the Casting of Spells Astrology, 60
Baby and Child Care, 175
Bach Flower Remedies, 94
Bachelor of Science, 58
Bachelor of Science degrees, 58
Bacon, Francis, 12, 316
Bad Science, 289
Bahrain, 174, 315, 327
Baltimore Orioles, 231
Banerjee, Anjan, 199
Barbour, Ginny., 197
Barnes, D. E., 203
Barrett, Dr Stephen, 60
Barrett, Stephen, 67, 69, 142, 278, 279, 280
Barrett, Stephen, 278
Barriaux, Marianne, 263
Barzilai, Nir, 214
Baum, Michael, 48
Baum, Michael, 42
Baum, *Professor Michael*, 40, 44, 51
Bayh–Dole Act, 206
Baylis, Roger, 280
BBC News West, 96
BBC news, September 16th 2010, 236
BBC. 26th October, 2006., 46
BBC's Food and Drink Program, 229
BBC's Panorama - Secrets of the Drug Trials, 258
BBC's Panorama - Seroxat Emails from the Edge" (2003), 258
BBC's Panorama - Taken on Trust, 258
BBC's Panorama - The Secrets of Seroxat, 258
BBC2 TV, 55
BBC2 TV -13th July 2006, 101
BBC's Today Program, 40
Beacon Bay, 28
Bear Stearns, 14
Beautifying Creams, 282
Beauty Elixirs, 282
Beauty specialist, The, 282
Bechler, Steve, 231
Beddington, John. Government Chief Scientific Adviser,, 108
Beeching, Dr Nick, 110
Behrens, Dr Ron, 102
Belfast, 283
Belfast Telegraph. The, 283
Belgium, 104
Bell Laboratories, 330
Bell's Telephones, 329
Belmont Report, 258
Belon, Philippe, 49
Bemer 3000, 276
Benbow, Alistair, 262
Benbow, Alistair, 261
Benbow, Alistair, 262
Benbow, Dr Alastair. Medical Director for GSK Europe, 261
Bender, Arnold, 244
Bender, David, 244, 245, 247
Bender, Professor Arnold, 228
Benson Harer Jr. W, 181
Benson, Dawn and David, 187
Benson, Eliza-Mae, 187
Bergman, David A., 333
Berk, R. A., Korenman, S. G. and Wenger, N. S., 204
Berman, Brian, 60
Berwick, Donald, 317, 327
Best available evidence, 292
Best, Mark, 316
Beta carotene, 167
Beta Carotene, 242
Beta-carotene, 245
Bextra, 208
Beyerstein, Barry, 62, 64
Bian shi, 123
BICOM, 277
Big Pharma, 257
Bio resonance therapy (BRT), 277
Biocybernetic medicine (BM), 277

Bioelectric functions diagnosis (BFD), 277
BioElectric Shield, 45
Bio-energy regulatory technique (BER), 277
Biofeedback, 279
Biofeedback CPT codes, 278
Bioforce AG, 47
Bioforce(UK), 47
Bioharmony, 21
Bio-identical hormone replacement therapy (BHRT), 27
Bioidentical hormone therapy, 303
Bio-identical" hormones, 27
Bio-Ionic System, 276
Biomeridian, 277
BioResonance Tumor Therapy, 276
Biosciences Federation, 46
BioSciences Federation, 46
Biotech Cell Information, 276
Bioterrain Management System, 276
Bio-Tron, 277
Birmingham, 283
Bjelakovic, Goran, 168
Black bears, 140
Black, Sir James, 42
Blackie Foundation Trust, 50
Blackie, Dr Margery, 50
Blair, Cherie, 45
Blair, Cherie, 45
Blair,Tony, 45
Bloemenkamp, D. G. et al[204], 215
Blood clots, 304
Bloodletting, 124
Bloomberg Markets. December 2005, 257
Blumenthal, David, 326
Blunden, Frances, 46
BMJ, 211
Bob Beck Protocol, 276
Body mass index, 298
Body mass index (BMI), 297
Boehringer Ingelheim, 206
Boerewors, 242
Boiron, 49
Bond Street, 282
Boots, 93, 105
Boots the Chemists, 92
Botox, 46
Botswana, 200
Bowen, Angela, 258
Bozzini, Philip, 11
Brahams, Malcolm, 285
Brannan, Stephen, 184

Braunwald, Eugene, 199
Breast cancer, 17, 297, 304
Breckenridge, Professor Alasdair. Chairman of the MHRA Agency Board, 44
Brewin, Dr Thurstan, 283
Brighton, 233
Bristol Myers, 206
Britain, 307
British Association for Psychopharmacology, 184
British Association of Homeopathic Veterinary Surgeons, 92
British Chiropractic Association, 37
British Dietetic and Diabetic Associations, 229
British Dietetic Association, 244
British Dietetic Association's Public Relations Advisor, 229
British General Medical Council, 203
British Health Food Manufacturers Association (HFMA), 239
British Homeopathic Association, 92
British Homeopathic Dental Association (BHDA), 92
British House of Commons Science and Technology Committee, 104
British Journal of Obstetrics and Gynaecology, 137, 188
British Medical Association, 46, 105, 108
British Medical Association (BMA), 89
British Medical Association Junior Doctors Committee, 90
British Medical Association's Junior Doctors Committee group's conference, 108
British Medical Journal, 50, 56, 133, 139, 188, 189, 196, 235, 242, 257, 260, 291, 317
British Medical Journal (BMJ), 182, 198
British Menopause Society, 303
British National Formulary, 308
British Pharmacological Society, 46, 49
British Pharmacological Society 2001, Bulletin of, 62
British Pharmacological Society, The, 44
British sausage, The. Uniquely Australian, 242
British School of Yoga, 229, 230
British Society for Integrated Medicine, 96
British Society of Gastroenterology, 199
Broad Street Pump, 291

Broadway shows, 268
Brooks Brothers, 289
Brunswick Medical Centre in Camden, 96
Bryans' test, 169
Bryomixol, 276
Buba,, 176
Bullivant's Natural Health Products, 23
Bunnythorpe, New Zealand, 265
Burton, LaVarne A. President of the Pharmaceutical Care Management Association, 267
Bush, The administration, 266
Byrd, Dr. Randolph, 66

C

Caesarean section, 293
Caesarean sections, 178
Cahi, Dr. Dick, 319
Calcium, 228, 247, 307
Calcium carbonate, 308
California, 31, 258
California teachers, 304
Cambridge Heart Antioxidant Study, 245
CAM-related systematic reviews, 58
Canadian Institutes of Health Research, 200
Canadian Medical Association Journal, 180
Cancer, 297
Cancer Act, 284
Cancer Act Section 4, 284
Cao Nanyan, 202
Capital University of Integrated Medicine, 278
Capitol Hill, 38
Capone, Al, 317
CARD, 174
Cardiovascular disease, 297
Cardiovascular Research Center at the University of Connecticut Health Center (UCHC), 213
Carter's Little Liver Pills, 276
Case for Using Industrial Quality Management Science in Health Care Organisations, The, 326
Case Western University, 26
Castor beans (ricin), 23
Cat's Claw, 276
Celebrex, 208
Celebritiesinfluencing medical treatment Steve McQueen, Larry King, Prince Charles, David Beckham, Roger Moore, Tom Cruise and Peter Sellers. Suzanne Somers and Oprah Winfrey and others, 26
Cellular Health, 276
Center for Bioinformatics and Computational Biology, 141
Center for Drug Evaluation and Research (CDER), 281
Center for Frontier Medicine in Biofield Science, 90
Center for Integrative Medicine (CIM), 40
Center for Integrative Medicine (CIM) within the University of Maryland School of Medicine, 60
Center for Integrative Medicine at the University of Maryland, 139
CenterWatch, 257
Chairman Mao, 128
Chalmers, Iain, 291
Chamberlain, Geoffrey, 209
Chamberlain, Professor Geoffrey, 188
Chandra, R K, 200
Change, 207, 315, 328
Changing Clinical Practice and Perceptions, 317
Chaparral, 276
Chapters from My Autobiography, 290
Charing Cross Hospital, 186
Charing Cross Hospital ethics committee, 186
Charlatanism, 291
Chelation therapy, 30, 39
Cheng, B. Q. et al, 198
Cherry-picking, 246
Chichester, 233
China, 105, 124, 126, 245
China National Knowledge Infrastructure (CNKI), 201
China Off, 102
China Sulph, 102
China's Medicine, 125
Chinese Communist Party, 124
Chinese Emperor and the Imperial Academy of Medicine, 124
Chinese Journal of Physiology., 125
Chinese Medical Association, 125
Chinese Medical Journal (CMJ), 125
Chinese medicine, 123
Chiropractic, 54
Chiropractic therapy, 169

Chiropractors, 279
Cholera, 291, 323
Cholesterol, high density lipoprotein (HDL), 296
Cholesterol, low density lipoprotein (LDL), 296
Chondroitin, 235
Chondroitin sulphate, 139
Christian Science, 68
Christian Science Publishing Society, 68
Christian Science Sentinel, 68
Christian Scientist school, 99
Christmas trees, 268
Cicutto, Lisa, 215
Cinchona bark, 102
Circulation, 208
cis.nci.nih.gov, 55
Clarence House, 44, 52
Clark, Susan, 18
Class III devices, 279
Claxton, Larry, 210
Clegg, D. O., 235
Cleveland Clinic, 186
Clifford, Max, 166
Climacteric, 302, 303
Clinical audit, 319
Clinical ecology/ environmental illness, 169
Clinical trials, 93, 291
Clomiphene, 306
CNKI Academic Integrity Research Center, 201
Cocculus, 88, 169
Cochrane CAM Field, 57
Cochrane CAM Field staff, 57
Cochrane Collaboration, 291
Cochrane Collaboration articles on pain, 133
Cochrane Collaboration reviews regarding acupuncture, 136
Cochrane Collaboration, The, 57
Cochrane Database of Systematic Reviews, 292
Cochrane for CAM Providers, 58
Cochrane Library, The, 57, 58
Cochrane Library's CENTRAL Register of Controlled Trials, 58
Cochrane Pregnancy and Childbirth Database, 293
Cochrane review, 41, 235
Cochrane Review on Acupuncture, Nausea and Vomiting .2009, 132
Cochrane Review on Acupuncture, Nausea and Vomiting .2011, 132
Cochrane Review on Acupuncture, Nausea and Vomiting. 2004, 132
Cochrane reviews, 208
Cochrane Reviews, 291
Cochrane reviews - antioxidant supplements, 168
Cochrane Systematic Reviews, 33
Cochrane, Archie, 291
Codman, Ernest, 328
Coffee enemas, 176
College of Physicians, 12
Collins, Catherine, 244
Colonic irrigation, 176
Colorectal cancer, 17
Colposcope, 11
Colquhoun, David, 49, 90, 92, 107, 169, 239
Colquhoun, David, 47, 48
Colquhoun, David, 56
Colquhoun, David, 58
Colquhoun, David, 62
Colquhoun, David, 87
Colquhoun, David, 92
Colquhoun, David, 107
Colquhoun, David, 237
Colquhoun, Professor David, 59
Colquhoun, Professor David, 59
Columbia University, 184
Columbia University's Rosenthal Center, 61
Colwyn, Lord, 49
Colwyn, Lord, 50
Commerce Commission, 265
Committee for the Ethical Aspects of Human Reproduction and Women's Health of FIGO, 183
Committee on Nutrition of the American Academy of Pediatrics, 228
Committee on Publication Ethics (COPE), 197, 203, 211
Commons Science and Technology Select Committee, 91
Commons science select committee, 108
Complementary and Alternative medicine, 30
Complementary and alternative medicine (CAM), 34
Complementary Healthcare: a guide for patients, 52
Complementary Therapies in Medicine, 58

Computerised electrodermal screening (CEDS), 277
Computerised electrodermal stress analysis (CDCSA), 277
Computron, 277
Congressional hearings into scientific misconduct, 195
Consensus, 134
Conservative Party, 107
Consumer Reports, 278
Consumer Safety Officer with the United States Food and Drug Administration's Office of Regulatory Affairs, 281
Consumers for Health Choice (CHC), 239
Continuous performance improvement, 328
Coody, Gary, 281
Cookson, Clive. Science Editor of the Financial Times, 197
Copenhagen University[18], 168
Copper, 247
Copper bracelet, 284
Coronary artery disease, 17
Coronary heart disease, 298
Coronary heart disease (CHD), 304
Cortisone, 21
Costain, Lyndel, 229
Council for Healthcare Regulatory Excellence, 95
Council for Healthcare Regulatory Excellence (CHRE), 90
Council for Responsible Nutrition, 232
Council for Scientific Medicine, 30, 39
Council of the European Communities, 104
Counterirritant techniques, 136
Counter-irritation, 134
Countess of Mar, The 30th, 49
Courtship Behaviour of Ostriches Towards Humans Under Farming Conditions in Britain, 14
Cox, 214
Cox-Brown, Tim, 262
Cranberry, 33
Cranial therapy allergy elimination techniques, 169
Cressey, Daniel, 197
Crohn's disease, 187
Cromwell, Oliver, 282
CrossCheck, 201
Croswell Doane, Bishop William, 87
Cruises, 268
Crump, Susan C., 100
Crystal Therapy, 283
CSA 2001, 277
Cultural Revolution, 125
Curare, 23
Cure for All Cancers, 276
Cyanide (in Sorghum and Prunus species), 23
Cyberonics, Inc., 184
Cyranoski, David, 202
Czech Republic, 104

D

Daily Mail, The, 103, 189, 237
Daily Telegraph -14th Feb., 2006, 56
Daily Telegraph -September 17th, 2010, 236
Dalton, Katherine, 21
Dangers of CAM, 53
Daniel 1: 1-16, 290
Danish Knowledge and Research Center for Alternative Medicines, 136
Darracott, Helen -Proprietary Association of Great Britain (PAGB) Director of Legal and Regulatory Affairs,, 109
Darsee, John, 199
Darwin, Charles, 276
Das, Dipak, 213
David, J and others, 139
Davis, Gary, 175
Dawkins, Richard, 170
Dawkins, Richard Dawkins, 276
De Deus, João (John of God),, 129
Deadly nightshade, 23
Death cap (amanita phalloides), 23
Deats, Mick, 235
Deats, Mick, 235
Declercq, Eugene. Professor of Maternal and Child Health at the Boston University School of Public Health in Massachusetts, 294
Deep venous thrombosis, 297
Deer, Brian, 187
Deming, Dr. W. Edward, 327, 329, 331
Deming, Dr. W. Edwards, 316
Denmark, 104
Dentists, 279
Department of Health, 41, 43, 44, 50, 102, 106, 107, 108, 239
Dermatology, 320
Dermatron, 277, 279, 280

Desktop Guide to Complementary and Alternative Medicine. An evidence-based approach, The, 32
Devathasan, Anna, 265
Devil's claw, 33
Devlin, Kate, 275
Devlin, Kate, 89, 170
DHA (Docosahexaenoic acid), 238
DiagnoMètre, 277
Dialbuy, 241
Diazepam (Valium), 186
Dietary change, 278
Dietary Supplement Health and Education Act, 231
Digestive System, 229
Digitalis, 23
DiOrio, Reverend Ralph, 69
Dioscorea villosa, 21
Diosgenin, 23
Diplomate of Acupuncture, 131
Directive 2001/83/EC, 104
Directive 92/73/EEC, 104
Director of the Service of Medical informatics of the Geneva University Hospitals, 55
Disease States, 229
Disraeli, Benjamin, 290
Disraeli, Benjamin Disraeli, 210
Distraction, 134
Divisional Manager of Cancer Services, 38
Docere, 320
Doctor's Dilemma, The, 12
Dolphin, Dr Tom, 90
Dolphin, Dr Tom, 108
Dominus, Susan, 188
Dorchester, 233
Doubt is our product, 248
Douglas, Catherine, 14
Dr Spock, 95
Dr. MacKenzie's Veinoids, 276
Droperidol, 56
Duchy Herbals detox remedy, 37
Dulcan, Dr. Mina, 260
Dunn, Laura, Professor of psychiatry at the University of California, San Diego, 258
Durban University of Technology, 106
Durham, 237
Durham Council, 237
Dutch government, 106
Dysbiosis, 169

E

Eames, Dr Sara, 111
East London, 28
ebandolier.com, 55
Ecclesiastes, I 10-11, 283
Echinacea, 40, 231
Eclosion, 277
Ectopic pregnancy, 188
E-Ferol, 244
Effective Care in Pregnancy and Childbirth, 293
ELAST, 277
Electrical resistance of the patient's skin, 277
Electro Dermal Resistance Analysis, 278
Electro Interestitial Scanner (EIS), 280
Electroacupuncture according to Voll (EAV), 277
Electroacupuncture according to Voll (EAV) devices, 277
Electrodermal screening (EDS), 277
Electrodermal testing (EDT), 277
Electrodiagnostic devices, 277
Electro-magnetic energy, 277
Electronic fetal heart rate monitoring, 293
Eli Lilly, 206, 266
Elliott, Austin, 46
Ellis, Chris, 320
Elsevier, 62
E-Lybra 8, 277, 278
Emeritus Professor of Paediatrics at the Mayo Clinic, 33
Emery, C. Eugene. Jr, 69
Endau, 23
Endocrine Society, The, 302
Endostatin, 14
English and South African cricket sides, 280
EPA (eicosapentaenoic acid), 238
EPFX, 280
Ephedra, 231
Epidural analgesia, 182, 293
Episiotomy, 293
Epsom salts, 230
Equazen, 237
Ernst, Edzard, 32, 53
Ernst, Professor Edzard, 55
Ernst, Professor Edzard, 35, 48, 54
Ernst, Professor Edzard, 42
Ernst, Professor Edzard, 52
Ernst, Professor Edzard, 56

Ernst, Professor Edzard, 58
Ernst, Professor Edzard, 93
Ernst, Professor Edzard, 96
Ernst, Professor Edzard, 100
Ernst, Professor Edzard, 106
Ernst, Professor Edzard, 111
Ernst, Professor Edzard, 135
Ernst, Professor Edzard, 138
Ernst, Professor Edzard, 141
Ernst, Professor Edzard, 170
Ernst, Professor Edzard, 170
Ernst, Professor Edzard, 275
Ernst, Professor Edzard Ernst, 94
Estrogen, 18, 296
Estrogen plus progestin (EPT), 298
Estrogen replacement therapy, 248
Estrogen replacement therapy (ERT), 20
Estrogen therapy (ET), 298
Europe, 124
European Council for Classical Homeopathy, 46
European Directive 2004/24/EC, 47
European Federation of Health Food Manufacturers, 245
European Food Safety Authority, 237
European Food Supplements directive, 45
European Medical Writers Association Guidelines for Medical Writers and Good Publication Practice for pharmaceutical companies, 207
European Menopause and Andropause Society, 302
European Menopause and Andropause Society, The, 302
European Union, 43, 102, 104, 105
European Union (EU) Food supplements directive. 2002, 239
European Union (EU) laws, 239
European Union leaders, 45
Evening Primrose Oil, 242
Evidence based medicine, 292, 327
Evidence- based medicine, 290
Evidence based patient choice, 327
Evidence-based guidelines, 319
Evidence-based Medicine, 289
Evidence-based patient choice, 292
Executive Board of the MHRA, 48
Executive Board of the MHRA members
  Professor Kent Woods, Professor Sir Alasdair Breckenridge, CBE, Professor Angus Mackay,OBE, Michael Fox, Shelley Dolan, Charles Kernahan, Garry Watts and Lisa Arnold., 48
Exeter University, 32
Exeter University Department of Complementary Medicine, 96
Exeter University Development Campaign, 93
Expectation, 134
Expert Group on Vitamins and Minerals, 245
Explore, 58
  The Journal of Science & Healing, 62
Explore. Contents of
  Acupuncture/Acupressure, Ayurveda, Biofeedback, Botanical or Herbal Medicine, Chiropractic, Consciousness, Creative Therapies, Diet/Nutrition/Nutritional Supplements, Environmental Medicine, Holistic Medicine/Nursing, Homeopathy, Indigenous Medical Practices, Manual Therapies, Mind-Body Therapies, Naturopathy, Osteopathic Medicine, Qigong/Tai Chi, Touch Therapies, Spiritual/Transpersonal Healing/Prayer, Tibetan Medicine, Traditional Chinese Medicine and Yoga, 62
Express Scripts, 267

F

Fabrication, 195, 198
Faculty of Homeopathy, 98, 107
Faculty of Homeopathy in Great Britain, 99
Fair Go, 265
Faith, 276
Faith Healers, The, 128
Faith healing, 30
Falsification, 195, 198
Fanelli, D., 204
Farnborough, 233
Farthing, Mike, 197
Fatigue, 134
FBI, 280
FDA, 105, 280
FDA Center for Devices and Radiological Health, 279

Federal Food, Drug, and Cosmetic Act, 236
Federal Trade Commission, 232, 280, 281
Federation of American Societies for Experimental Biology Journal, 61
Fedorowicz, Zbys, 327
Felig, Philip, 199
Felkin, R. W., 178
Feminine Forever, 295
Feng shui, 45
Feng-shui, 45
Fentanyl, 56
Fields, Howard, MD, PhD, 134
Finland, 245
Fish oil, 237
Fisher, Dr. Peter, 59
Fisher, Peter, 102
Fisher, Peter, 58
Fisher, Sir Ronald, 18
Fishman, Alfred P., 61
Fleming, Alexander, 12
Flint, Caroline, 107
Flint, Caroline. Minister of State at the Department of Health, 106
Flonase, 263
Florida Board of Governors, The, 62
Florida State University, 61
Florida State University predicted future map
　chiropractic medicine, Yeti Foundation, School of Astrology, Institute of Telekinesia, Department of ESP studies, College of Homeopathic Medicine, Bigfoot Institute, Faith Healing, Foundation for Prayer Healing Studies, School of UFO Abduction Studies, School of Channelling and Remote Sensing, Creationism Foundation, Tarot Studies, Palmistry, College of Dowsing, Past Life Studies, Crop Circle Simulation Studies., 62
Fluoride, 228
Fly agaric, (muscarine), 23
Folic acid, 228, 247
Food and Drug Adminisration Top Heath Frauds
　unproven treatment for cancer, arthritis and AIDS, instant weight loss schemes, fraudulent sexual aids, quack baldness remedies and other appearance modifiers, false nutritional schemes, unproven use of muscle stimulators and candidiasis hypersensitivity, 276
Food and Drug Administration, 169, 184, 231, 232, 236, 240, 244, 257, 258, 264, 275, 281, 299
Food and Drug Administration (FDA), 27
Food and Drug Administration (FDA), 184
Food and Drug Administration Advisory Panel, 208
Food and Drug Administration in the United States, 295
Food and Drug Administration in the USA, 276, 297
Food and Drugs Administration (FDA), 43
Food Combining, 229
Food Labelling Regulations 1984, 242
Food makers and Supplements, 233
Food Marketing Institute, 267
Foods Standards Agency, 245
Forbes, Dr Alec, 243
Forest, 282
Forest Pharmaceuticals, 282
Forever Young, 284
Forticel tea, 276
Foundation for Integrated Medicine, 43
Fowler, Neil, 238
Fox, Alissa. Policy director for the Blue Cross and Blue Shield Association, 267
Foxglove, 23
Fracastoro, 315
France, 104, 125
Francis, Roger, 309
Frankel, Mark, 202
Franks, Stephen, 306
Fraudulent cancer products, 281
Free dinners, 268
Free lunches and conflicts of interest., 173
Free radicals, 242
French, 106
frequency generators, 280
Friedlander, Edward R., 98
Friedlander, Edward R., 100

G

Gale, Thomas, 13
Galileo, 171
Gall Bladder Flush, The, 229
Gallstones, 229
Galton, Francis, 65
Galvanometers, 277

Galvanotherapy, 277
Gardner, Martin, 15
Garlic, 232
Garrow, John, 240
Garrow, Professor John, 241
Garrow, Professor John, 239
Gasoline, 268
Geim, Andre, 14
Geissbühler, Professor Antoine, 55
Geller, Uri, 128
Gelsemium sempervirens, 50
General Chiropractic Council, 90, 95
General Dental Council, 90
General Medical Council, 90, 95, 96, 187, 189, 199, 200, 244
General Medical Council (GMC), 261
General Medical Council in the United Kingdom, 188
General Osteopathic Council, 90, 95
General Practitioner, 101
Georgia, 258
Germany, 104, 105
Gerson Method, 277
Gerson's diet, 170, 276
Gertel, Art, 212
GetwellUK, 52
gGerm theory of disease, 315
Ghana, 175
Ghost authorship, 207
Ghost writing, 207
Gibson, Owen, 166
Ginger, 33
Ginkgo, 33, 231
Ginkgo biloba, 32, 174, 231
Ginkgo Biloba, 232
Ginkgo Information Centre, 174
Ginseng, 232
Glasgow Homeopathic Hospital, 92
Glaxo builds bonny babies, 265
Glaxo Wellcome, 206
Glaxo Wellcome chair of medical journalism, 206
GlaxoSmithKline, 263, 264
GlaxoSmithKline (GSK), 258, 259
GlaxoWellcome and SmithKline Beecham plc, 265
Gleason, Dr. John, 185
Glucosamine, 139, 235
Goat serum, 174
God Men in India, 128
Godlee, Dr Fiona. Editor in chief *British Medical Journal (BMJ)*, 196

Godlee, Fiona, 50
Godlee, Fiona, 260
Gold standard of research based evidence, 291
Goldacre, Ben, 230, 289
Goldacre, Ben, 15, 87, 165
Goldacre, Ben, 237
Goldacre, Ben, 237
Goldacre, Ben, 244
Golden Femur award, 309
Goldman Sachs, 14
Golf Course Management, 59
Gore, Al, 203
Gore, Al, 195
Gorski, Dr., 25
Gorski, Dr., 25
Gøtzsche, Peter, 210
Gøtzsche, Peter, 212
Government Accountability Office, 232
Government Accountability Office', 232
Government of Zimbabwe MDG Status Report, 2010, 322
GP Associates, 52
Grant, W.V., 69
Great Ormond Street Hospital, 108
Greater Dallas-Fort Worth Council Against Health Fraud, 25
Green, Dr. Saul, 167
Greene, Mrs. Janet, 66
Groote Schuur Hospital, Cape Town, 319
Gross, Dr Barbara, 22
Gross, Dr. Barbara, 24
Guardian, The, 103
Guardian, The, 45
Guardian, The, 237
Guardian, The, 263
Guardian, The -April 1st, 2006, 56
Guardian, The February 12, 2007, 166
Guardian, The. 14 July 2006, 103
Guest and ghost authorship, 207
Guest authorship, 207
Gulf News, 178
Gulf War Syndrome, 186
Gut, 199, 211
Guyatt, G. H., 289

H

Habituation, 134
Haemorrhage, 294
Hagan, Dr Robert, 110
Hahnemann Hospital in Liverpool, 92

Hahnemann, Samuel, 87
Hahnemann, Samuel's, 93
Hain, Peter, 52
Hair Restorers, 282
Hall, Harriet, 130
Hamburg, Margaret, 236
Hamilton, Cindy, 212
Hammonds, Tim., 267
Han Dynasty, 123
Han, Dr., 127
Hand-cleansing between patients, 318
Hannes, Sir William, 13
Harkin, Senator Tom, 40
Harkin, Tom, 38
Harmon, Katherine, 231, 232
Harris, Dr Evan, 103
Harris, Dr. Evan, 44
Harris, Gardiner, 268
Harris, Roy, 233
Harris, Sue, 50
Harris, William S., 66
Harvard Medical School, 57
Harvard Medical School's Center to Assess Alternative Therapy for Chronic Illness, 61
Harvard Medical School's Osher Institute, 61
Harvard University, 199
Hastings, Max, 45
Hatha yoga, 34
Hawthorn, 33
Hazuga, Rachel, 280
He, Haibo, 201
Healing astrology, 284
Healing Crisis, The, 229
Health and Food Fair, 283
Health and Medicines Act 1988, 285
Health Care Commission, 96
Health Notification Service, 25
Health On the Net Foundation, 55
Health or Hoax: The Truth about Health Foods and Diets, 228
Health Protection Agency, 102
Health Restoration Program, 277
Health Screening UK Ltd. (HSL), 233
Health Show, 283
Health Supplements Information Service, 244
Healthpoint Ltd, 282
HealthWatch, 94, 229, 283
HealthWatch Award, 2005, 32
HealthWatch newsletter, 14

HealthWatch Newsletter, 285
HealthWatch, Honorary Secretary, 239
Healy, David. Professor of psychiatry at Cardiff University, 263
Heart and Estrogen/progestin Replacement Study (HERS), 300
Heart disease, 304
Helios, 101
Helios in Covent Garden, 101
Helms, J. M., 136
Hemila, H., 246
Hemophilus meningitis, 100
Henderson, Mark, 103
Henderson, Mark, 42, 91
Hendrik Schön, Jan, 204
Henk, Dr. Michael, 17
Her Majesty, the Queen, 50
Her Majesty's Revenue and Customs (HMRC), 268
Herbal formulations, 298
Herbal medicines, 30, 234
Herbal remedies, 234
Herbal roulette, 21
Herbal Viagra, 234
Herbert, Victor, 128
Herceptin, 42
Hercules, 241
Here and Now, 283
Hertfordshire Trading Standards Department, 240
Hettie, Ben Goldacre's dead cat, 165
Heuss, Thender, 326
Hewitt, Patricia, 93, 108
High colonics, 46
High Quality Women's Health Care: A proposal for change, 315
Hindmarch, Ian. Professor of Human Psychopharmacology at the University of Surrey, 174
Hip fractures, 297
Hirsutism, 306
HIV, 110
Hodgkin's disease, 69
Hodgkinson, Neville, 186
Hoffman, Dr. Beverly, 21
Holford, Patrick, 230
Holford, Patrick, 230
Holistic Healing Plan, 93
Holistic physicians, 279
Holland and Barrett, 232, 233
Holt microwave treatment, 277
Home Birth Raises Risk for Baby, 294

Home births, 293
Homemark, 281
Homeopathic "mumbo jumbo",, 109
Homeopathic malaria prophylaxis, 100
Homeopathic products, 279
Homeopathic Prophylaxis, 97
Homeopathic remedies, 278
Homeopathy, 30, 87, 169, 284
Homeopathy and its Kindred Delusions, 57
Homeopathy in South Africa, 106
Homeopathy, Masters degree, 106
Homoeopathic Gazette of Leipsig, 89
Homoeopathic Medicine, Archives of, 89
Homoeopathy, Annals of Clinical, 89
Honesty, 198
Hoorman, et al. v. SmithKline Beecham Corp, 263
Hope, Jenny, 303
Hormone replacement therapy, 295, 304
Hormone replacement therapy (HRT), 17, 295, 308
Hormone Replacement Therapy and Heart Disease Prevention, 304
Hormone therapy (HT), 297
Hormones, 17
Horny Goat Weed, 166
Horse chestnut, 33
Horse's urine, 26
Horton, Richard, 257, 291
Hospital for Tropical Diseases, 102
Hot flashes, 298
Hot flushes, 298
House of Commons Science and Technology Select Committee, 197
House of Lords, 48, 49
Hu Nan Aimin Pharmaceutical Ltd, 234
Huangdi Neijing, the *Classic of Internal Medicine (History of Acupuncture)*, 123
Huangdi Neijing, the legendary Yellow Emperor's *Classic of Internal Medicine (History of Acupuncture)* which was compiled around 305–204 BCE, 123
Hughes, Ian, 186
Human Genome Project, 292
Human Medicines Regulations, The, 109
Hunt, Lord, 239
Hurley, Dan, 239
Hwang Woo Suk, 207
Hwang Woo-Suk, 204
Hydrogen peroxide, 167
Hydroxyhomosildenafil, 234
Hynes, Marcella, 241

Hypericum 2000 + L-Tyrosine, 23
Hyperventilation, 186
Hypothalamus, 305

I

IgNobel Prizes, 13
Illinois Attorney General, 26
Illinois Food, Drug and Cosmetic Act, 26
Immunisation, 95
Immunisations, 98
Immuno-Augmentative Therapy, 277
Imperial College London, 103
Independent, The, 55
Independent, The - 20 Feb, 2007, 45
Independent, The - January 2006, 165
Independent, The 1st August, 2006, 169
Independent, The. 17th September, 2010, 236
India, 105
Indian ayurvedic medicine, 45
Indian Grass Therapy, 283
Infections, 294
Inflammatory bowel disease, 187
Ingelfinger rule, The, 209
Ingelfinger, Franz J., 209
Inside Out, 233
Instinctotherapy, 277
Institute for Aging and Health at Newcastle University, 309
Institute of Food Science and Technology, 228
Institute of Medicine in the United States, 328
Institute of Medicine in the United States (IOM), 307
Institute of Optimum Nutrition, 230
Institutional review boards (IRBs), 257
Insulin sensitising agents, 306
Insurance company, 280
Integrated Health Associates, 52
Interactive Query System (IQS), 277
Internal Revenue Service (IRS), 263
International Academy of Bioenergetic Practitioners, 279
International Committee of Medical Journal Editors (ICMJE), 210
International Committee on Publication Ethics, 201
International Conference on Population and Development (Cairo 1994), 320
International Hospital of Bahrain, 178

International Journal for Quality in Health Care, 317
International Journal of Cardiology, 201
International Menopause Society, 302
International Menopause Society, The, 302
International Osteoporosis Foundation, 302
Interro, 277, 278
Iowa Women's Health Study, 247
Iridology, 169, 284
Iron, 228, 247
Iron Deficiency, 229
Isbell, Brian, 58
Iscador products, 91
Islington Tribune of 11th May 2007, The, 37
Issels Whole Body Therapy, 277
Italy, 99, 280
I-Tronic, Kindling, 277
Ivy Restaurant in London WC2, 174

J

Jackson, John P., 141
Jacobs, Adam, 212
Jacobs,Joseph, 38
Japan, 99, 106, 329
Japan's Order of the Sacred Treasure, Second Class in 1960, 330
Jarvis, Katie, 97
Jarvis, Mrs, 240
Jason Winters tea, 277
Jazz Pharmaceuticals, 185
Jesus Christ, 128
Jha, Alok, 103
Jia Yi Jian, 234
Jofre, Shelley, 259
John, Sir Elton, 239
Johnson & Johnson, 265
Joint Commission, 328
Joint Commission (TJC), 328
Joint Commission for the Accreditation of Healthcare Organizations, 328
Joint Commission International (JCI), 328
Joint Commission on Accreditation of Healthcare Organizations (JCAHO), 328
Joint Commission on Accreditation of Hospitals (JCAH), 328
Joint Commission Resources, 328
Jomanda, 96

Josling, Mr Peter, 174
Journal of Alternative and Complementary Medicine, 58
Journal of Clinical Oncology, 198
Journal of the Academy of Child and Adolescent Psychiatry, 260
Journal of the American Medical Association, 17, 231, 258, 265
Journal of the American Medical Association (JAMA), 198
Journal of the International Association for the Study of Pain, 133
Journal of the Royal Society of Medicine, 47, 186
Journal of Zhejiang University — Science, 201
Juran Trilogy, 316
Juran, Dr Joseph, 316
Juran, Joseph, 327
Juran, Joseph, 329

K

Kahura, Uganda, 178
Kaiser Permanente, 268
Kassirer, J. P., 31, 212
Kava, 33
Kehrer, Ferdinand Adolf, 178
Keller, Professor Martin. Head of Psychiatry at Brown University, 258, 260
Kennedy, Donald, 207
Kenneth Walker, 12
Kenton,Leslie, 24
Kenya, 264
Kenyon, Dr Julian, 96
Khalik, Madjide, 241
Khunpradit and others, 183
Khuu, Duke, 320
Killing Us Softly The Sense and Nonsense of Alternative Medicine, 304
Kinesiology, 169, 229
King Nebuchadnezzar, 290
King, *John R*, 56
King's Fund,Chief economist, 43
Kings College Medical School, 200
Kings Fund, The, 130
Knipschild, Paul. Professor of Epidemiology at the University of Maastricht, 246
Konstam, Dr., 208
Koocher, G., 212

Kovacs, Peter, 304
Kuhlman, Katherine, 69

L

Lacerations, 294
Laetrile, 38, 170, 275, 277
Laffel, Glenn, 326
Lahore, 236
Laing Foundation of the U.K, 134
Lancet, 98, 187, 188, 211
Lancet, The, 103, 198
Lancet, The, 257
Lancet, The, 291
Lancet,*The*, 198
Lang, Andrew, 289
Langdon, Dr. Michelle, 96
Lansley, Andrew, 107
Lateef, Riz, 59
Lead, 23
Lee, Dr Hyangsook, 138
Lee, Dr. John R., 24
Lee, Dr. John R., 20
Leeds University Maternity Audit Project, 317, 318
Leeuwenhoek, 315
Lehman Brothers, 14
Lerner, Martin, 38
Les Trois Frères, 11
Lex Regia, of 715–673 BC, 178
Liberal Democrats, 44
Lichtleiter, 11
LichtwerPharma, 174
Lignocaine, 234
Lilly, 206
Limbic stress assessment (LSA), 277
Lincoln, Abraham, 289
Lind, James, 290
Linden, Tom, 206
LISTEN, 278
LISTEN System, 277
Littlejohns, Professor Peter, 43
Littlewood, J. E., 165
Liverpool Department of Homeopathic Medicine, 92
Lock, Stephen, 200
Lock, Stephen, 196
London Evening Standard -May 16th 2006, 51
London School of Hygiene and Tropical Medicine, 101
London Stock Exchange, 265

London, Dr. William M., 32
London's Science Museum, 289
Los Angeles, 264
Low birth weight, 294
Low risk patients, 294
Luxembourg, 104

M

Macmillan group, The, 202
Magnesium, 247
Magnetar, 14
Magnetic wristbands, 280
Mail-order companies, 241
Mainini, Simona, 45
malaria, 110
Malaria, 102, 323
Malawi, 101
Mammography, 300
Mander, Michael, 242
Mann, Felix, 136, 142
Mao Tse-tung, 125
Marigold products, 91
Marketed Unapproved Drugs -Compliance Policy Guide (CPG), 281
Marketing practices, 266
Marshall, E., 38
Martindale, 21
Maslow, Abraham, 326
Mason, Paul, 174
Massachusetts Medical Society, 268
Master of Surgery degree, 199
Master's Degree in Complementary and Alternative Medicine, 61
Maternal Mortality Ratio (MMR), 322
Mathias, King of Hungary, 13
Matrix Physique System, 277
Maturitas, 302
Maves, Dr. Michael D. executive vice president of the American Medical Association, 266
Mayo Clinic, 27, 67
Mbeki, Thabo, 175
McCall-Smith, Alexander or, 200
McCartney, Sir Paul, 239
McGarrity, Professor Thomas O., 205
McGill University, 26
McKeith Research Ltd., 166
McKeith, Dr. Gillian, 165
McKeith, Gillian, 176
Mead, Elaine, 98

Measles, mumps and rubella (MMR) vaccine, 187
Medawar, Charles, 261
Medawar, Peter, 188
Medawar, Peter, 262
Médecins Sans Frontières, 264
Medicaid, 263, 266
Medical Consultant of Signalysis Ltd, 243
Medical Defence Union, 187
Medical Devices Agency (MDA), 43
Medical Director of the Bristol Cancer Help Centre, 243
MEDICAL QUACKERY, 173
Medical Recall Notice, 25
Medical Register, 187
Medical Research Council, 46, 291
Medicare, 266, 267
Medicine and Healthcare products Regulators Agency (MHRA), 43, 166, 235, 258
Medecines Act, 243
Medicines Act 1968, 109, 242
Medicines Act, 1968, 46
Medicines Act, Section 80(1)(b), 243
Medicines and Healthcare products Regulatory Agency (MHRA), 104
Medicines and Healthcare Products Regulatory Agency (MHRA), 258
Medicines and Healthcare Products Regulatory Agency.MHRA., 263
Medicines Control Agency (MCA), 43
Meditations, 315
Medline, 47
MEDLINE, 34
Medscape, 305
Melchart, D, 138
Melton, Lisa, 167
Memorial Sloan-Kettering Cancer Center, 167
Memorial University of Newfoundland, 200
Menopausal Hormone Therapy - Global Consensus Statement, 302
Menopause, 300
Mental Health America, 206
Merck, 208
Merck & Company, 266
Meridian energy analysis (MEA), 277
Meridian Energy Analysis Device (MEAD, 277
Meridians, 123
Merrill Lynch, 14

meta-analysis, 293
Metformin, 306
Mexican Riviera, 45
Mexican wild yam, 21
Mexico-United States-Canada Health fraud working group, 281
MHRA, 44, 46, 50, 109, 234, 236
MHRA Assessment Team Manager, Licensing Division, 50
MHRA, Chief Executive, 47
MHRA's Regulatory Excellence program, 109
MHRA's, 50
Michaels, David, 248
Michal, Carl A., 294
Midazolam, 56
Migliaccio, Steve, 175
Millecam, Sylvia, 95
Millenium Declaration, The, 321
Millenium Developmen Goal Action Plan.(MDG), 322
Millennium Development Goals (MDGs), 321
Millennium Development Goals by the year 2015, 322
Millennium Development Goals Summit, 2010, 321
Mind, 258
Mind to let, 19
Minister for Health, 285
Minister for Northern Ireland, 52
Miracle cures, 165
Miracle shampoo, 240
Miracle Wild Yam Cream, 26
Miraculous" cancer cures, 30
Mirror, The, 237
Miss America, 100
Mister, Steve, 232
Mitochondria, 167
MMR vaccination, 95, 187
MMR vaccine, 97
Moore, Harriet, 283
MORA, 277
Morinda citrifolia or Noni, 240
Moses, 128
Moxibustion, 123
MRC Clinical Sciences Centre, Hammersmith Hospital, 237
MSAS, 277
Mt. Sinai School of Medicine, 128
Mugabe, Robert, 322
Multivitamin tablets, 247

Multivitamin-mineral supplementation, 228
Multivitamins, 247
Munneche, Dr., 89
Murdoch, James, 263
Myocardial infarction (MI), 301

N

Namibian Medical Association, 207
Nathanson, Dr Vivienne, 108
Nathanson, Dr Vivienne. British Medical Association's director of science and ethics,, 97
National Academy of Sciences, 199, 204
National Association of Certified Professional Midwives, 295
National Association of Health Stores (NAHS), 239
National Cancer Institute, 131
National Center for Complementary and Alternative Medicine, 38, 141
National Center for Complementary and Alternative Medicine (NCCAM), 33, 38, 131
National Childhood Vaccine Injury Act of 1986, 100
National Commission for the Protection of Human Research Subjects, 258
National Council against Health Fraud, 32, 229
National Council Against Health Fraud, 34, 141, 142
National Federation of Spiritual Healers., 50
National Fraud Information Center, 280
National Health Fraud Coordinator, 281
National Health Service, 38, 42, 45, 52, 57, 90, 96, 107, 180, 235, 284, 292, 315, 317
National Health Service (NHS), 104
National Health Service Centre for Reviews and Dissemination from the University of York, 59
National Health Service of the United Kingdom, 135, 141
National Health Service, Highland, 98
National Hospital for Neurology, 108
National Institute for Clinical Excellence, 56
National Institute for Clinical Excellence - NICE, 43

National Institute for Clinical Excellence (NICE), 180
National Institute for Health and Clinical Excellence (NICE), 43, 236
National Institute of Drug Abuse, (NIDA) held a Consensus Conference on Acupuncture, 133
National Institute of Health, 39, 133
National Institute of Health (NIH), 40
National Institute of Health's National Center for Complementary and Alternative Medicine, 135
National Institute of Health's Office of Alternative Medicine (NIH's OAM), 38
National Institutes of Health, 90, 232, 291, 303
National Institutes of Health (NIH), 33
National Institutes of Health (NIH) Center of Excellence, 60
National Institutes of Health in the United States, 296
National Pharmaceutical Association, 284
National Secular Society, The, 38
Natra Gest, 23
Natrum Muriaticum, 103
Natural bioidentical hormones, 26
Natural Causes, 239
Natural Herbal Research, 241, 242
Natural history of disease, 134
Natural Hormones, 25
Natural Therapists' Approach to Health, 229
Nature, 201, 202
Nature Chemical Biology, 198
Nature Communications, 202
Nature Neuroscience, 184
Nature News and Comment, 197
Nature Publishing Group, 184
Nature Publishing Group (NPG), 202
NCCAM, 57
Neill, Anna. Investigation Manager - GMC, 262
Nelsons Coldenza, 50
Nelsons Pharmacy, 101
Nemeroff, Charles B., 183
Nemeroff, Charles, B., 184
Neolithic, 123
Netherlands, 99, 293
Nettle, 33
Neuhauser, Duncan, 316
Neurontin, 185
Neuropsychopharmacology, 183

Neuroscience Group at Imperial College London, 237
Nevada Clinic, 278
New Age spirituality, 45
New England Journal of Medicine, 31, 209, 257, 291
New England Journal of Medicine (NEJM), 182
New Era Products, 91
New Labour Member of Parliament for the Don Valley constituency in South Yorkshire, 106
New York Presbyterian Hospital/Weill Cornell Medical Center, 232
New York State, 264
New York Times, 129
New York Times business section, 174
New Zealand, 14, 307
New Zealand's Commerce Commission. Fair Trading Act, 265
Newborn babies, 294
Newbury, 233
Newcastle University, 14
News of the World, The, 319
Newsnight, 101, 102
Newsweek, 32
Newsweek's Misleading Report on Alternative Medicine, 32
NHS Constitution, 104
NHS Direct website, 41
Niacin, 244
Nicholson, Jack, 292
Nijmegen, 96
Nissen, Dr. Steven, 186
Nixon, Dr Peter, 186
Nixon, President Richard, 258
Nixon, President Richard, 126
No. 1 Ladies' Detective Agency, 200
Nobel peace prize, 246
Nobel prize, 243
Nobel prize in chemistry, 246
Nobel prize-winners, 39
NoCold-Max cold and flu remedy ... homeopathic, 44
Nohl, Johannes, 280
Nolen, William M.D, 69
Nolen, William. MD, 128
Noni juice, 240
Noni-juice, 240
Norplant, 177
North American government agencies, 281

North American Menopause Society, 302, 305
North American Menopause Society (NAMS), 298
North West College of Homeopathy in Manchester, 60
North Yorkshire Country Council, 240
North Yorkshire Trading Standards Department, 241
Norton, Amy, 137
Novartis, 208
Novella, Steven, 40, 141
Novum Organum, 1620, 316
Nutraceuticals, 91
Nutrition, 200
Nutrition consultants, 229
Nutrition Society, 228

O

O'Donnell, E., 305
Oberon, 277
Observer, The, 318
Observer, The-18th Dec, 2005, 106
Office of Alternative Medicine, 39
Office of Alternative Medicine (OAM), 33, 133
Office of Medical Applications of Research (OMAR), 133
Office of Research Integrity (ORI), 213, 214
Office of Scientific Integrity, 213
Offit, Dr. Paul, 304
Offit, Dr. Paul[24], 26
Olive oil, 230
Oman, 98
Omega, 277
Omega 3, 237, 238
Omega Vision, 277
Operative delivery, 293
Oral provocation and neutralisation, 169
Organisational inertia, 317
Orion Bioscan, 280
Orion System, 277
Orphan Medical, 185
Oscillococcinum, 88
Osteoarthritis, 235
Osteoarthritis Research Society International, 139
Osteomalacia, 246
Osteopathy, 169, 284
Osteoporosis, 17, 246, 297

Osteoporotic fractures, 307
Otago University, 14
Owens, Michael, 184
Oxford, 291
Oxley, Melanie, 102
Oxley, Melanie, 100
Oxygen radicals, 167
Oxygenation therapies, 277
Ozone, 167

P

Packaged Facts, 233
Packham, Chris, 233
Packham, Chris, 233
Paediatric surgery in Bristol, 318
Paediatric Surveillance Unit, 53
Pakistan, 236
Pakuranga College in Auckland, 265
Palmistry, 57
Panay, Dr Nick, 303
Panorama, 260, 262, 263
Paracetamol, 244
Parade, 127
Pareto Chart, 316
Pareto Principle, 316
Pareto, Vilfredo Pareto, 316
Park, Robert, 170
Parker, Peter, 129
Pasteur, 315
Pasvol, Professor Geoffrey, 103
Patwardhan and Patwardhan, 332
Pauling, Linus, 168
Pauling. Linus, 246
Paxil, 263, 264
Paxil CR (paroxetine), 263
PDCA (plan–do–check–act, 316
Pearce, Malcolm, 188, 189
Peebles, Roger J. and Debra L., 26
Peer review, 212
Pegasus Publications, 174
Pendulums, 229
Penning, Mike M.P, 107
Peppermint, 33
Pertussis, 99
Peters, Sir Keith, 42
Peters, Tim, 199
Petitti, Diana, 304
Pfizer, 184, 206, 208, 265, 266
Pharmaceutical companies, 257, 266
Pharmaceutical Companies, 257
Pharmaceutical company gifts, 265

Pharmaceutical Research and Manufacturers of America, 266
Pharmacia, 208
Pharmacotherapy, 208, 209
Pharmacotherapy Board of Directors and Scientific Editor Council, 208
Pharmacotherapy Board, The, 209
Phazx, 278
Phazx Systems, 278
Phazx,, 277
Philippine Islands, 127
Philips, 326
Physiological Society, 46, 109
Phytochemicals, 240
Picrotoxin, 88, 169
Placebo, 280
Plagiarism, 195, 214
Plague epidemics, 280
Plan, Do, Study, Act (PDSA), 316
Plan-Do-Check-Act cycle, 330
Plant estrogens, 298
Poehlman, Eric, 213
Point testing. EAV, 277
Poison ivy, 23
Policy and procedure guidelines, 327
Polycystic ovary syndrome, 306
Polycystic ovary syndrome (PCOS), 306
Polynesian cultures, 240
Popoff, Peter, 69
Popularity of CAM, 54
Porcari, John, 280
Posner, Gary P., 127, 128, 129
Power Balance, 280
Power Balance magnetic wristband, 280
Power Balance magnetic wristband, 280
Prayer, 30
Prayer and CAM, 65
Premanand, B., 128
Premarin, 25
Premature, 294
President of the National Academy of Sciences, 195
President of the Royal College of Obstetricians and Gynaecologists, 188
Primary Care Trusts, 105
Prince Charles, 37, 43, 45, 51, 61, 170, 276
Prince of Wales, 42, 44, 240
Prince, Richard, 309
Prince's Foundation for Integrated Health, 52
Prince's Foundation for Integrated Health, 51

Princess Anne Hospital, Southampton, 47
Princess Diana, 45
Princess Elizabeth Orthopaedic Hospital, 96
Product Licences of Right (PLR), 43
Professional golfers, 280
Professor Ennis, Madeleine, 49
Professor Michael Baum, Professor Frances Ashcroft, Professor Sir Colin Berry, Professor Gustav Born, Professor Sir James Black, Professor David Colquhoun, Professor Peter Dawson, Professor Edzard Ernst, Professor John Garrow, Professor Sir Keith Peters, Mr Leslie Rose, 42
Professor of Complementary Medicine, 32
Professor savages homeopathy, 106
Progest, 23
Progesterone, 21
Progesterone, 18
Progesterone cream, 25
Progesterone,, 20
Progestin, 18
Prognos, 277
Prophylactic anticoagulation in surgery, 318
Prophyle, 277
Prostatic hyperplasia, 231
Protective amulets, 280
Providence Journal, 69
Psychic healers, 67
Psychic surgery, 277
Public Library of Science (PloS), 197
Public Library of Science (PLoS), 207
Punctos III, 277
Punjab Institute of Cardiology (PIC), 236
Punjab province, 236
Puri, Professor Basant, 237
Pyrénées, 11

Q

Qigong, 123
Quacksalver, 11
Quackwatch, 60, 88, 141, 276
quackwatch.org, 55
Quality control, 317
Quality improvement, 317
Quality of life, 298
Quality planning, 317
Quantum Medical Consciousness Interface (QMCI) System, 280

Queen Anne, 13
Queen Elizabeth, 65
Queenie Lane, 14
Quietlynn Ltd, 241

R

Radical Defence, 242
Radionics (psionic medicine, dowsing), 169
Radium Hospital, The, 198
Radon, 23
Ramírez, Orlando Ruiz, 178
Ramírez, Inés, 178
Ramsey, David. President of the University of Maryland, Baltimore, 134
Randi, James, 69, 128
Randi, James Educational Foundation, 66
Randomised controlled trials, 291
Rath, Matthias, 175
Raviglione, Dr Mario, 110
Read,, 13
Reagan, Ronald, 183
Redundant publication, 196
Rees, Lord of Ludlow, 49
Rees-Mogg, Jacob, 37
Reflexology, 284
Reflexology (zone therapy), 169
Regional Health and Diet Centre, 241
Regional Health and Diet Centre (RHDC), 240
Regression to the mean, 134
Regulation of homeopathy, 104
Reidenberg, Marcus M., 232
Reiki, 40
Reiki massages, 46
Reinforcement, 134
Relman, Dr. Arnold, 31
Renewed Balance, 23
Renner, John H., 229
Rescuing Science from Politics, 205
Research Fellowship in the Centre for Complementary Health Studies, 93
Research misconduct, 195
Resorts in exotic places, 268
Reston, James, 129
Reuters Health Information from New York. February 2011, 137
Ri Fang Ho, Doctor of Chinese Medicine and Member of the British Acupuncture Council, 283
Ribena, 265

Richardson, Dr Alex, 237
Ridge, Dr Keith, Chief Pharmaceutical Officer, 93
Ritual, 134
Robin Hood effect, The, 319
Rofecoxib (Vioxx), 208
Roger II of Sicily, 13
Rose, Louis, 68
Rosenfeld, Dr. Isadore, 129
Rosenfeld, Dr. Isadore, 127
Rosenfeld, Dr. Isadore, 129
rosenthal.hs. columbia.edu., 55
Ross, J. S., 208
Ross, Paula. Chief executive of the Society of Homeopaths, 110
Routine examination of diabetic feet, 318
Routledge, Professor Philip, 44
Rowlinson, Peter, 14
Royal and Ancient golf club of St. Andrews, 174
Royal Children's Hospital in Melbourne, 53
Royal College of General Practitioners, 46
Royal College of Obstetricians and Gynaecologists, 293
Royal College of Obstetricians and Gynaecologists in the United Kingdom, 315
Royal College of Paediatrics and Child Health, 53
Royal College of Pathologists, 46
Royal Courts of Justice in London, 186
Royal Free Hospital in London, 187
Royal Free Hospital Medical School, 187
Royal Liverpool University Hospital, 110
Royal London Homeopathic Hospital, 102
Royal London Homeopathic Hospital (RLHH), 90
Royal London Homeopathic Hospital, Clinical Director, 59
Royal London Homoeopathic Hospital, 92
Royal London Hospital for Integrated Medicine, 92
Royal Marsden Hospital, 17
Royal Pharmaceutical Society, 21
Royal Pharmaceutical Society (RPS), 94, 243, 244
Royal Pharmaceutical Society code on Medicines, Ethics and Practice, 94
Royal Pharmaceutical Society's (RPS) Statutory Committee, 242
Royal Society of Health and Hygiene, 228

Royal Society of Medicine, 46
Royal Society, The, 46
Royal Society, The, 56
Rubin, Professor Peter, 189

S

Sackeim, Harold, 184
Salami publishing"., 210
Salusa 45, 276
Salzberg, Steven, 40, 141
Sampson, W, 133, 134
Sampson, W., 127, 128, 129
Sampson, Wallace, 141
Sampson, Wallace I., 39
Sanatogen, 276
Santa Claus, 130
Saudi Arabia, 320
Saville Row, 290
Saw palmetto, 33
Saw Palmetto, 231
SB Pharmco Puerto Rico Inc in Cidra, Puerto Rico, 264
Scandinavia, 307
Schein, M. and Paladugu, R., 215
Schering-Plough, 266
Schiefe, Richard T, 209
Schimmel, Helmut, 277
Schmidt, Katya, 94, 100
Schwartz, Lisa, 206
Schwarz Pharma, 282
Schwarz, Joe, 26
Science, 207
Science Based Medicine, 141
Science Editor, The Times 23rd May 2006, 42
Science of Alternative Medicine, The, 32
Science of Alternative Medicine. The, 32
Science-Based Medicine, 40
Scientific American, 202, 233
Scientific Freedom, Responsibility and Law Program at the American Association for the Advancement of Science (AAAS), 202
Scientific Review of Alternative Medicine, 30, 133, 142
Scientific Review of Alternative Medicine and Aberrant Medical Practices, 39
Scientist, The, 184
SCIO, 280
Scottish Conservative politicians, 166
Seasilver, 277

Seaweed, 238
Second World War, 285
Self Diagnostic Procedures, 229
Self-styled nutritionists, 279
Sellers, Peter, 127
Selman, Sherril, 24
Senate Finance Committee investigation, 184
Sense about Science, 46, 101
Sense About Science, 110
Seroxat, 258, 260, 261, 264
Seroxat(Paroxetine), 258
Seven Deadly Diseases, 330
Shandong University School of Medicine, 198
Shang Dynasty (1600–1100 BCE, 123
Sharif, Shahbaz, 236
Shark cartilage, 32
Shark Cartilage, 277
Shark fin, 170, 275
Shaw, Bernard, 12
Shaw, Charles D, 318
Shaw, Charles D., 317
Shekelle, Paul G., 231
Sheldrake, Rupert, 65
Shepherd, Dr Charles, 243
Shewhart cycle, 316
Shewhart, Walter Andrew, 316, 327, 329, 330
Shi-chi text, 124
Shropshire Crown Court, 241
Shropshire Trading Standards officers, 241
Shufelt, Chrisandra, 305
Sibutramine, 234
Signalysis Ltd, 243
Signalysis Ltd, of Stroud, Gloucestershire, 242
Sildenafil, 234
Silverman, Steve, 27
Simon Fraser University, 62
Singh, Dr Ram B, 198
Singh, Simon, 37, 141
Singh,*Simon*, 56
Skin prick testing, 279
Skin resistance, 279
Skrabanek, P and McKormick, J, 129
Sky News, 19, 319
Sky News - 8th January, 2012, 175
Sloan-Kettering Institute, 199
Slutsky, Robert, 199
Smallwood Inquiry 2005, 35

Smallwood Report, 41, 43, 52
Smallwood report on The Role of Complementary and Alternative Medicine in the NHS, 43
Smallwood, Christopher, 43
Smith, Professor Steve, 52
Smith, Richard, 196, 199, 203, 210, 257
Snake Oil, 276
Snitz,Beth, 231
Snow, John, 291
So Good Soya Essential Omega 3 drink, 238
Social Audit Ltd, 261
Society of Homeopaths, 100, 102
Soil Association, 166
Solgar Vitamins, 52
Solicitor General, 285
Solomon, Dr Neil MD, PhD, 240
Solvay Pharmaceuticals, 267
Soman, Vijay, 199
Some Notes on Management in a Hospital, 331
South African Advertising Standards Authority, 281
South African consumers, 281
South African Department of Health, 106
South African Government, 175
South African Menopause Society (SAMS), 297
South African sausage, 242
South West Kent Primary Care Trust (PCT), 91
Southampton, 233
Southern California Evidence-Based Practice Center, 231
Soybeans, 26
Spagyrik, 243
Spagyrik therapy, 242
Speedslim CP-2000, 241
Spellman, Kenneth, 243
Spellman, Rosemary, 243
Spitzer, Eliot. New York State Attorney General, 264
Split ends, 276
Split-ends, 282
Spock, Dr. Benjamin, 175
Sporting events, 268
Spot Removers, 282
Squibb, 206
St George's Hospital, 188
St George's Hospital Medical School, 188, 189

St John's Wort, 33
St. Bartholomew's Hospital, 13
St. John's wort, 34, 231
St.Thomas's Hospital, 13
Standish-White, Mike, 319
Stanford University, 141
Stanford University Medical Center, 265
Stanford, Clare, 184
State attorney general, 280
State licensing board, 280
Stelfox, H. T., 203
Stellenbosch University, 21
Steroids, 232
Stickler, Gunnar B., 33
Stiegman, Albert, 61
Stinging nettles, 23
Stockholm effect, 134
Stone Age, 123
Stop TB department - WHO, 110
Story of Medicine, The, 315
Story of Medicine, The, 12
Straus, Steven. M.D. NCCAM Director, 39
Strokes, 304
Strychnine, 23
Student Notes, 93
Study 329, 259, 260, 261
Subfertility, 306
Sudbø, Jon, 198
Sugar Menace, The, 229
Suggestion, 134
Summerlin, William, 199
Sun Xiongyong, 201
Sunday Telegraph, The, 18
Sunday Times, 186
Sunday Times, The, 45, 187
Sunday Tribune - 8th August 2004, 170
Sunday Tribune 8th August 2004, 275
Suo, Jenny, 265
Superoxide dismutase (SOD), 167
Supplements, 228
Sutcliffe, Thomas, 45
Swan, Rita and Douglas, 68
Swaziland, 174
Swaziland Health Ministry, 175
Sweden, 308
Swiss Government, 104
Sykes, Kathy, 90
Sykes, Kathy, 55
Syncrometer, 277
System of Profound Knowledge, 330
Systematic reviews, 291

T

Tadalafil, 234
Tai Sophia Institute of Applied Healing Arts, 60
Tang, 125
Taub, Arthur, 128, 141
Taverne, Lord, 49
Taverne, Lord Dick, 46
TB, 110
Teesside Crown Court, 241
Ten red flags, 15
Tennessee, 31
Tesco's Healthy Living pomegranate juice, 238
Tessman, Irwin, 66
Thallium, 23
Thallon, James, 91
Thames Valley University, 60
Thatcher, Margaret, 45, 183
The 10
  23 campaign, 105
The Antioxidant myth, 167
The Black Death, 280
The Bucket List, 292
The Consensus Conference, 134
The General Medical Council, 96, 188
The Minister of State, 50
The New England Journal of Medicine, 198
The Shop, 317
The Times, 40
The Times 10th July, 2002, 17
The Wizard of Oz, 128
Therapeutic touch, 30
There's no remedy for the Prince of Quacks, 51
Thrombo-embolic disease, 17
Thyroid hormones, 240
Tian Li, 234
Tijuana, 38
Timely thrombolytics in myocardial infarction, 318
Times, The, 103
Times, The, 237
Titus, S. L. et al[2], 195
Tobacco, 23
Tobyward, 242
Tobyward Ltd, City Trading Ltd, 241
Toft Hill school, 237
Tooth Fairy, 26
Tooth Fairy science, 130
Top Health Frauds, 275, 276

Total consumption poverty line (TCPL), 322
Trachtenberg, Alan. MD, 133
Trade descriptions Act 1968, 242
Trading Standards offences, 241
Traditional Chinese Medicine, 283
Traditional Chinese medicine (TCM), 234
Traditional Chinese medicine. TCM, 123
Traditional Herbal Registration (THR), 234
Transcutaneous electrical stimulation (TENS), 135
Travel Clinic, 101
Trends in Pharmacological Sciences (2005), 106, 111
Trick or Treatment, 135
Tshabalala-Msimang, Manto, 175
Tsinghua University, 202
Tuberculosis, 323
Tunbridge Wells Homeopathic Hospital, 91
Turnitin, 202
Twain, Mark, 210
Twain, Mark, 290
Two Feathers Healing Formula, 277
Tygerberg Hospital, 21

U

U.S. Congress, 33
U.S. Department of Justice, 264
U.S. News & World Report. February 17, 1997, 88
U.S. Office of Research Integrity (ORI), 195
U.S. Office of Research Integrity (ORI), 195
U.S. Preventive Services Task Force, 228
UK Corporate Citizenship Index. 2006., 265
UK Medicines Act 1968, 43
UK report on Dietary Reference Intakes, 245
UK Research Integrity Office (UKRIO), 197
UK. Commons Health Committee, 293
Ullman, Dana, 61
Ultrafemme, 21
Ultraviolet blood irradiation, 277
Unichem, 94
Union Jack, 242
United Kingdom, 104, 319
United Kingdom Department of Health, 42, 55
United Nations, 321
United States, 99, 131
United States congressional inquiry, 203
United States Federal Trade Commission, 281
United States Food and Drug Administration, 26, 131
United States Food and Drug Administration., 27
United States Medical Licence in 1993, 240
United States National Institutes of Health, 141
United States National Science Foundation, 31
Universal access to contraception, 322
Universities and CAM, 58
Universities in the United Kingdom, 55
University College London, 244
University College London Hospital, 38
University of Arizona, 90
University of Bern, Switzerland, 235
University of California, 199
University of California San Francisco, 204
University of California, San Diego, 204, 304
University of California, San Francisco, 134
University of Cape Town, 173
University of Connecticut, 213
University of Edinburgh, 200, 204
University of Health Sciences College of Osteopathic Medicine in Kansas City, 98
University of Johannesburg, 106
University of Lincoln, 14, 60
University of London, 199
University of Maryland, 141
University of Maryland Center for Integrative Medicine, 57
University of Maryland Medical Center in the USA, 60
University of Maryland School of Medicine, 40
University of New Mexico, 14
University of North Carolina, 206
University of Nottingham, 189
University of Oslo, 198
University of Pennsylvania, 60, 265
University of Salford, 60
University of Southampton, 47
University of St Andrews, 110
University of Westminster, 59
Unlicensed individuals, 279

Uranium, 23
US Commission on Research Integrity, 195
US Department of Justice, 244
US National Cancer Institute, 167
US National Institutes of Health, 179
US Physicians' Health Study, 245
US/Canadian reports on Dietary Reference Intakes, 245
USA, 105
USA Department of Health and Human Services, 266
USA Food and Drug Administration's Consumer Updates page, 27
USA Government's drug safety advisers, 261
Utian, Wulf, 26

V

Vaccinations, 97
Vaccine Roulette, 100
Vagus nerve stimulation (VNS) device, 183
Vale Practice, 102
Vale Practice in East Dulwich, 101
Van der Merwe, Professor Kobie, 21
Van't Hoff, Dr. William, 53
Vanishing Creams, 282
Vantage, 277
Vardenafil, 234
Variation, Intended, 331
Variation, Unintended, 331
Vega machine, 232, 233
Vega MRT (Matrix Regeneration Therapy), 169
Vega test, 169, 233
Vega testing, 169, 279
Vegans, 229
Vegatest, 96, 277, 278
Vegatest I device, 279
Vegetarians, 229
Venus Pill, The, 295
Veterinarians, 279
Viagra, 234
Vickers, Andrew J., 52
Victor-Vitalpunkt Diagnose, 277
Viegas, Dr. Marisa, 95
Vine, Jeremy, 258
Vioxx, 208
Virgin Mary, 128
Viridian Trace Mineral Complex, 45
Vistron, 277
Vital energy, 123

Vital energy (chi or qi), 123
Vital forces, 93
Vitamin A, 244, 247
Vitamin B6, 244, 247
Vitamin C, 168, 230, 246, 265, 277
Vitamin D, 229, 244, 246, 247, 307
Vitamin E, 167, 244, 245
Vitamin supplements, 247, 278
Vitamins, 228
Vitamins and Minerals, 229
Vitel 618, 277
Voice of Young Science Network, 110
Voll, Reinhold, 277
Voll, Reinhold, 277
Voltaire, 87
Von Stift, Dr. Andreas Josef, 11
Vyas, Bharti, 45

W

Wager, Elizabeth, 197, 207, 210
Wager, Elizabeth, 52
Wager, Elizabeth, 212
Wagner, Marsden, 181
Wagner, Wendy, 205
Wakefield, Andrew, 100
Wakefield, Doctor Andrew, 187
Walker, Kenneth, 12, 315
Warren, Richard, 293
Warren, Richard. Honorary Secretary of the Royal College of Obstetricians and Gynaecologists, 292
Washington DC, 202
Washington Post, 40
Wax, J. R. and others, 294, 295
Wax, J. R. and others, 293
Weekly Telegraph, 89, 187
Weekly Telegraph, The July 7-13th 2010, 294
Weight gain, 298
Weight loss, 306
Weir, 208
Weissmann Gerald, 61
Weleda Flower essence, 91
Wells, Mrs Jacqueline, 243
Wendell Holmes, Dr. Oliver, 57
Wendell Holmes, Oliver, 88
West Kent Primary Care Trust, 91
Western Electric Company Inspection Engineering Department, 329
Western Electric Hawthorne plant in Cicero, Illinois, USA, 316

Western Institutional Review Board (WIRB), 258
Westminster University, 58
What to do About Stress, 229
What's the Alternative, 18
Wheatgrass, 277
Wheen, Francis, 51
Which?, 238
Which? magazine, 50
Whiskas, 168
White, Jamie, 103
Whitehead, Stephen, 109
Whole body Hyperthermia, 277
Why the National Center for Complementary and Alternative Medicine (NCCAM) Should Be Defunded, 39
Wickmaratne, Renuka, 45
Wikipedia, 123
Wild Pink Yam, 166
Wild Yam, 21
Wild Yam (Dioscorea), 21
Wild Yam Cream, 24, 25
Wild Yam extract, 23
Wild yams, 26
Wilkinson, Anna, 14
Willis, Phil, 91
Wilmshurst, Peter, 197
Wilson, Robert, 295
Winston, Lord, 91
Witty, Andrew, 264
Women's Health Initiative, 17, 20, 95, 303
Women's Health Initiative (WHI), 300, 305
Women's Health Initiative Calcium/Vitamin D Supplementation Study, 307
Women's Health Initiative Limited Access Dataset, 307
Women's Health Initiative Memory Study (WHIMS), 299
Women's Voices 1994, 320
Women's' Institute, 174
Women's Health Initiative (WHI), 296, 301
Won, J. et al, 198
Woodcock, Dr. Janet. Acting Deputy Commissioner for operations of the Food and Drug Administration, 268
Wooding, David, 180
Woods, Professor Kent, 47
Woods, Sir Kent, 109
Woodsd, Professor Kent, 263
Woolley, Karen, 212
World Health Organisation, 51, 102, 182, 244, 259
World Health Organisation (WHO) 2005 report, 135
World Health Organisation assembly in Geneva, 43
World Health Organization, 141
World Health Organization (WHO), 110
World Health Organization global survey, 2005, 178
World Health Organizations, 179
World War II, 329
Worts and All, 231
WOW factor, 326
Wrinkle Smoothers, 282
Wyeth, 18, 206, 207

X

Xyrem, 185

Y

Yale, 265
Yale School of Medicine, 40
Yale University, 199
Yang, 124
Yang Wei, 201
Yeoman, Fran, 91
Yew, 23
Yin, 124
Yohimbe, 33
Yoshida, T, 305
You Are What You Eat presenter, The, 166
Yuehong, 201
Yuehong Zhang, 201

Z

Zero Balancing, 283
Zhang, Yun, 198
Zhejiang University (ZJU), 201
Zimbabwe, 131, 176, 307, 322
Zinc, 247
Zink, 326
ZYTO, 277